MEDICAL RESIDENT'S MANUAL

WILLIAM J. GRACE, M.D., F.A.C.P.

Director, Department of Medicine, St. Vincent's Hospital and Medical Center of New York; Professor of Clinical Medicine, New York University School of Medicine.

RICHARD J. KENNEDY, M.D., F.A.C.P.

Associate Director of Medicine, St. Vincent's Hospital and Medical Center of New York; Clinical Professor of Medicine, New York University School of Medicine.

FRANK B. FLOOD, M.D., F.A.C.P.

Chief Cardiologist, St. Joseph's Hospital, Yonkers, New York; Attending Physician, Yonkers General Hospital.

MEDICAL RESIDENT'S MANUAL

Third Edition

ACC

APPLETON-CENTURY-CROFTS
Educational Division/Meredith Corporation
New York

72 73 74 75 76/10 9 8 7 6 5 4 3

Library of Congress Catalog Card Number: 75-110106

Third Printing

PRINTED IN THE UNITED STATES OF AMERICA

390-50431-9

CONTRIBUTORS

Helen M. Anderson, M.D. *Chief of Hematology*	Hematology
Harry Bartfeld, M.D. *Chief of Rheumatology*	Rheumatic Disorders
Godfrey Burns, M.D. *Medical Resident*	Defibrination Syndrome
Joseph A. Chusid, M.D.	Neurology
Fritz A. Freyhan, M.D. *Attending Psychiatrist*	Psychotherapeutics
Nancy E. Gary, M.D. *Chief of Nephrology*	Nephrology
John J. Gregory, M.D. *Assistant Director* *Cardiopulmonary Unit*	Cardiac Pacemakers
Michael J. Lepore, M.D. *Chief of Gastroenterology*	Gastronenterology
James Mazzara, M.D. *Fellow* *Cardiopulmonary Laboratory*	Electrolyte Disorders, Serum Proteins, Immunoglobulins, Hyperlipoidemia, Vasculitis
Albert Maniscalco, M.D. *Senior Medical Resident*	Cardiogenic and Septic Shock, Bacterial Endocarditis
Anthony E. Maniscalco, M.D.	Psychotherapeutics
Lawrence Nastro, M.D. *Senior Medical Resident*	Antibiotics
Charles A. Ribaudo, M.D.	Pulmonary Disease
Leonard Stutman, M.D. *Chief of Coagulation Laboratory*	Coagulating Mechanisms
Iven S. Young, M.D. *Chief of Endocrinology*	Endocrinology

PREFACE

Rapid advances in medicine have prompted the preparation of this Third Edition of the Medical Resident's Manual. Basically it follows the aims originally set forth and, hopefully, strikes a balance between the diagnosis and treatment of major conditions encountered most often in everyday resident practice.

This edition has been largely rewritten by the generous contributions of the members of both the attending and senior resident staff of the Department of Medicine of the St. Vincent's Hospital and Medical Center of New York. To those who have written major sections of this edition we acknowledge our gratitude in the list of contributors.

Our gratitude and appreciation goes to Sister Anthony Marie FitzMaurice, S.C., Administrator, who, during her twenty-five years at St. Vincent's Hospital, has been a continuing source of encouragement and inspiration.

WILLIAM J. GRACE
RICHARD J. KENNEDY
FRANK B. FLOOD

PREFACE TO THE FIRST EDITION

As characteristic of the medical resident as his curiosity, his questions, and his dedication is the loose-leaf notebook he carries. The book is his private medical text in which he notes clinical pearls, rules of thumb, diagnostic clues, seldom used and easily forgotten procedures that are of importance in emergencies, dosage of drugs, key references, summaries of his reading, and many unanswered questions that arise during his busy day. The notebook grows with time and experience, becoming more and more a reference source from which, after a careful history and physical examination, the vast number of problems encountered in resident practice are approached.

This manual is the outgrowth of many residents' notebooks. In it we endeavored to include the "heart of the matter" as it pertains to the resident in hospital practice. It is not intended to be a textbook but rather a *vade mecum* in which the resident may readily locate brief descriptions of clinical states, clues to diagnosis, and selected laboratory tests necessary to further substantiate a clinical impression arrived at by history, physical examination, logical reasoning, and experience. We have emphasized particularly those problems which from teaching experience have been found to offer difficulty. In the manual we have aimed to select and synopsize much material scattered in recent medical literature. Most topics are concluded with an up-to-date and readily available key reference that may be consulted for further study of a subject. Many commonly used abbreviations have been employed throughout the book for the sake of brevity.

We are grateful to the many members of the house and attending staff of St. Vincent's Hospital. Their encouragement and advice have been invaluable in the preparation of this manual.

FRANK B. FLOOD
RICHARD J. KENNEDY
WILLIAM J. GRACE

CONTENTS

TABLES OF NORMAL VALUES

BLOOD

HEMATOLOGIC VALUES

Hemoglobin	
males	14-18 g/100 ml whole blood
females	12-16 g/100 ml whole blood
Hematocrit	
males	40-54%
females	37-47%
Erythrocytes	
males	5.4 ± 0.8 million/mm^3
females	4.8 ± 0.6 million/mm^3
Leukocytes	5,000-10,000/mm^3
segmented neutrophiles	54-62%
bands	3-5%
basophiles	0-0.75%
eosinophiles	1-3%
monocytes	3-7%
lymphocytes	25-33%
Platelets	150,000-450,000/mm^3
Reticulocytes	0.5-1.5%
Erythrocytes sedimentation rate	20 mm or less per hour (Westergren)
Bleeding time	6 min (IVY)
Clotting time	6-12 min (Lee-White)
Clot retraction	4+ in 2 hr
Recalcification time	80-180 sec
One-stage prothrombin time	14 sec
Partial thromboplastin time	45 sec
Prothrombin consumption	21 sec
Fibrinogen	275 mg per 100 ml ± 50, ± 100 1 S.D. 2 S.D.
Fibrinolysins (serial plasma clot lysis time)	0 at the end of 24 hr
Euglobulin lysis time	More than 2 hr. (Van Kaulla modification)

BLOOD CONSTITUENTS

Acetone	0.3-2.0 mg per 100 ml
Albumin	3.5-5.5 g per 100 ml
Ammonia	40-70 mcg/ml
Amylase	40-180 units
Antistreptolysin-O titer	Less than 200 Todd units (serial titers suggested)
Ascorbic acid	0.4-1.5 mg per 100 ml
Base, total	142-160 mEq/L
Bilirubin	
total	Up to 1.1 mg %
direct	Up to 0.4 mg %
indirect	Up to 0.6 mg %
Blood volume	Approx. 8% of body weight
Bromsulphalein (BSP)	Less than 5% retention/45 min
Blood urea nitrogen (BUN)	10-20 mg per 100 ml
C-reactive protein	0
Calcium	9-11 mg per 100 ml (do serum protein also); 4.5-5.5 mEq/L
Carbon dioxide (CO_2)	
content	22-31 mEq/L
Carotene	70-200 μg per 100 ml
Catecholamines	
norepinephrine	2.43 μg/L of plasma
epinephrine	0.22 μg/L of plasma
Chloride	100-106 mEq/L
Copper	70-140 μg per 100 ml
Cholesterol	150-280 mg per 100 ml (esters: 50-65%)
Cholinesterase	0.5 pH units/hr or more
Creatinine	1-2 mg per 100 ml
Ethanol (medicolegal)	0.15% unfit to drive 0.3-0.4% marked intoxication 0.45-0.6% coma
Fibrinogen	200-400 mg/100 ml
Glucose	70-110 mg per 100 ml
Iodine, protein-bound (PBI)	4-8 μg per 100 ml
Iron	50-150 μg per 100 ml
Iron-binding capacity	150-300 μg per 100 ml
Lactic acid dehydrogenase	Under 680 units/ml of serum (fractionation is of value)
Lipase	Less than 2 units
Lipids, total/serum	450-850 mg/100 ml
Lipid partition	
blood cholesterol	150-280 mg/100 ml
cholesterol esters	50-65%
phospholipids	9-16 mg/100 ml

total fatty acid	190-420 mg/100 ml
neutral fat	0-200 mg/100 ml
Magnesium	1.5-2.5 mEq/L
Methemoglobin (adults)	Approx. 0.1 g per 100 ml
Nitrogen, nonprotein (NPN)	20-40 mg per 100 ml
Osmolality	285-295/L/mOsm
Oxygen saturation, arterial	94-100%
Phosphatase, acid	0.5-2.0 units total Up to 7 units prostatic portion
Phosphatase, alkaline	2.0-4.5 Bodansky units Up to 13 King-Armstrong units
Phosphorus	3.0-4.5 mg per 100 ml
Potassium	3.5-5.0 mEq/L
Protein	6-8 g per 100 ml (total)
albumin	3.5-5.5 g per 100 ml
globulin	1.5-3.5 g per 100 ml
paper electrophoresis	
alpha 1	0.13-0.29 g per 100 ml (5-8% of total)
alpha 2	0.31-0.89 g per 100 ml (8-13% of total)
beta	0.48-1.06 g per 100 ml (11-17% of total)
gamma	0.63-1.77 g per 100 ml (15-25% of total)
Pyruvic acid	1.0-2.0 mg/100 ml
Salicylate	
therapeutic	20-25 mg per 100 ml
toxic	Over 30 mg per 100 ml
Serotonin	0.08-0.22 μg/ml of serum
Sodium	132-144 mEq/L
Transaminase	
SGOT	10-40 units
SGPT	5-35 units
Urea nitrogen	10-15 mg per 100 ml
Uric acid	2.5-7.2 mg per 100 ml

CARDIOPULMONARY

	PRESSURE	O_2 SATURATION % OF NORMAL	VOLUME %
Venous pressure, arm	80-120 mm H_2O	–	
Right atrium	2-3 mm Hg	74 ± 4	14.00 ± 0.75
Right ventricle	25/2 mm Hg	74 ± 4	14.00 ± 0.75
Pulmonary artery	25/10 mm Hg	74 ± 4	14.00 ± 0.75
Pulmonary capillary	5-14 mm Hg	–	
Left atrium	2-12 mm Hg	97 ± 1	18.00 ± 1.00

HEART CHAMBER SAMPLES (O_2 CONTENT)

(Step-up values)

Pooled vena caval–right atrial O_2 diff.	Less than 1.9 vol %
Right atrial–right ventricular O_2 diff.	Less than 0.9 vol %
Right ventricular–pulmonary artery O_2 diff.	±0.5 vol %

MISCELLANEOUS

Mitral valve area	4-6 cm^2
Circulation time (decholin), arm-tongue	10-16 sec

PULMONARY FUNCTION

Maximum breathing capacity (average)	
young male	86-144 L/min
young female	47-114 L/min
Vital capacity	
15-34 years	2.7-4.9 L
35-49 years	3.3-5.2 L
50-59 years	2.2-5.4 L
Timed vital capacity	
1st second	75% of total
2nd second	85% of total
3rd second	95% of total

The following table gives the P_{CO_2} in mm Hg when the pH and total CO_2 are determined:

pH \ CO_2 mm/L	5	10	20	30	40	50	
7.10	15	30	61	91	121	152	
7.20	12	25	49	74	98	123	
7.30	10	20	40	59	79	99	
7.40	8	16	32	48	64	80	P_{CO_2} values
7.50	6	13	26	38	51	64	
7.60	5	10	20	31	41	51	

If a P_{CO_2} value above the dotted line is obtained, this indicates inadequate ventilation, and the patient should be treated with a respirator.

Normal Values

pH	7.36 to 7.44
P_{CO_2}	34 to 46 mm Hg
Total CO_2	24 to 33 mmole/L

CEREBROSPINAL FLUID

Cells	0-5 mononuclear cells/mm^3
Character	Clear, colorless
specific gravity	1.005-1.009
Chloride	120-130 mEq/L
Glucose	45-80 mg per 100 ml (approx. ½ of blood sugar)
Pressure (reclining)	70-200 mm H_2O
Protein	15-45 mg per 100 ml
Transaminase (SGOT)	5-21 units/ml

Note: Usually, grossly bloody CSF will not clot in the test tube.

GASTROINTESTINAL

GASTRIC ACIDITY

AVERAGE VALUES—12 HOURS OVERNIGHT COLLECTION.

	VOLUME	FREE HCl mEq/L (OR CLINICAL UNITS)
Normals	581	29
Duodenal ulcer	1,000	61
Gastric ulcer	600	21
Zollinger-Ellison syndrome	1,000+	100+

AVERAGE VALUES—HOURLY COLLECTION.

	VOLUME	pH	FREE HCl mEq/L
Normal	20-60	1.5-3.0	20-30
Duodenal ulcer	60-100	1.2-0.5	30-60

MALABSORPTION TESTS

Serum carotene	70-200 μg per 100 ml (Best simple test for sprue)
d-Xylose test	Fasting subject given 25 g d-xylose; average 5 hr output over 4 g
idiopathic malabsorption	Output less than 2.5 g/5 hr
secondary malabsorption	Output 2.5-4 g/5 hr
Triolein and oleic acid I^{131}	Compare blood and fecal counts
normal	4th, 5th, & 6th hr blood specimens average more than 10% of the administered dose; less than 5% of dose in stool during a 2-3 day period
Stool fat, total	Up to 6 g/24 hr

Qualitative examination of stool for fat droplets

Also. Glucose tolerance test, prothrombin time, Schilling test, serum calcium.

LIVER FUNCTION TESTS

Bromosulphalein	5% or less after 45 min
Cephalin flocculation	2+ or less
Portal pressure (splenic pulp)	Under 280 mm H_2O
Prothrombin time	70-100% of normal control; approx. 13 sec
Thymol turbidity	0-4 units
Transaminase (SGPT)	5-30 units
Urobilinogen	
urine	0.0-0.4 mg/24 hr
feces	50-280 mg/24 hr

RENAL FUNCTION TESTS

Clearance tests (corrected to 1.73 sq m body surface area)	
Glomerular filtation rate (GFR)	
inulin clearance	100-150 ml/min
mannitol clearance	120-130 ml/min
endogenous creatinine clearance	100-120 ml/min
endogenous urea clearance	50-75 ml/min
Renal plasma flow (RPF)	
Para-aminohippurate (PAH) clearance	400-600 ml/min
Filtration fraction (FF)	17-23%

$$FF = \frac{GFR}{RPF}$$

Phenolsulfonphthalein Test (PSP)

$>$25% of dye excreted in 15 min

$>$65% of dye excreted in 60 min

Maximum concentration (after 12 hr of dehydration)	
Specific gravity	$>$1.028
Maximum dilution	$<$1.003
Maximal Diodrast excretory capacity TM_D	
males	43-59 mg/min
females	33-51 mg/min
Maximal glucose reabsorptive capacity TM_G	
males	300-450 mg/min
females	250-350 mg/min
Maximal PAH excretory capacity TM_{PAH}	80-90 mg/min

URINE

Albumin	$<$100 mg/24 hr

Test	Normal value
Aldosterone	
in urine	6-16 μg/24 hr
total adrenal production	100-300 μg/24 hr (isotope dilution)
Bacterial count	Over 10,000 colonies/ml usually due to infection, less than 10,000 to contamination
Calcium	0.1-0.3 g/24 hr
Sulkowitch	Normal average 1+
Casts	0-400/12 hr
Cathecholamines	
epinephrine	Under 10 μg
norepinephrine	Under 100 μg/24 hr
Copper	70 mcg/24 hr output
Corticosteroids	
17-hydroxy	male 5-15 mg/24 hr female 4-10 mg/24 hr
17-keto	male 8-25 mg/24 hr female 5-15 mg/24 hr
Creatine	Less than 100 mg/24 hr
Creatinine	1.0-1.7 g/24 hr
Epithelial and white blood cells	32,000-1,000,000/12 hr
Erythrocytes	0-425,000/12 hr
5-Hydroxyindoleacetic acid	208 mg/24 hr (mephenesin may interfere)
Lead	Up to 120 μg/24 hr
Phenolsulfonphthalein (PSP)	25% or more in 15 min
Phosphorus	Approx. 1 g/24 hr
Porphobilinogen	0/24 hr
Potassium	2.5-3 g/24 hr
Serotonin	60-160 μg/24 hr
Sodium	4.2-5 g/24 hr (180-220 mEq)
Sugar	0/24 hr
Uric acid	0.5-1.0 g/24 hr
Urobilinogen	Up to 1.0 Ehrlich units/2 hr or 0.0-4.0 mg/24 hr
Vanillyl mandelic acid (VMA)	1.8-8.4 mg/24 hr
Vitamin B_{12} (Schilling)	8-38% oral dose/24 hr
Volume	800-1,600 ml/24 hr

THE ANGIOCARDIOGRAM
FRONTAL PROJECTION

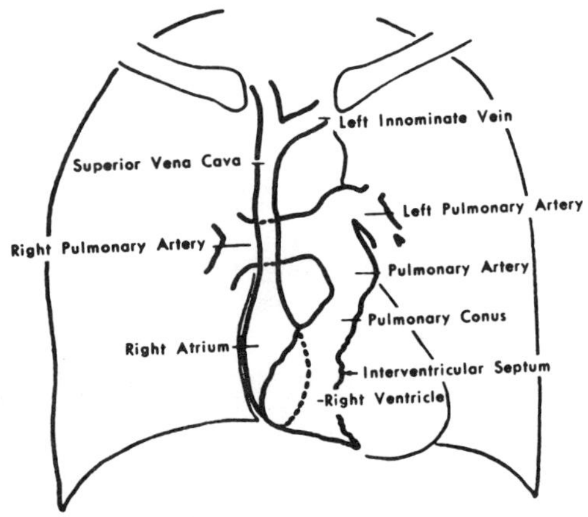

Right Heart

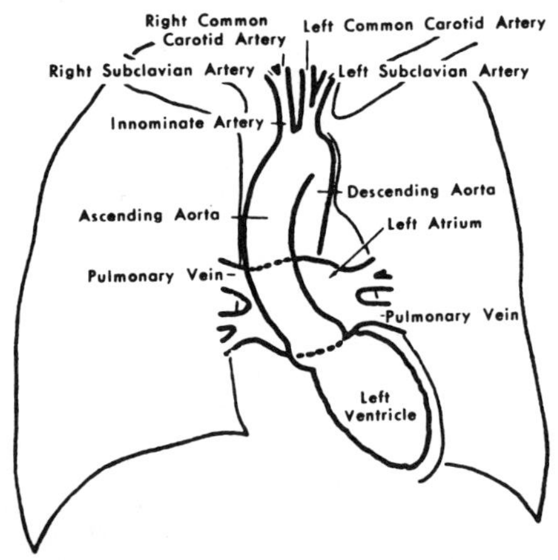

Left Heart

From Dotter, C. T., and Steinberg, I., 1952. Angiocardiography, Paul B. Hoeber. Courtesy of the American Heart Association, Inc.

LEFT LATERAL PROJECTION

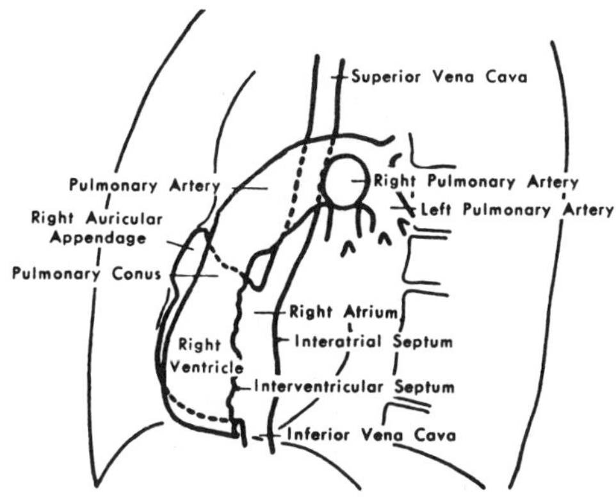

Right Heart

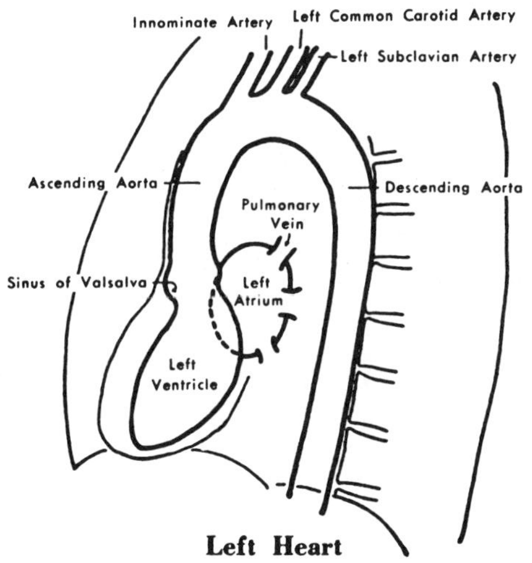

Left Heart

LEFT ANTERIOR OBLIQUE PROJECTION

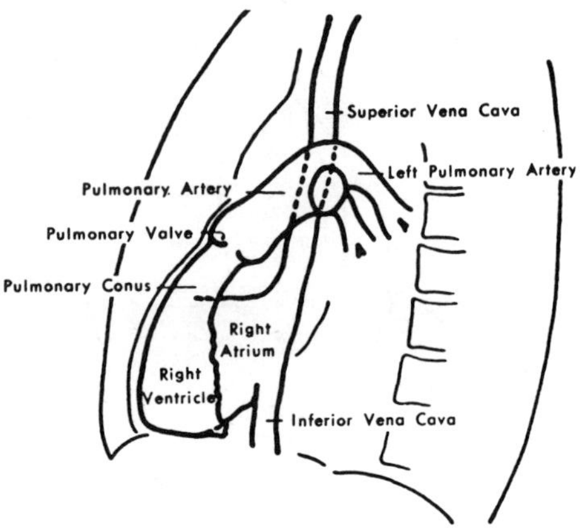

Right Heart

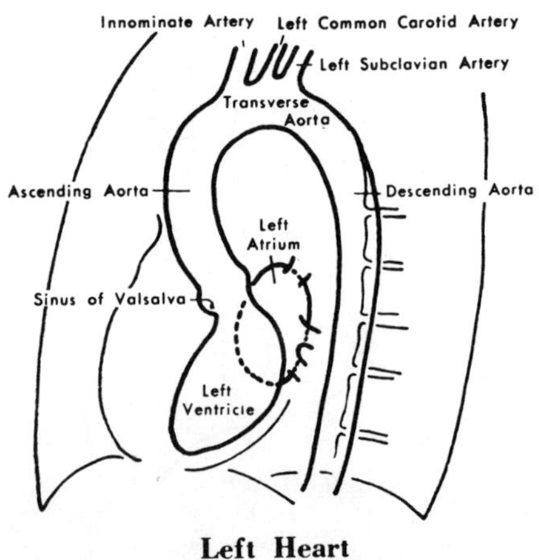

Left Heart

RIGHT ANTERIOR OBLIQUE PROJECTION

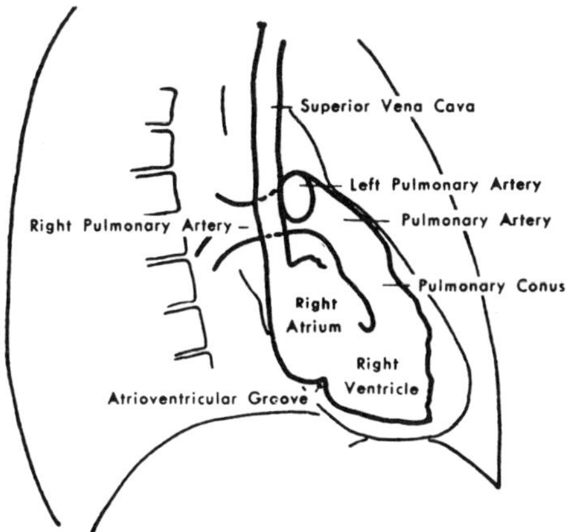

Right Heart

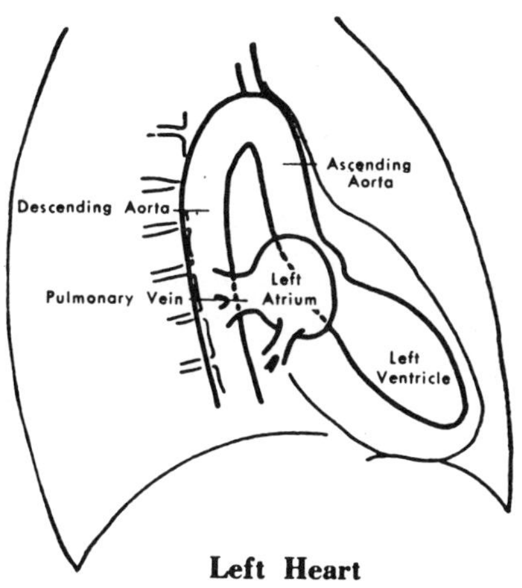

Left Heart

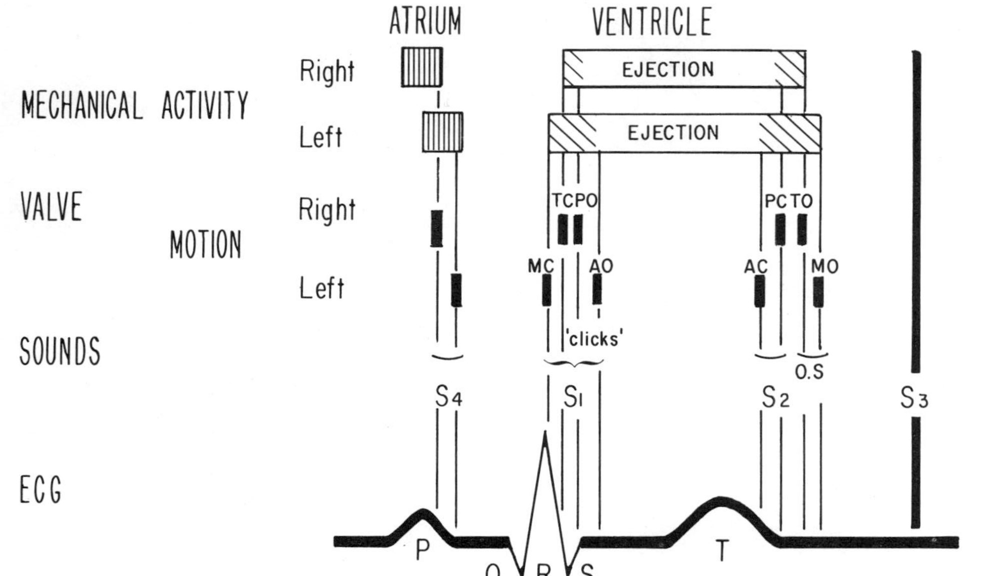

Schematic relationship between electrical and mechanical events and heartsounds. OS represents the opening snap of the mitral or tricuspid valve. "Clicks" are produced by tensing and opening of the aortic or pulmonic valve. S3 represents the ventricular gallop or filling sound produced by the A-V valve of the involved ventricle. S4 is the atrial gallop. (From Hurst and Logue, 1966. The Heart. Courtesy of Blakiston Division, McGraw-Hill Book Company.)

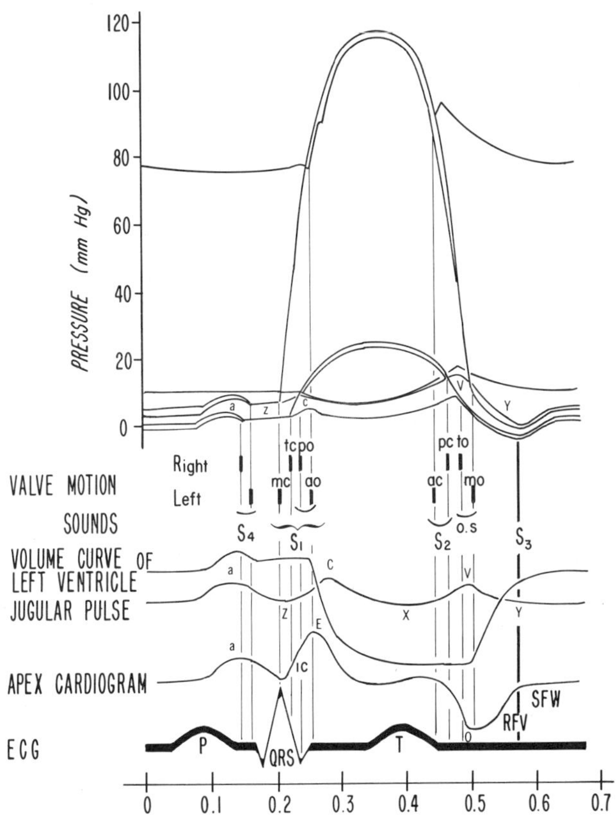

Diagram of the cardiac cycle showing the pressure curves of the great vessels and cardiac chambers, valvular events and heart sounds, left ventricular volume curve, jugular pulse wave, apex cardiogram and electrocardiogram. Valve motion: MC and MO, Mitral "Closure" and opening; TC and TO, tricuspid "closure" and opening; PC and PO, pulmonic "closure" and opening; TC and TO, tricuspid closure and opening; O.S., opening snap of A-V valve(s). Apex cardiogram: IC, isovolumetric contraction wave; IR, isovolumetric relaxation wave; o, opening of mitral valve; RFW, rapid filling wave; SFW slow filling wave. (From Hurst and Logue, 1966. The Heart. Courtesy of Blakiston Division, McGraw-Hill Book Company.)

MEDICAL RESIDENT'S MANUAL

ADAMS-STOKES SYNDROME

Adams-Stokes attacks are due to acute cerebral ischemia on the basis of a sudden change in cardiac rate. Symptoms of an attack vary from slight dizziness or weakness to unconsciousness with or without convulsions. This broad range of symptoms is included in the syndrome because their appearance depends on the duration of the common mechanism–namely, inadequate cerebral perfusion due to a critical decrease in cardiac output.

The most common immediate causes of Adams-Stokes attacks are the ventricular tachyarrhythmias (ventricular tachycardia, ventricular flutter and fibrillation, and chaotic heart action). Ventricular tachycardia was identified in 67 percent of Dressler's cases. Ventricular asystole, complete heart block, or advanced degrees of AV block with an unstable ventricular pacemaker, contrary to opinions before the advent of cardiac monitoring, occupy a secondary etiologic role. Among the lesser degrees of block the unstable Mobitz second-degree type is prone to proceed to a more advanced degree of block with subsequent appearance of Adams-Stokes seizures.

Adams-Stokes attacks most commonly occur as complications of chronic coronary artery disease or as manifestations of the arrhythmic disturbances associated with acute myocardial infarction; they occur infrequently in congenital heart disease and the various forms of myocarditis and digitalis toxicity.

The treatment of Adams-Stokes syndrome is discussed under the heading "Cardiac Pacing."

REFERENCES

Crosby, R. S., et al. Complete heart block. Amer. J. Cardiol., 17:190, 1966.

Dressler, D. Observations in patients with implanted pacemakers. Amer. Heart J., 68:19, 1964.

Grace, W. J., et al. Use of the permanent subcutaneous transvenous pacemaker in Adams-Stokes syndrome. Amer. J. Cardiol., 18:888, 1966.

ADDISON'S DISEASE AND ADRENAL INSUFFICIENCY STATES

ETIOLOGY

A. Secondary adrenocortical insufficiency
   Most commonly associated with panhypopituitarism but rarely associated with an isolated deficiency of corticotropin secretion.
   1. Tumor—craniopharyngioma (more common in preadolescents), chromophobe adenoma (more common in adults).
   2. Postpartum pituitary necrosis (Sheehan's syndrome).
   3. Hypophysectomy.

B. Primary adrenocortical insufficiency
   1. Idiopathic—over 50 percent of cases.
   2. Tuberculosis.
   3. Waterhouse–Freidrichsen syndrome (the fulminating form of meningococcemia associated with purpura and bilateral adrenal hemorrhage).
   4. Other infections (staphylococcemia, histoplasmosis, coccidioidomycosis, cryptococcosis, blastomycosis).
   5. Metastatic cancer (bronchogenic and breast are most common).
   6. Hormone withdrawal after prolonged steroid therapy.
   7. Hemorrhage (traumatic, surgical, secondary to anticoagulant therapy).
   8. Other (amyloid, hemochromatosis, syphilis, congenital).

DIAGNOSIS

HISTORY AND PHYSICAL FINDINGS

1. Weight loss 100%
2. Weakness 100%
3. Pigmentation 90%
4. Vitiligo 15%
5. Hypotension 50%
6. Anorexia, nausea, vomiting.
7. Loss of body hair.
8. Fatigue, nervous and mental irritability.
9. Dizziness, syncope.
10. Muscle aching.
11. Abdominal or back pain.
12. Cold intolerance.
13. Weak voice.
14. Small heart.
15. Hyperpyrexia (crisis).
16. Coma (crisis).
17. Calcification of the pinna.

LABORATORY FINDINGS

1. Decreased urinary 17-hydroxy- and 17-ketosteroids.
2. Decreased response to ACTH stimulation as measured by urinary 17-hydroxysteroids. Twenty-five units of aqueous ACTH given intravenously in 500 ml of normal saline over an 8-hour period should lead to a three- to fivefold increase over the control level of 17-hydroxysteroids. A gradual sustained increase in 17-hydroxysteroids when the ACTH test is repeated over 2 days is seen in patients with secondary adrenal insufficiency.
3. *Metyrapone (Metopirone)* test employs an 11-β-hydroxylase inhibitor which decreases subsequent cortisol production calling forth endogenous ACTH secretion and adrenal stimulation. The test is performed by measuring control urinary 17-hydroxysteroids and 17-ketosteroids. Metopirone tablets–250 mg–3 tablets QID $\times$ 6 doses are given. Twenty-four-hour urinary 17-hydroxysteroids and 17-ketosteroids are measured on the second day of drug administration. Normal patients have at least a twofold increase in 17-hydroxysteroids and a 5.0-mg increment. This is a useful test in patients with ACTH responsiveness. Lack of response to ACTH indicates primary adrenal failure.
4. Water test–1,500 ml of water are given in 15 minutes after an overnight fast. If the urinary output is less than 1,000 ml in 5 hours, water tolerance is impaired.

TREATMENT

CRISIS. Management consists of the administration of hydrocortisone, intravenous fluids (dextrose and saline), and if necessary vasopressors.

1. Hydrocortisone hemisuccinate 100 mg, I.V., stat., plus
2. Hydrocortisone hemisuccinate 100 mg in 1,000 ml glucose in saline 5 percent, over 4 to 6 hours, plus
3. Cortisone acetate 50 to 100 mg, I.M., q. 4 h.
4. Vasopressors (Levophed, Neosynephrine, etc.) if severe hypotension is present.
5. Treatment of cause (meningococcemia, pneumonia, etc.).
6. Additional 5 percent glucose in saline may be given up to 2.5 liters per 24 hours.
7. As improvement occurs, hydrocortisone is discontinued, and cortisone gradually tapered over a number of days.
8. Hourly vital signs, intake-output, and electrolytes should be carefully followed.
9. Morphine and barbiturates are contraindicated.

PREPARATION OF PATIENT FOR SURGICAL REMOVAL OF ADRENAL GLANDS AND PREPARATION OF ADDISONIAN PATIENT FOR SURGERY.

1. For 24 hours prior to surgery give 50 mg of cortisone q. 6 h.
2. During the operation a continuous drip of 5 percent glucose in saline containing 100 mg of hydrocortisone is given.
3. Day of surgery 50 mg of cortisone, q. 6 h., I.M., and 2,000 ml of 5 percent dextrose in saline are given.
4. Subsequently, cortisone is reduced over a 7-10 day period to a maintenance dose (25-37.5 mg). 9-α -fluorohydrocortisone (Florinef) is added to maintain the systolic blood pressure at 110 mm or above. This is generally accomplished by a dose of 0.1 mg P.O. 110 mm Hg daily.

MAINTENANCE THERAPY.

1. Cortisone 12.5 mg b.i.d. to t.i.d., or hydrocortisone, 10 mg b.i.d. to t.i.d.
2. 9-α -fluorohydrocortisone, 0.05 mg to 0.1 mg q.d.

NOTE

Deaths have occasionally been reported with ACTH stimulation. We, therefore, recommend infusing sodium chloride with the aqueous ACTH and placing the patient on dexamethasone for the ACTH gel stimulation test.

REFERENCES

Dunlop, Sir D. Eighty-six cases of Addison's disease. Brit. Med. J., October 12, 1963.

Gold, E. M., Kent, J. R., and Forshan, P. H. Clinical use of a new diagnostic agent, methopyrapone (SU-4885) in pituitary and adrenocortical disorders. Ann. Intern. Med., 54:175, 1961.

Mead, R. K. Autoimmune Addison's disease. New Eng. J. Med., 266:583, 1962.

Paris, J. Pituitary–adrenal suppression after protracted administration of adrenal cortical hormones. Proc. Mayo Clin., 36:305, 1961.

ALCOHOLISM

The patient with chronic alcoholism is subject to a number of disorders in addition to those with which he presents. Besides the alcoholic patient's complaints, which call for the usual type of differential diagnosis, the resident must always keep in mind that the alcoholic patient may have

1. Active liver disease (hepatitis, subacute or chronic active hepatitis, or cirrhosis of the liver).
2. Malnutrition, hypoproteinemia, hypogammaglobulinemia.
3. Anemia from repeated blood loss through varices, gastritis, or hemorrhoids, or hemolytic anemia because of hyperlipemic cirrhosis (Ziev's syndrome).

In addition, the patient with severe chronic alcoholism has a significant alteration in his resistance mechanisms and in his ability to tolerate stress. Often enough, the mechanisms by which bacteria are controlled are sorely impaired in such individuals and only the physician's constant attention to sputum and blood cultures may reveal the infecting organism, but not the nature of the defect in the resistance system. The correction of malnutrition and hypoproteinemia necessary to overcome serious disease should not be overlooked.

The chronic alcoholic may develop one of many clinical syndromes: delirium tremens, Korsakoff's syndrome, Wernicke's syndrome, grand mal seizures, or the acute wet brain syndrome.

DELIRIUM TREMENS. This begins after the withdrawal of alcohol. It is seen in an alcoholic patient who, because of illness or injury, has been admitted to a hospital. It may begin within a few days after the drinking has stopped. The early signs are tremors and restlessness. Later the patient becomes delirious; he is disoriented in time and place. Finally, the delirium is associated with terrible fears and visual hallucinations.

The clinical picture is striking. The patient is frightened, terrified, trembling, restless, subject to hallucinations, and generally drenched with perspiration. Fever and even hyperpyrexia may occur, hypotension may appear, and episodes of uncooperativeness and even violence are the rule. Mortality reaches 20 percent without therapy. These symptoms may mask a serious underlying disease, such as acute infections, pancreatitis, and fat embolism, which frequently precipitates the delirium tremens. Sedation is the therapeutic keynote. Fluid balance and caloric intake are accomplished by giving intravenous glucose and saline. There is little reason to believe that high doses of glucose intravenously will provide anything more than calories.

TREATMENT OF ACUTE ALCOHOLISM.

1. Examine for and treat complicating infections and trauma.
2. Hydrate with oral fluids. About 10 percent require 5 percent D/W I.V. to which 20 mEq K per liter is added.
3. Barbiturates are effective in controlling restlessness and agitation. The doses range between 32 mg q 4 h. P.O. to 165 mg of sodium phenobarbital I.M. q. 2-3 h. For severe agitation pentobarbital 50 mg I.V. over a 5-minute period may be necessary. Diazepam (Valium) 5 mg I.V. repeated in ½ hr is also effective.
4. In the acutely psychotic patient chlorpromazine (Thorazine) 50 mg I.M., q. 6 h. may be substituted for pentobarbital.
5. To control seizures sodium amytal I.V. followed by sodium dilantin 250 mg I.M.
6. No restraints. Keep room well lighted.
7. Give vitamin B complex preparation I.M. q. d.

KORSAKOFF'S SYNDROME. Korsakoff's syndrome is marked by disorientation, memory loss, confabulation, retrograde falsification, and peripheral neuropathy.

WERNICKE'S SYNDROME (Superior Hemorrhagic Polioencephalopathy). Wernicke's syndrome is manifested by mental and emotional deterioration, eye signs consisting of constricted pupils and impairment of extraocolar movements, tremors of the hands, and progressive mental deterioration.

GRAND MAL SEIZURES. The chronic alcoholic is subject to grand mal seizure especially on withdrawal of the alcohol. The seizures may also be associated with a postseizure state of delirium, disorientation, and hallucinations. The seizure is usually brief but may recur and last for weeks. Postictal states are also usually of short duration, but may persist for days or weeks.

ACUTE BRAIN SWELLING. The acute "wet brain" syndrome is characterized by protracted coma. There may be high fever; the mortality rate is high. Treatment consists of general supportive measures, and, in the presence of normal urinary output, the administration of hypertonic solutions. Hypertonic urea 30 percent (Urevert) is frequently valuable.

BLOOD ALCOHOL LEVELS

Blood alcohol is frequently determined for medicolegal reasons. The following levels are approximate indications of "intoxication."

BLOOD LEVEL (percent)	SUBJECTS INTOXICATED (percent)
.05-.10	7-10
.15-.20	22-34
.25-.30	80-100
.35-.40	95-100
.45 plus	100

Fatal dose: 0.5 to 0.9 percent (5 to 9 mg/L).

REFERENCES

Freeman, R. M., and Pearson, E. Hypomagnesemia of unknown etiology. Amer. J. Med., 41:645, 1966.

Hoff, E. C. Newer concepts of alcoholism and its treatment. Quart. J. Stud. Alcohol, 1(suppl.):160, 1961.

Schultz, J. D. Treatment of alcoholism in a general hospital. Quart. J. Stud. Alcohol, 1(suppl.):85, 1961.

ALDOSTERONISM

Primary aldosteronism, the syndrome of mineralocorticoid excess, is produced by certain tumors (95 percent) or hyperplasia (5 percent) of the adrenal cortex. The principal action of aldosterone is exerted on the renal tubule to retain sodium and chloride ions and to promote the excretion of potassium and hydrogen ions. Regulation of aldosterone secretion is normally mediated through the renin-angiotensin system which is primarily responsive to changes in intravascular fluid volume; secondarily by changes in body sodium and potassium and, to a lesser degree, by ACTH.

DIAGNOSIS

Diagnosis is suggested by findings of hypertension, weakness, hypokalemia, and the finding of increased urinary aldosterone.

HISTORY AND PHYSICAL

1. Polyuria, polydipsia.
2. Weakness, frequently episodic.
3. Tetany.
4. Severe headache.
5. Paresthesias of the face, hands, and feet.

6. Hypertension, moderate to severe.
7. Edema is unusual.
8. Chvostek and Trosseau signs may be present.
9. Cardiac enlargement may be present.

LABORATORY

1. Hypokalemia (serum K usually below 3.0 mEq/L), which is alleviated by the administration of spironolactone and rigorous sodium restriction.
2. Slight hypernatremia and hypochloremia, with alkalosis. The CO_2 content is elevated above 25 mEq/L.
3. Alkaline urine (pH consistently above 6.0).
4. Normal 17-hydroxy- and 17-ketosteroids are present in primary aldosteronism, in contrast to Cushing's syndrome.
5. Plasma volume is increased, in contrast to other forms of hypertension in the absence of heart failure.
6. Increased urinary aldosterone is present on a normal salt diet. Sodium deprivation itself may give rise to very high aldosterone levels. Administration of deoxycorticosterone leads to little suppression of aldosterone tumor, while normal patients or those with secondary hyperaldosteronism have significant suppression.
7. Plasma renin low or absent.
8. Intermittent or persistent proteinuria.
9. Large volumes of low specific gravity urine unresponsive to vasopressin or water restriction.
10. Hyperkaluria.
11. Decreased renal function, especially tubular reabsorption of water.
12. Arteriography and venography for visualization of the adrenals.

SECONDARY ALDOSTERONISM

Excess excretion of aldosterone is also associated with congestive heart failure, cirrhosis with ascites, nephrosis, toxemia of pregnancy, malignant hypertension and a low-sodium diet. The serum sodium is usually decreased (less than 136 mEq/l) and the renin is normal or elevated.

REFERENCES

Biglieri, E. G., Slaton, P. E., Jr., Kronfield, S. J. and Schambelan, M. Diagnosis of an aldosterone-producing adenoma in primary aldosteronism; An evaluative maneuver. J.A.M.A., 201:510, 1967.

Conn, J. W. Aldosteronism in man, Part I. J.A.M.A., 183:775, 1963.

—— Aldosteronism in man, Part II. J.A.M.A., 183:871, 1963.

——Rovner, D. R., and Cohen, E. L. Normal and altered function of the renin-angiotensin-aldosterone system in man: Application in clinical and research medicine. Ann. Intern. Med., 63:266, 1965.

Davis, J. O., et al. Bilateral adrenal hyperplasia as a cause of primary aldosteronism with hypertension, hypokalemia and suppressed renin activity. Amer. J. Med., 272:1189, 1965.

Editorial: Preoperative diagnosis of primary aldosteronism. Amer. J. Med., 41:855, 1966.

AMYLOIDOSIS

Definition: A disease state produced by the deposition of hyaline proteinaceous substance in various tissues. Three clinical types have been described but there is increasing evidence of considerable overlap among the categories.

PRIMARY AMYLOIDOSIS. The deposit may be found in any tissue or organ. It is most frequently seen in the heart and blood vessels. Abnormalities are often found in the plasma cells of the bone marrow in this condition. A familial history may exist.

SECONDARY AMYLOIDOSIS. Deposition here occurs in the liver, spleen, adrenals, and kidneys. It is associated with rheumatoid arthritis, osteomyelitis, chronic ulcerative colitis, regional enteritis, Hodgkin's disease, lymphosarcoma, chronic TB, cirrhosis, and chronic nephritis. A high percentage of patients with familial Mediterranean fever eventually develop amyloidosis.

"PARAMYLOID". Amyloidosis is associated with multiple myeloma in 15 percent of cases. This possibly may be related to or identical with primary amyloid.

DIAGNOSIS

HISTORY AND PHYSICAL

The diagnosis of amyloidosis will never be made unless the disease is kept in mind. Intractable congestive heart failure with cardiomegaly but without hypertension or valvular lesions is a common presenting manifestation. The nephrotic syndrome is also a common manifestation.

Symptoms and findings depend upon the organ or organs

involved. In 81 cases of primary amyloidosis, the following occurred:

Weakness, fatigue	20%	Macroglossia	25%
Anorexia, weight loss	(most cases)	Hepatomegaly	50%
Dyspnea	10%	Splenomegaly	10%
Paresthesias of hands	6%	Lymphadenopathy	15%
Nausea, vomiting	5%	Skin lesions	30%
Ankle edema	12%	Congestive heart failure	30%
Purpura	31%		

LABORATORY FINDINGS

1. Most helpful is biopsy of gingiva, skin, liver, rectum, or kidney.
2. Ophthalmologic biomicroscope examination of vitreous opacities, when present, may show amyloid.
3. Serum protein electrophoresis may show an "M spike," or hypogammaglobulinemia, or other abnormality.
4. Anemia is frequently present.
5. Proteinuria is often found, and Bence Jones protein may be present in those cases associated with a plasma cell dyscrasia.

ANEMIA

ETIOLOGY

1. Excessive destruction or loss of red cells
   a. Blood loss anemia.
   b. Hemolytic anemia.
2. Insufficient supply of certain substances
   a. Iron deficiency.
   b. B_{12} deficiency.
   c. Folic acid deficiency.
3. Defective function of the bone marrow
   a. Anemia of infection.
   b. Bone marrow failure due to chemicals, drugs, or physical agents.
   c. Myelophthistic anemia (infiltration of the marrow with neoplastic cells, leukemia, myelofibrosis).
   d. Idiopathic aplastic anemia.
   e. Anemia associated with uremia, rheumatoid arthritis, chronic disease.
   f. Sideroachrestic (sideroblastic) anemia.

DIAGNOSIS

1. History, with special attention to
   a. Clues concerning possible sources of blood loss (G.I., G.U., GYN., blood donations)
   b. Family history including racial and national origin
   c. Duration of anemia
   d. Dietary history (especially in children)
   e. Presence of other disease.
2. Physical examination.
3. Laboratory studies.
   a. Examination of peripheral smear (red cell morphology, presence of abnormal forms, etc.).
   b. Reticulocyte count.
   c. Stool examination for occult blood.
   d. BUN.
   e. Bone marrow examination including stain for hemosiderin.
   f. Serum iron and iron-binding capacity.

DISEASE	SERUM IRON	IRON-BINDING CAPACITY
Iron deficiency	↓	↑
Pregnancy	↓	↑
Acute infections	↓	↓
Chronic infections	↓	↓
Viral hepatitis	↑	↓
Hemochromatosis	↑	↓

DIFFERENTIAL DIAGNOSIS OF THALASSEMIA MINOR AND IRON DEFICIENCY ANEMIA

	COOLEY'S ANEMIA	IRON DEFICIENCY
Spleen	±	0 to +
Serum Fe++	normal or ↑	↓
Bone marrow hemosiderin	abundant	↓ to absent
Target cells	++	occasional
Response to Fe++ ℞	0	++++
Hemoglobin	A2 or HbF ↑	normal

IRON DEFICIENCY ANEMIA

Iron deficiency anemia is usually due to chronic blood loss. Gastrointestinal loss in males and obstetrical, menstrual, or gastrointestinal loss in females accounts for over 90 percent of cases. In growing children, iron deficiency may result because of inadequate dietary intake.

Approximately 10 ml of blood–stool positive for occult blood.
Approximately 60-80 ml of blood–black stool.

IRON THERAPY. Ferrous sulfate tabs., USP, contain approximately 60 mg of elemental iron. Of this about 10 percent is absorbed through the gastrointestinal tract. Iron-dextran complex may be used for parenteral administration, but because of possible side effects (skin rash, fever, anaphylaxis) it should be employed only when oral therapy has failed or absolutely cannot be tolerated. Clinical and hematologic response occurs at the same rate regardless of the route of administration, if dosage is adequate.

REFERENCES

Barry, W. E., et al. Refractory sideroblastic anemia, clinical and hematologic study of ten cases. Ann. Intern. Med., 61:1029, 1964.

Council on Foods and Nutrition. Iron deficiency in the United States. J.A.M.A., 203:407, 1968.

Ellis, L. D., et al. Marrow iron, an evaluation of depleted stores in series of 1,332 needle biopsies. Ann. Intern. Med., 61:44, 1964.

Movitt, E. R., et al. Idiopathic true bone marrow failure. Amer. J. Med., 34:500, 1963.

MEGALOBLASTIC ANEMIAS

Megaloblastic anemias	respond to
Pernicious anemia	B_{12}
Malabsorption	B_{12}; or folic acid; or both
Liver disease	Folic acid
Dilantin therapy	Folic acid
D. latum infestation	Eradication of worm; B_{12}
Blind loop syndrome	Antibiotics; B_{12}
Pregnancy	Folic acid
After total gastrectomy	B_{12}
Associated with hemolysis	Folic acid

TREATMENT

1. Pernicious anemia: B_{12} 200 μg I.M. daily for one week, then 100 μcg I.M. every four weeks.

2. Folic acid deficiency: 5 mg t.i.d.

REFERENCE

Silber, R. Recent developments in non-Addisonian megaloblastic anemias. Seminars in Hematology. 1:250, 1964.

ANTIBIOTICS AND OTHER ANTIMICROBIALS

The appropriate use of these agents may be lifesaving; their indiscriminate use can lead to tragedy. The problem of the resistant staphylococcus and of "hospital infections" is related largely to the overuse of antibiotics. Sufficient studies have been performed to indicate that prophylactic use of antibiotics is fraught with danger. Antibiotics will not prevent pneumonia in heart failure, in bulbar polio, in barbiturate overdoses, or in other patients with coma; they will not prevent postoperative infections or urinary infections in patients with indwelling catheters. Indeed, the physician in these situations is then confronted with a resistant organism, in addition to taking the added risk of the untoward effects of these drugs.

Antibiotic prophylaxis in adults is universally accepted in only one situation: prevention of rheumatic fever. In epidemics caused by the sensitive Type A meningococcus, sulfonamides are generally used and, in some areas, antibiotics have been recommended for families in which one member incurs a Group A streptococcal pharyngitis.

Finally, the use of antimicrobials in upper respiratory infections, "flu," etc., is mentioned only to be condemned. The vast majority of these infections are viral in etiology. The risk of "secondary invaders" in viral infections is considerably overestimated.

AMPHOTERICIN B

Active against *Coccidioides immitis, Histoplasma capsulatum, Cryptococcus neoformans, Blastomyces dermatitides, B. brasiliensis,* and some species of *Candida.*

UNTOWARD EFFECTS. Anorexia, vomiting, headache, fever and chills occur frequently. Salicylates, antihistamines and steroids may be required to alleviate symptoms. Azotemia may occur and is the chief limiting factor of this drug. It appears to be dose-related and reversible on stopping therapy. However, permanent renal damage may occur.

DOSE. Used only intravenously: 0.25 mg/kg of body weight daily initially; diluted to 0.1 mg/ml of glucose/water solution (*not saline*). This dose is gradually increased up to as high as 1.5 mg/kg daily, or to the highest level not accompanied by toxic manifestations. Since amphotericin B is very slowly excreted, patients on the higher doses may be given the drug on alternate days if necessary. Duration of therapy averages 4 to 8 weeks at full doses. Intrathecal therapy may be required for cryptococcal meningitis.

BACITRACIN

Recommended for topical use only, because of renal toxicity.

CEPHALOTHIN

Bactericidal with a broader spectrum than penicillin; effective against almost all gram-positive organisms. An excellent antibiotic in patients allergic to penicillin although occasionally cross allergenicity may occur.

UNTOWARD EFFECTS. Pain on deep I.M. injection; phlebitis after I.V. administration. Hypersensitivity reactions, e.g., urticaria and skin rash.

DOSE. Must be given I.V. or I.M. in doses of 4-12 g q.d. depending on severity of infection or may be given in full dosage in presence of renal impairment.

CHLORAMPHENICAL

Effective against nearly all the gram-positive and gram-negative bacteria, all the rickettsiae and larger viruses (lymphogranuloma-psittacosis group); particularly valuable in salmonella infections (especially extraintestinal infections). *Chloramphenical is bacteriostatic.*

UNTOWARD EFFECTS. Bone marrow depression which is dose-related and reversible by discontinuing drug may occur. Rarely, aplastic anemia, which is almost always fatal, may occur. Nausea, vomiting, diarrhea and superinfections may complicate its use.

DOSE.

1. Oral: The usual oral dose is 250 to 500 mg, q.i.d.
2. Parenteral: 1.0 g, q.d., in divided doses.

COLISTIN

(Colymysin)

Bactericidal against gram-negative organisms, especially *Pseudomonas.*

UNTOWARD EFFECTS. Paresthesias, dizziness. Impaired renal function may occur in patients with prior renal disease.

DOSE. Usually 2-3 mg/kg I.M. q.d. In severe infections with normal renal function 5 mg/kg I.M. q.d. may be given. With decreased renal function the dose must be decreased. Must be given intrathecally in the treatment of meningitis.

ERYTHROMYCIN AND ERYTHROMYCINLIKE ANTIBIOTICS

(Carbomycin, Oleandomycin, Spiramycin)

These antibiotics have completely overlapping activity. Erythromycin is by far the superior of the group, effective against almost all gram-positive cocci and bacilli and gram-negative cocci.

GENTAMYCIN

Bactericidal in action with a broad spectrum. Useful in urinary tract infections.

UNTOWARD EFFECTS. Irreversible vestibular damage may occur especially in patients with impaired renal function who are unable to excrete the drug. Azotemia and proteinuria may occur.

DOSE. 0.4 mg/kg q. 6 h. I.V. or I.M.

KANAMYCIN

This antibiotic is related in its spectrum and toxicity to both streptomycin and neomycin. It is bactericidal and effective against many gram-positive cocci and gram-negative bacilli.

UNTOWARD EFFECTS. Renal damage. Eighth cranial nerve damage.

DOSE. Kanamycin is absorbed from the gastrointestinal tract in negligible amounts.

1. Oral: 500-1,000 mg, q.i.d.
2. Parenteral: 500 mg, b.i.d., is the average dose. If renal disease is present, an initial dose of 1.0 g followed by 0.5 g q. 2-3 d. is given.

LINCOMYCIN

(Lincocin)

Effective against gram-positive organisms and "resistant" staphylococci.

DOSE.

1. Oral: 2 g daily.
2. Parenteral: I.M., 600 mg, b.i.d.; I.V., 600 mg, q. 8-12 h.

NEOMYCIN

Most common applications are in preoperative bowel preparation and hepatic coma. It is active against many gram-negative and gram-positive bacteria, and is most effective against the particularly troublesome trio: *Proteus, Pseudomonas,* and *Staphylococcus.* It is useful also as an aerosol in chronic lung infections, and orally in bacterial diarrheas.

UNTOWARD EFFECTS. Deafness occurs in about 20 percent of patients treated with parenteral neomycin, and is irreversible. Nephrotoxicity and neurotoxicity may also occur. Malabsorption from the small intestine may appear after prolonged use.

DOSE.

1. Oral: 1.0 g, q.i.d.
2. Parenteral: 0.5 g in 500 ml saline solution I.V., b.i.d.

NILIDIXIC ACID

(NegGram)

Used for acute and chronic urinary tract infections. Very low tissue and serum levels obtained. Therefore, it should not be used for systemic infections.

DOSE. Oral: 2-4 g daily.

NITROFURANTOIN (FURADANTIN)

The nitrofurans have a limited usefulness and only in acute urinary tract infections. They produce little serum or tissue levels of drug and are rapidly excreted; hence, they are not useful for systemic diseases or deep-seated lesions.

DOSE. Oral: 50-100 mg q.i.d.

NOVOBIOCIN

Spectrum of activity is similar to penicillin. Rarely used because of the high frequency of untoward effects. See "Erythromycin" or "Penicillin."

NYSTATIN

For infections caused by *Candida albicans (Monilia).*

Nystatin is poorly absorbed from the gastrointestinal tract, and, therefore, is of no value in systemic moniliasis. Nystatin has been used, with generally poor results, against infections caused by other yeasts, fungi and molds.

DOSE.

1. For intestinal moniliasis 500,000 units, t.i.d., may be used.
2. Nystatin gargles are helpful for oral moniliasis (100,000 units, q.i.d.).
3. Vaginal preparations are also available.

PENICILLIN

Penicillin is the most remarkable of the antibiotics. Its safety and usefulness are unsurpassed.

It is effective against gram-positive cocci—e.g., pneumococci, streptococci, and staphylococci. There are almost no resistant pneumococci or streptococci.

Some strains of staphylococci are penicillin-resistant due to their capacity to produce penicillinase. The semisynthetic penicillins are useful for such infections. In the face of a serious staph infection of mixed or "resistant" type, a combination of biosynthetic and semisynthetic penicillins is to be used.

UNTOWARD EFFECTS. In sensitized allergic individuals the range of reactions varies from urticaria to acute anaphylactoid reactions with death. For this reason, a careful allergic history must be taken on every patient in whom the use of penicillin is indicated. This is of greater value than scratch or conjunctival tests, which may be falsely negative. Penicillin is perhaps best avoided in patients with bronchial asthma. The safety of the semisynthetic penicillins for such allergic persons has not yet been demonstrated.

In those cases where penicillin administration is vital for life—for example, subacute bacterial endocarditis due to *Streptococcus viridans*—100 million or more units of penicillin have been successfully administered per day to patients with known sensitivity. The administration of steroids (prednisolone, 15 mg, q. 6 h.) and/or Dimetane (4 to 8 mg, q. 4 h.) has successfully prevented reactions in these patients even though penicillin was continued for 6 weeks in these massive doses.

TYPES.

Biosynthetic: Penicillin G and V. Both are penicillinase susceptible and are not useful in the infections due to "resistant" or penicillinase-producing staphylococci. Dose: 300,000-600,000 units, I.M., b.i.d.; oral dose: 200,000 units t.i.d.

Semisynthetic:

A. Penicillinase susceptible
   1. Have a spectrum and limitations as penicillin G (Tynallin; Alpen; Chemipen; Maxipen; Darcil; Semopen).
   2. "Broad spectrum" penicillin. Ampicillin (Polycillin). Use for gram-positive organisms as in penicillin G. Also useful for *Hemophilus. E. coli.* and *Shigella.* Dose: 1 g, q. 4 h.

B. Penicillinase-resistant penicillins (I.V. or I.M. or oral)
   1. Methicillin (Staphcillin) (parenteral only) 1 g q. 4-6 h. Higher doses may be given in severe infections.
   2. Oxacillin (Prostaphlin) 0.5 g q. 4-6 h. Oxacillin is best

absorbed on an empty stomach and should be given 1 hour before meals.

3. Nafcillin (Unipen). Dose: 1 g q. 4 h.

POLYMYXIN B

Very rarely used. See "Colistin."

RISTOCETIN

(Spontin)

Effective against gram-positive organisms, gram-negative diplococci and *Mycobacterium tuberculosis.* At present, the main use is in coccal septicemias and particularly enterococcal endocarditis. The average dose is 1.0 g, q. 12 h., given intravenously in 100 ml 5 percent glucose in water over a 15- to 30-minute period. In endocarditis, this is continued for two weeks.

SPIRAMYCIN

See "Erythromycin."

STREPTOMYCIN

Active against both gram-positive bacteria and mycobacteria and slightly active against some rickettsias. Its major usefulness is in the treatment of tuberculosis. To a lesser extent, it is of aid against gram-negative bacteria and as a second antibiotic either for synergism or to help reduce resistant variants.

It is also of value in Friedländer's pneumonia and in subacute bacterial endocarditis due to resistant streptococcus in combination with penicillin.

UNTOWARD EFFECTS.

1. Vestibular damage with vertigo and deafness. The latter is most frequent with dihydrostreptomycin, and for that reason dihydrostreptomycin has fallen into disrepute. Although the toxic effects are permanent, patients learn to compensate for the vertigo. Vestibular damage may occur after as little as 10 g of streptomycin.
2. Skin rashes, drug fever, transient paresthesias, and eosinophilia have also been reported. Resistant strains develop quickly and thus streptomycin is usually used in combination with another antibiotic.

DOSE. The usual dose is 0.5 g, q.d. or b.i.d. I.M. (see also "Tuberculosis").

SULFONAMIDES

The treatment of choice in meningococcal meningitis, and of value in bacillary dysentery and urinary tract infections. Sulfonamides are active against many gram-positive and -negative organisms, but have been replaced to a large degree by penicillin.

UNTOWARD EFFECTS. Occur in about 1 to 5 percent of patients.

1. Nausea, vomiting.
2. Fever.
3. Headache, dizziness.
4. Hematuria, oliguria or anuria.
5. Skin rashes.
6. Anemia, leukopenia, or agranulocytosis.
7. Hepatic damage.
8. Vasculitis.

DOSE. Prophylactic:

1. In cases of exposure to meningococcal infections: sulfadiazine or sulfisoxazole (Gantrisin), 2 g, stat., or 0.5 g, b.i.d., for 2 days.
2. Against Group A streptococcal infections, either of the above drugs, 1.0 g, daily.
3. Against urinary tract infection in patients with indwelling catheters. This therapy is to be condemned. With or without antimicrobials over 90 percent of patients with catheters indwelling for 3 days or more will develop infection. If prophylaxis is employed, the physician is then more likely to be faced with a resistant organism.

Therapeutic: The usual dose is 1.0 g q.i.d., of sulfisoxazole (Gantrisin) or sulfadiazine: or 1.0 g a day of the longer-acting dimethoxysulfadiazine (Madribon). Another long-acting derivative, sulfamethoxypyridazine, has been associated with a high degree of untoward effects.

TETRACYCLINES

(Chlortetracycline, Oxytetracycline, and Tetracycline)

The activity of the three may be considered identical. They are bacteriostatic. Spectrum of activity includes nearly all the gram-positive and -negative bacteria, all the rickettsia, and the larger viruses (lymphogranuloma-psittacosis group).

UNTOWARD EFFECTS.

1. Nausea, vomiting, diarrhea with or without monilial overgrowth. Resistant staphylococci may overgrow the normal flora in tetracycline-

treated patients and produce the severe and often fatal staphylococcal enterocolitis.

2. Photosensitivity reactions have been reported with the newer tetracycline derivative demethylchlortetracycline.
3. Systemic lupus erythematosus (SLE) may be aggravated by any of the tetracyclines.
4. Fanconi-like syndromes have been reported from use of "outdated" tetracyclines.
5. Yellowing of teeth in infants.
6. Azotemia due to interference with anabolism of proteins. This may cause difficulty in patients who already have impaired renal function.

DOSE. The usual oral dose is 250 mg, q.i.d. Intramuscular or intravenous dose averages 100-200 mg, q.i.d.

TRIACETYLOLEANDOMYCIN

See "Erythromycin."

VANCOMYCIN

Main field of usefulness is against the staphylococci.

UNTOWARD EFFECTS. Ototoxicity, especially in patients with impaired renal function. Fever, chills, nausea, urticaria, rashes, and thrombophlebitis.

DOSE. Intravenous preparations only: 500 mg, q. 6 h., as intermittent or continuous infusion.

REFERENCES

Butler, W. T. Pharmacology, toxicity and therapeutic usefulness of Amphoteracin B. J.A.M.A., 195:371, 1966.

Christie, A. B. Treatment of typhoid carriers with Ampicillin, Brit. Med. J., 1:1609, 1964.

Eickhoff, T. C., et al. Clinical evaluation of Nafcillin in patients with severe staphylococcal disease. New Eng. J. Med., 272:699, 1965.

Hewitt, W. L. The penicillins. J.A.M.A., 185:118, 1963.

Klein, J. O., and Finland, M. The new penicillins. New Eng. J. Med., 269:1019, 1963. *Continued,* New Eng. J. Med., 269:1074, 1963. *Concluded,* New Eng. J. Med., 269:1129, 1963.

Kunin, C. L. A Guide to Use of Antibiotics in Patients with Renal Disease. Ann. Intern. Med., 67:151, 1967.

MacKay, D. N., et al. Serum concentrations of colistin in patients with normal and impaired renal function. New Eng. J. Med., 270:394, 1964.

Med. Clin. N. Amer., 48:255, 1964.

Petersdorf, R. G., and Plorder, J. J. Colistin–a reappraisal. J.A.M.A., 183:123, 1963.
Seelig, M. S. The role of antibiotics in the pathogenesis of candida infections. Amer. J. Med., 40:887, 1966.

ANTICOAGULANTS

INDICATIONS

Acute myocardial infarction.
Long-term management of postmyocardial infarction.
Acute thrombophlebitis.
Rheumatic heart disease with emboli.
Acute and chronic peripheral arterial insufficiency.
Recurrent pulmonary emboli.
Frostbite.
Central retinal vein and artery thrombosis.

Reports indicate that anticoagulants have also been used with varying degrees of success in angina pectoris, acute cerebral thrombosis or insufficiency, congestive heart failure, polycythemia vera, in crush injuries, chronic recurrent thrombophlebitis, and primary pulmonary artery hypertension.

CONTRAINDICATIONS

Coagulation disorders and hemorrhagic states.
Severe liver disease with hypoprothrombinemia.
Active duodenal ulcer.
Chronic ulcerative colitis.
Pericarditis.
Renal disease with bleeding diathesis.
SBE.
Late pregnancy.
Hypertension (produces cerebral hemorrhage).
Cerebral hemorrhage and postoperative brain or cord surgery.

Save possibly for the first and last of these, the contraindications are relative, and should be weighed against the severity of the primary disease.

PREPARATIONS

HEPARIN

PROCEDURE.

1. Perform Lee-White clotting time.
2. Heparin, 7,500 units, I.V.
3. Recheck clotting time after 4 hours.
4. Continue heparin at a dose sufficient to keep clotting time 2 to 3 times the control. This will range between 5,000 and 7,500 units, I.M., q. 6 h.
5. If bishydroxycoumarin or a related drug is also employed, heparin may be discontinued when the prothrombin time reaches 25 seconds.
6. If bleeding develops (hematuria, rectal bleeding, and epistaxes most common), the effect of heparin may be quickly reversed by I.V. protamine in the same dose as the last dose of heparin.
7. Other rare side effects include alopecia and anaphylaxis.

COUMARIN DERIVATIVES

PROCEDURE.

1. Prothrombin time stat. and q.d.
2. If a normal time is obtained initially dicoumarol 300 mg, or Coumadin 25 mg, P.O., is given.
3. On the following day, the usual dose is 100 to 200 mg dicoumarol or 10 to 25 mg Coumadin.
4. Subsequent daily doses are regulated depending on the prothrombin time, with a maintenance dose to keep the prothrombin time approximately 2 to 2.5 times the control. The usual maintenance dose of Coumadin is 5 to 10 mg.
5. When the prothrombin time is stable at this level, the frequency of determination may be gradually decreased to one- or two-week intervals.
6. If bleeding appears, the intravenous administration of vitamin K_1 (Mephyton) in a dose of 10 to 50 mg will reverse the hypoprothrombinemia in approximately 3 to 6 hours. The lower doses appear preferable because of the possibility of producing hypercoagulable states at the larger doses. Hykinone and Synkavite (menadione derivatives) may also be employed at doses of approximately 75 mg I.V.; however, these agents do not act as promptly.

COMMENTS

1. Long-term or lifelong continuous anticoagulant therapy following myocardial infarction appears to be associated with a significantly

lower death rate according to some authors. Recently some evidence has been presented to challenge this opinion and the former wide-spread use is no longer routine. A cooperative and observant patient is a prerequisite for this therapy.

2. Patients on long-term or outpatient therapy should carry an identification card indicating that they take anticoagulants.
3. Dental surgery has been safely performed in an anticoagulated patient.
4. The one-stage prothrombin time may be prolonged by heparin. If a patient is on both heparin and a coumarin compound, prothrombin determination should be drawn just before heparin administration or be performed by the two-stage test.

REFERENCES

Conrad, L. L., Kyriacopoulos, J. D., Wiggins, C. W., and Honick, G. L. Prevention of recurrences of myocardial infarction. Arch. Intern., Med., 114:348, 1964.

Symposium: Anti-coagulation. Amer. J. Med., 33:619, 1962.

INAPPROPRIATE ANTIDIURETIC SYNDROME

Inappropriate ADH syndrome should be suspected in patients with hyponatremia and hypo-osmolality.

SYMPTOMS

With significant lowering of serum sodium, anorexia, nausea, vomiting followed by apathy, confusion, and coma may develop. Edema is characteristically absent.

LABORATORY FINDINGS

1. Hyponatremia and hypochloremia.
2. Hypo-osmolality.
3. Urine hypertonic in relation to plasma.
4. Normal renal, cardiac, and adrenal function.

ETIOLOGY

1. Carcinoma of the lung (oat-cell or anaplastic type most common).

2. Central nervous disorders – meningitis, trauma, brain tumors.
3. Acute intermittent porphyria, myxedema.

TREATMENT

Restriction of fluid intake.

REFERENCE

Bartter, F. C., and Schwartz, W. B. The syndrome of inappropriate secretion of antidiuretic hormone. Amer. J. Med., 42:790, 1967.

APEX CARDIOGRAM (ACG)

The apex cardiogram and its relation to the cardiac cycle have been well standardized by use as a reference tracing in phonocardiography, by changes due to various pathologic conditons (especially valvular heart disease), and by the simultaneous recording of ventricular pressures during cardiac catheterization.

There are four, easily recognized reference points in the apex cardiogram: the "A" wave discussed below, the "E" point, normally the highest point of the tracings, the "O" point and the "F" point or summit of the rapid-filling wave (RFW). The "E" point represents the opening of the aortic valve and therefore separates isometric contraction from the ejection phase. The "O" point correlates well with the opening of the mitral valve (therefore corresponding in time with the opening snap in mitral stenosis) at which point the impulse of the heart on the chest wall is least. As the ventricle fills, a positive deflection is again present in the ACG terminating in the "F" point which coincides with the normal or pathologic third heart sound (S3).

The normal ACG consists of four phases:

1. "A" Wave. This represents ventricular filling due to atrial contraction. It is a small wave (less than 20 percent of the total or E-O height) occurring 0.08 to 0.12 second after the P wave of the ECG and is simultaneous with or slightly precedes the ORS complex. It coincides with the fourth heart sound or presystolic (atrial) gallop.
2. Systolic phase. Extends from the end of the "A" wave to the "O" point. It consists of an initial positive deflection followed by a negative deflection after the "E" point and usually has a plateau before a final negative deflection to the "O" point.

3. Rapid filling phase. Extends from the "O" point to the "F" point. This represents the rapid filling wave following the opening of the mitral valve and terminates when ventricular pressure begins to rise due to compliance of the left ventricle. During this phase, 50 to 75 percent of ventricular filling takes place with S3 occurring at its terminus, the "F" point.
4. Slow filling phase. Extends from the "F" point to the beginning of the "A" wave and represents the remainder of the passive filling phase of diastole.

REFERENCE

Tafur, E., et al. The normal apex cardiogram. Circulation, 30:381, 1964.

ASCITES

(See also Cirrhosis)

Ascites refers to the presence of free fluid within the abdominal cavity in clinically detectable amounts. *Causes* are essentially five in number:

1. HEPATIC AND PORTAL. The usual cause is Laennec's cirrhosis. Obstruction of the hepatic veins (Budd-Chiari syndrome) from any cause may result in ascites. Severe malnutrition with avitaminosis, echinococcus, and other parasitic diseases may cause ascites, but are extremely rare causes in this country.

2. CARDIAC. Right heart failure secondary to left failure or pulmonary disease, tricuspid valvular disease, and chronic constrictive pericarditis.

3. RENAL. Outstanding is the nephrotic syndrome with its six major causes:

a. Glomerulonephritis.
b. Diabetic nephropathy.
c. SLE.
d. Amyloid disease.
e. Renal vein obstruction.
f. "Pure" lipoid nephrosis.

4. NEOPLASTIC. Tumors most frequently producing ascites are those of the liver, pancreas, stomach, ovary, and kidney. Sarcomas, leukemias, and lymphoma also may cause ascites.

5. RARE CAUSES. Include tuberculous peritonitis and Mediterranean fever (periodic peritonitis).

REFERENCES

Liebowitz, H. R. Hazards of abdominal paracentesis in the cirrhotic patient, Part I, N.Y. J. Med., June 1, 1962; Part II, N.Y. J. Med., June 15, 1962; Part III, N.Y. J. Med., July 1, 1962.

Snell, A., et al. Panel: Ascites. Gastroenterology, 38:129, 1960.

ASTHMA

Definition: A disease characterized by increased responsiveness of the trachea and bronchi to various stimuli and manifested by a widespread narrowing of the airways that changes in degree either spontaneously or as a result of therapy.

CAUSES

Primarily, hereditary predisposition plus allergy (extrinsic asthma) or infection (intrinsic asthma). Precipitating factors are physical or chemical respiratory irritants or certain kinds of emotional tension. The following table provides approximate figures on causes. It should be noted that in about 10 to 20 percent of patients no definite cause can be ascertained.

Infants (age 1 to 5)	Infection	90%
	Foods rarely primary	
Children (age 5 to 15)	Inhalants	70%
	Infection	5%
	Both	15%
	Foods	1%
Adults (age 15 to 40)	Inhalants	50%
	Infection	10%
	Both	25%
	Foods and drugs rare alone	
Adults (over 40)	Inhalants	10%
	Infection	40%
	Both	40%
	Foods	rare

PATHOLOGY

1. Plugs of packed mucus block many of the terminal bronchioles.

2. The goblet cells are increased in size and number.
3. Marked thickening and irregularity of the basement membrane are present.
4. The smooth muscle of the preterminal bronchioles are hypertrophied.
5. An inflammatory infiltrate composed of mononuclear cells and eosinophiles is found in the submucosa and between the hypertrophied muscle bundles.

DIAGNOSIS

HISTORY AND PHYSICAL

1. Wheezing, which can frequently be heard without the stethoscope.
2. Cough.
3. Dyspnea.
4. Chest tightness.
5. Evenly distributed musical rales.
6. Diminution of breath sounds.

LABORATORY

(No laboratory test is diagnostic)

1. Eosinophilia may be present.
2. Sinus x-rays may show polyps.
3. Chest x-rays (emphysema, pneumonitis, etc.).
4. Venous pressure may help differentiate from cardiac asthma.

TREATMENT

1. Allergy: skin testing and appropriate desensitization or removal from environment.
2. Infection: appropriate antibiotics.
3. Symptomatic, acute:
   Epinephrine: 0.2 to 0.3 ml of 1:1,000 solution, subcutaneously
   Bronchodilator aerosols (Vaponephrin, Isuprel, etc.)
   Aminophylline: 0.25 to 0.5 g, I.V., slowly
   Oxygen, preferably humidified
   Sedation, chloral hydrate 0.5 to 1.0 g, P.O., every 4 to 6 hours. Barbiturates or tranquilizers may be employed.
   Fluids, 2 to 3 liters, q.d., of 5 percent dextrose in water.
4. Avoidance of specific antigen by environmental control.

The following drugs, though not commonly used, are promising in the control of asthma for they act after antigen-antibody interaction.

1. Diethylcarbamazine (Hetrazan) inhibits the release of SRS-A.
2. Disodium chromoglycate (Intal). Pretreatment with this drug inhibits the release of histamine.

Ether anesthesis is *not* recommended since it increases acidosis.

STATUS ASTHMATICUS

This is associated with a steadily rising arterial CO_2 tension, increasing O_2 unsaturation and a fall in pH.

1. Corticosteroid therapy should be intensive, e.g., 100 mg of Solu Cortef I.V. q. 6 h.
2. Parenteral fluids.
3. Molar lactate or sodium bicarbonate I.V. to combat acidosis.
4. Endotracheal tube or tracheostomy.
5. Use of the piston type respirator. The volume-cycled respirator is required in preference to the automatic pressure-cycled apparatus.
6. Use of curariform drug, e.g., I.V. gallamine triethiodide to paralyze respiratory muscles – this is used in desperate cases.

Sedation is not emphasized here. More patients with asthma die of oversedation than anything else.

In severe cases bronchoscopy may be lifesaving.

Epinephrine is best avoided here because of tachyphylaxis.

Morphine is contraindicated in asthma.

Antihistamines are of little or no use, and may inspissate the mucus.

MAINTENANCE

Potassium iodide, saturated solution, 10 to 15 gtt., q.i.d. This is the best single drug in chronic asthma.

Tedral tablets, 1 q. 6 to 8 hours, p.r.n.

Aminophylline suppository h.s.

PROGNOSIS

It is generally appreciated that death in acute asthma is not a rarity. Mortality rates over 10 percent have been reported in *status asthmaticus.*

REFERENCES

Ferguson, M., and O'Brien, M. M. Unexpected death in bronchial asthma: a warning sign with a clinicopathologic correlation. Ann. Intern. Med., 53:1163, 1960.

Lopez, M., Frauhlm, W., and Lawell, F. C. Double blind study of disodium chromoglycate in bronchial asthma. J. Allerg., 41:89, 1968.

Mallen, M. S. Treatment of intractable asthma with diethyl carbamazine citrate. Amer. Allergy. 23:534, 1965.

Middleton, E., Jr. Anatomical and bio-chemical basis of broncheal obstruction in asthma. Amer. Intern. Med., 63:695, 1965.

BARBITURATES AND OTHER SEDATIVE DRUGS

(Chloral hydrate and Paraldehyde*)

These drugs allay excitement, reduce motor activity, and most importantly induce sleep when insomnia is not due to a definite cause, such as pain, pruritus, or dyspnea.

The liver is the chief site of metabolic degradation of all of the barbiturates; and in the presence of severe hepatic disease barbiturates are markedly potentiated in effect. About 20 percent of barbital and phenobarbital are excreted by the kidneys, and are thus contraindicated in the presence of advanced renal disease.

USE

The principal indications for use include sudden stress situations, hypertension, potentiation of analgesic drugs, insomnia, and control of convulsions and suppression of epileptic seizures.

AMOBARBITAL

(Amytal)

An intermediate acting barbiturate which is effective for 4 to 6 hours. The usual oral dose is 60 to 100 mg.

BARBITAL

A long-acting barbiturate. Excitement and other outward

*See also Tranquilizers

effects are infrequent. The usual dose is 300 mg h. s.

CHLORAL HYDRATE

This agent is one of the most effective, least expensive, and least toxic agents in the sedative-hypnotic group. It undoubtedly deserves more use than it receives at present.

Chloral hydrate, unlike many other drugs of the group, can be given to patients of all ages. It is rapidly effective, producing an effect in 10 to 15 minutes. Sleep induced usually lasts 5 to 8 hours.

Detoxification occurs in the liver and excretion is via the kidneys. Large amounts should be avoided in the presence of hepatic or renal disease.

UNTOWARD EFFECTS. Mucous membrane irritation leading to gastric distress may occur. The drug is best avoided in the presence of peptic ulcer and alcoholism.

DOSE. The usual dose is 0.5 to 1.0 g, P.O.

DIAZEPAM

(Valium)

Action similar to chlordiazepoxide (Librium) but in smaller doses. It is useful in relieving tension and anxiety states and in acute alcoholic withdrawal with acute agitation, tremor, impending or actual delirium tremens and hallucinosis. The dose is 5 to 10 mg I.V. or I.M. which may be repeated in 3 to 4 hours. Orally 2 to 10 mg may be given t.i.d. or q.i.d.

PARALDEHYDE

Paraldehyde is useful in controlling severe insomnia in the presence of marked excitement or frank delirium, and is particularly applicable in the presence of hepatic or renal disease and in the alcoholic. Onset of action occurs in 10 to 15 minutes; metabolism occurs mainly in the liver, where the drug is degraded to acetaldehyde and then into CO_2 and water. In the presence of liver disease, degradation occurs more slowly, but larger amounts are then excreted by the lungs. Paraldehyde is thus contraindicated in the presence of advanced pulmonary disease, especially if there is coexistent liver pathology. Renal excretion is minor, hence the drug is useful in the presence of the various nephropathies. Paraldehyde in oral form produces mucous membrane irritation and is best avoided in the presence of esophagitis, gastritis, and peptic ulcer. It produces a disagreeable odor within the general vicinity of its use.

The usual oral dose is 8 to 10 ml, mixed with juice and ice. Intramuscularly, 4 to 8 ml may be given.

The therapeutic range is broad, however, and an oral dose of 20 to 30 ml, or an intramuscular dose of 10 to 15 ml, may be used in difficult situations without great risk.

PENTOBARBITAL

(Nembutal)

This is a relatively short-acting barbiturate. Currently, Nembutal and Seconal are popular for use as sedatives at bedtime. The usual dose is 100 mg, h.s.

PHENOBARBITAL

Cerebral depression is more outstanding with phenobarbital than other barbiturates. Thus this drug is most likely to be associated with confusion, excitement, and disorientation among a geriatric population. Otherwise, as a mild sedative, phenobarbital remains unsurpassed. The usual dose is 15 to 30 mg, 2 to 4 times a day.

SECOBARBITAL

(Seconal)

A rapid-acting barbiturate with onset within 20 to 30 minutes after oral dose, and effect for 2 to 4 hours. The usual oral dose is 100 mg, h.s.

ADDICTION

If any of the barbiturates are used daily in large doses for a period of 3 to 6 months or longer, habituation or even addiction may ensue. Serious withdrawal effects may occur when the drug is discontinued, and gradual tapering is desirable. During withdrawal, 200 mg of pentobarbital or a short-acting equivalent every 4 to 6 hours may be given. This is reduced by about 100 mg daily.

OVERDOSAGE

See "Drug Poisoning Treatment."

BLEEDING AND CLOTTING DISORDERS

BLEEDING DISORDERS

A careful history is the most important part of any evaluation of a bleeding disorder. Easy bruisability or bleeding following tooth extractions, T&A, or trauma may furnish an important clue. Family history, use of drugs, swelling of joints, epistaxis, etc., are all important historic points.

In the physical examination, particular attention is directed to the skin, mucous membranes, liver, and spleen.

Table 1 summarizes the common bleeding disorders that may be tentatively diagnosed by a selected group of coagulation determinations. These are tourniquet test, bleeding time (IVY), clotting time, fibrinogen level, platelet count, one-stage prothrombin time, activated partial thromboplastin time, and thrombin-clotting time.

The results of these tests can be available within one and a half hours in an emergency, and a method of therapy can then be devised before more complicated assays are performed.

COMMONLY TREATED COAGULOPATHIES

1. Overdosage with warfarin or warfarin-like drugs with a diminution in Factors II, V, VII, and X respond within 6 hours to parenteral administration of vitamin K_1 oxide.
2. Bleeding secondary to cirrhosis of the liver associated with low fibrinogen, shortened euglobulin lysis time, shortened plasma clot and whole clot lysis time will respond well to EACA (ϵ-aminocaproic acid), 0.5 g intravenously and then 1.0 g P.O. or I.V. q. h. times 8 doses or until the patient stops bleeding. If the diagnosis is uncertain or if the administration of EACA is extended, heparin therapy should be instituted to prevent thrombosis or embolus secondary to disseminated intravascular coagulation.
3. Heparin therapy is used to prevent the effects of disseminated

CONGENITAL AND ACQUIRED COAGULATION DEFICIENCIES

Tests:	TOURNIQUET TEST (Rumple-Leed)	CLOTTING TIME (Lee-White)	BLEEDING TIME (IVY)	CLOT RETRACTION
Deficiency State / Normal Values:	0-5 petechia	6-12 min	6 min or less	complete in 24 h
AHF, Mild (Factor VIII)	negative	n. to prolonged	normal	normal
AHF, Severe (Factor VIII)	negative	prolonged	normal	normal
PTC, Mild (Factor IX)	negative	n. to prolonged	normal	normal
PTC, Severe (Factor IX)	negative	prolonged	normal	normal
PTA (Factor XI)	negative	normal	normal	normal
Hageman Trait (Factor XII)	negative	prolonged	normal	normal
Von Willebrand's	sometimes positive	n. or prolonged	n. or prolonged	normal
Thrombocytopenia	positive	normal	n. or prolonged	abnormal
Stuart-Prower (Factor X)	negative	n. or prolonged	n. or prolonged	normal
Factor V	negative	n. or prolonged	n. or prolonged	normal
Factor VII	negative	normal	n. or prolonged	normal
Prothrombin	negative	n. or prolonged	n. or prolonged	normal
Fibrinogen	negative	prolonged	prolonged	abnormal

Abbreviations: n. = normal

CONGENITAL AND ACQUIRED COAGULATION DEFICIENCIES (continued)

PLATELET COUNT	PROTHROMBIN TIME	PARTIAL THROMBOPLASTIN TIME	STYPVEN TIME	THROMBOPLASTIN GENERATION TIME
150,000-400,000	12-14 sec	<45 sec	25-30 sec	7-12 sec
normal	normal	abnormal	normal	abnormal corrected by adsorbed plasma
normal	normal	abnormal	normal	abnormal corrected by adsorbed plasma
normal	normal	abnormal	normal	abnormal corrected by serum
normal	normal	abnormal	normal	abnormal corrected by serum
normal	normal	abnormal	normal	abnormal corrected by serum & adsorbed plasma
normal	normal	abnormal	normal	abnormal corrected by serum & adsorbed plasma
normal	normal	normal to prolonged	normal	normal or abnormal corrected by adsorbed plasma
decreased	normal	normal	normal	abnormal corrected by normal platelets
normal	abnormal	abnormal	abnormal	abnormal corrected by serum
normal	abnormal	abnormal	normal	abnormal corrected by adsorbed plasma
normal	abnormal	normal	normal	–
normal	abnormal	abnormal	normal	–
normal	abnormal	–	–	–

intravascular coagulation which presents with a low fibrinogen level (under 150 mg per 100 ml), a low platelet count, a low prothrombin level, and depression of Factors V and VIII. This syndrome of diffuse intravascular coagulation (consumption coagulopathy) is characterized by a hemorrhagic diathesis and thrombosis. Common entities causing the condition are abruptio placenta and placenta previa (obstetrical), transfusion reactions, malignancies, viral hemorrhagic fever, meningococcemia, leukemia, cardiac surgery and acute interstitial pancreatitis. There are two ways in which heparin may be used in this situation, i.e., approximately 7,000 to 10,000 units of heparin intravenously every 6 hours or 800 to 1,000 units of heparin every hour. The dosage is a function of the patient's response and a favorable response is indicated by a return of the prothrombin time, partial thromboplastin time, thrombin-clotting time, Factors V and VIII, and fibrinogen to normal levels. In addition, if the Lee-White clotting time is abnormally long, administration of I.V. heparin will paradoxically shorten the clotting time to a normal level.

4. Emergency therapy of hemophilia (Factor VIII). After a presumptive diagnosis is made, the bleeding patient should be treated with either cryoprecipitate or glycine precipitated antihemophiliac factor (AHF). Fresh frozen plasma can be used if the aforementioned substances are not available. The principles of therapy are based on 1) the degree and extent of bleeding, and 2) the initial AHF (Factor VIII) level of the patient. If the level is below 5 percent or if the patient is bleeding extensively, one should attempt to raise the AHF level to 30 to 50 percent.

Laboratory monitoring with assays is necessary to indicate the effective levels reached. In this way, the dosage and spacing of infusions are judged.

APPROXIMATE DOSAGE SCHEDULE

	FRESH PLASMA FRESH FROZEN PLASMA DRIED IRRADIATED PLASMA	CRYOPRE- CIPITATE	GLYCINE PRECIPITATE AHF
70 kg Adult	4 units initially and then 2 units q 12 hours	8-10 bags initially and then 4-5 bags q 12 hours	4 bottles initially and then 2 bottles q 12 hours
Child	20 ml/kilo initially and 10 ml/kilo q 12 h.	2 bags per 12 kilo initially and 1 bag/12 kilo q 12 h.	2 bottles/24 kilo and 1 bottle/24 kilo q 12 h.

COAGULATION MECHANISM

Blood coagulation is an adaptive mechanism and two systems, the extrinsic and the intrinsic systems are available. Tissue damage releases a tissue factor and a phospholipid which in the presence of a stable Factor (VII) activate Factor X. The intrinsic system comes into play when the surface of a vessel is damaged. Then a "cascade" sequence is activated which eventually transforms Factor X into the activated form. When there is vessel damage, platelets aggregate and eventually phospholipid is released. Both systems thus activate Factor X and provide a source of phospholipid. Then, in the presence of calcium ions and Factor V, Factor II (prothrombin) is converted to thrombin, and soluble fibrinogen (Factor I) is converted to insoluble fibrin. There are many checks and balances in these systems. In addition to procoagulant activity, there are antithromboplastins, antithrombins (i.e., heparin), and fibrinolysins which control the extent of clot formation and eventually lead to clot lysis.

REFERENCES

Wintrobe, M.M.: Clinical Hematology, Philadelphia, Lea & Febiger, 1967.

Biggs, R. and MacFarlane, R.G: Human Blood Coagulation, Philadelphia, F.A. Davis Co., 1962.

Quick, A.J.: Hemorrhagic Diseases and Thrombosis, 3 ed., Philadelphia, Lea & Febiger, 1966.

MacFarlane, R.G.: The Basis of the Cascade Hypothesis of Blood Clotting, Thrombosis, Diathesis Haemorrhagica, 15:591–602, 1966.

Roberts, H.R. and Brinkhous, K.M.: Blood Coagulation and Hemophiliod Disorders, Postgraduate Medicine, 43:114–121, May 1968.

INTRAVASCULAR HEMOLYSIS

The intravascular destruction of red cells is abnormal and is accompanied by hemoglobinemia. The normal plasma hemoglobin level may vary from one laboratory to another but the normal concentration is never higher than 3 mg per 100 ml and with good spectrophotometry less than 1 mg per 100 ml. When intravascular hemolysis takes place, in addition to the elevations in plasma hemoglobin, one may get oxidation of the heme moiety to the ferri(met-) form with the formation of methemalbumin. To summarize the role of intravascular heme pigments in hemolytic disease: initially during hemolysis, the released hemoglobin is bound to haptoglobin to form hemoglobin-haptoglobin complex. This latter material is rapidly removed from the plasma and if haptoglobin synthesis is not accelerated, haptoglobin is depleted. Then, in the absence of sufficient haptoglobin, the hemoglobin exists in the plasma in the free state and the heme equilibrates among globin, albumin and hemopexin (β-1-globulin). This distribution occurs depending on the state of oxidation of the heme and the ligands of the heme iron. Normally, no more than 5 mg per 100 ml of benzidine-stainable pigment is present in plasma; this includes hemoglobin and the various protein-bound heme compounds.

REFERENCES

Dallman, P. R., and Pool, J. G. Current concepts: Treatment of hemophilia with Factor VIII concentrates. New Eng. J. Med., 278:199, 1968.

Marder, V. J., and Shulman, N. R. Major surgery in classic hemophilia using Fraction I. Amer. J. Med., 41:56, 1966.

CONSUMPTION COAGULATION AND FIBRINOLYSIS

(Defibrination Syndrome, Disseminated Intravascular Coagulation)

In some disease states, acute activation of the clotting mechanism takes place with consumption of Factors I, II, V, VIII, and platelets. This may result in disseminated intravascular coagulation and disruption of hemostasis. Most often this entity presents as a mild to moderate bleeding disorder but this primary active consumption of clotting factors may be accompanied by a secondary rebound phenomenon called fibrinolysis or excessive digestion of fibrin and fibrinogen. Fibrinolysis most often coexists only as a secondary manifestation with primary consumption of clotting factors, but on very rare occasions fibrinolysis may be the primary cause of an obscure bleeding disorder.

Since digestion of clotting factors may take place during primary fibrinolysis because of activation of the fibrinolytic system, it becomes difficult to differentiate between primary consumption of clotting factors with secondary fibrinolysis and primary fibrinolysis. It is necessary to differentiate between these

SCHEMATIC OF MECHANISM OF BLOOD COAGULATION

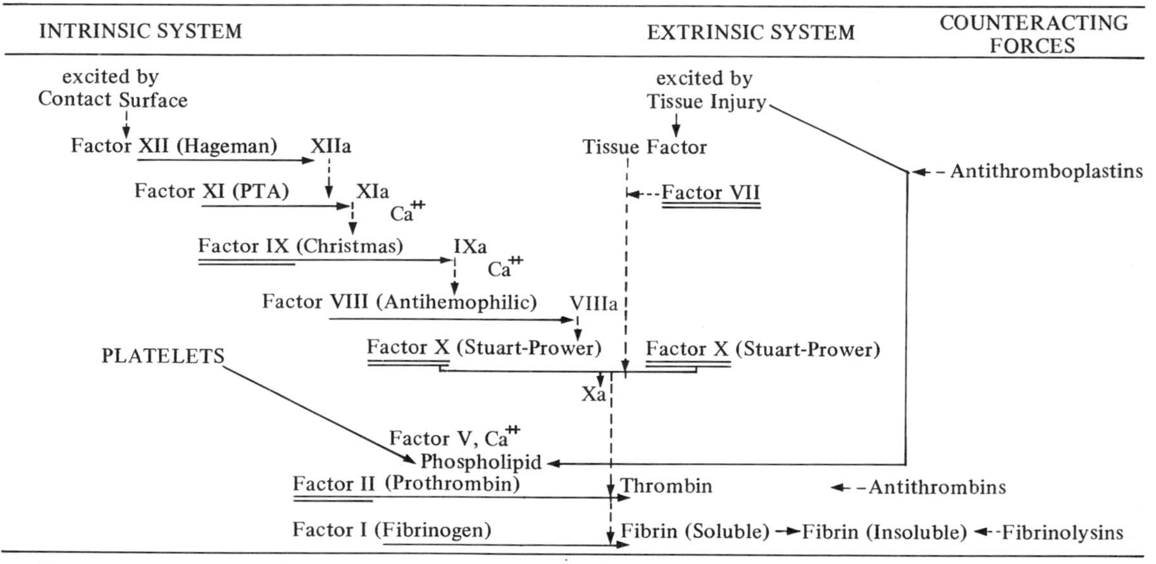

Scheme of blood coagulation, somewhat simplified, but based primarily on the "cascade" hypothesis of MacFarlane. An interrupted line indicates activity while a continuous line indicates transformation. The underlined Factors II, VII, IX and X are lowered in anticoagulant therapy (Dicoumarin-like drugs). A substance with "a" refers to the activated product.

two conditions because they represent life-threatening situations and therapy is different in each.

THERAPY

The specific treatment for consumptive coagulopathy is heparin – the recommended dose is between 5,000 units to 10,000 units q. 6 hrs. I.V.

The recommended therapy for primary fibrinolysis is ϵ-aminocaproic acid, 3-5 g I.V., or 0.5-1.0 g q. 1 h. until hemorrhage is controlled.

DIFFERENTIAL TESTS

TEST	CONSUMPTION OF FACTORS AND SECONDARY LYSIS	PRIMARY FIBRINOLYSIS
Blood clot	small friable	complete clot dissolution
Blood smear	low platelets fragmentation of red cells	normal platelets, normal red cells
Fibrinogen	low	low
Factor V, VIII	low	low
Prothrombin	low	low
Degradation of fibrin products	present	present in high titer
Euglobulin lysis time	normal	very rapid
Serial thrombin time	normal or abnormal	abnormal
Cryofibrinogen	present	absent

REFERENCES

Lasch, Hans-Gotthard Heene, L. D. Pathopathy. Clinical man and therapy of consumption – coagulopathy (Verbrauchskoagulopathie). Amer. J. Cardiol. 20:381, 1967.

Rodriguez-Erdmann, F. Bleeding due to increased intravascular blood coagulation. Hemorrhagic syndromes causes by consumption of blood-clotting factors (consumption coagulopathies). New Eng. J. Med., 273:1370, 1965.

Rosner, F., and Ritz, N. D. The defibrination syndrome. Arch. Intern. Med., 117:17, 1966.

Sherry, S. Fibrinolysis in health and disease. Resident Physician, February, 1968.

Verstraete, M., et al. Excessive consumption of blood coagulation components as cause of hemorrhagic diathesis. Amer. J. Med., 38:899, 1965.

DISEASES ASSOCIATED WITH BLEEDING (DIATHIASIS) CAUSED BY CONSUMPTION OF CLOTTING FACTORS AND SECONDARY FIBRINOLYSIS – RARELY PRIMARY

INFECTION	SHOCK	OB-GYN	HEMATOLOGIC	SURGERY	MISCELLANEOUS
Gram-negative sepsis	Septic	Abruptio placentae	Acute leak	Extensive operation	Cancer disseminated lungs breast stomach colon pancreas prostate ovary
Viral septecemia	Hemorrhagic	Septic abortion	Reticulum cell sarcoma	Lungs	Dissecting aneurysm
Hemorrhagic fevers	Anaphylactic	Amniotic fluid embolism	Thrombosis	Stomach	Burns
Rocky mountain spotted fever	Trauma	Retention of fetal material	Thrombotic purpura	Pancreas	Chemicals
Malaria			Purpura fulminans	Prostate	Liver disease
			Acute hemolytic crisis	Cardiopulmonary bypass	
			Transfusion reaction		
			Hemolytic uremic reaction		

BONE DISEASES

The following table outlines the chemical abnormalities found in certain diseases that frequently affect bone.

DISEASE	Ca^{++}	PO_4	ALKALINE PHOSPHATASE	TOTAL PROTEIN	URINE Ca^{++}	MISCELLANEOUS
Primary hyperparathyroidism	↑	↓N	N↑	N	↑N	A disease of "stones, bones, abdominal groans, and psychic moans" (St. Goar).
Secondary hyperparathyroidism ("renal rickets")	↓	N↑	↑	N or ↓	↓	Serum pH↓.
Osteomalacia with ↓Ca^{++} absorption	↓ or N	N or ↓	↑	N or ↓	↓	Steatorrhea may be present.
Hypoparathyroidism	↓	↑	N	N	O	Usual cause: post thyroidectomy.
Osteoporosis	N	N	N	N	N or ↑	X-rays show diffuse demineralization.
Polyostotic vibrous dysplasia	N	N	N or ↑	N	N	Bones may show enlargement on x-ray.

Paget's disease of bone	N	N	↑ to ↑↑	N	N or ↑	Alkaline phosphatase may be 2-3 times normal.
Multiple myeloma	N or ↑	N, ↑ or ↓	N or ↑	↑ or N	N or ↑	Serum electrophoresis may show "M" protein. Osteolytic—never osteoblastic—lesions on x-ray.
Metastatic malignancy	N or ↑	N, ↑ or ↓	N or ↑	N	N or ↑	
Malignancy without osseous metastasis	↑	N↓	N↑	N	N↑	Tumor produces parathyroid hormone-like or vitamin D-like substance.
Xanthomatosis	N	N	N or ↑	N	N or ↑	Histocytosis-X (Letterer-Siwe, Hand-Schüller-Christian Eosinophilic granuloma).
Sarcoid	↑ or N	N or ↑	N or ↑	N or ↑	↑	Chest x-ray usually shows bilateral adenopathy.
Vitamin D intoxication	↑	↑ or N ↓	N or ↑	N	↑	History of vitamin ingestion.

REFERENCE

Goldhaber, P. Some current concepts of bone physiology. New Eng. J. Med., 266:870, 1962; 266:924, 1962.

BRAIN ABSCESS

Most cerebral abscesses are diagnosed for the first time at autopsy.

DIAGNOSIS

HISTORY AND PHYSICAL

1. Headache and fever are seen in the majority of patients.
2. Vomiting occurs in about half of cases.
3. Seizures occur in a third.
4. Hemiparesis or hemiplegia.
5. Hemiparesthesia.
6. Cerebellar symptoms.
7. Diplopia.
8. Personality changes and irritability.
9. Signs and symptoms vary with the site of the abscess.

LABORATORY

1. Skull x-ray.
2. L.P.
3. Brain scan.
4. Electroencephalography.
5. Cerebral angiography is the procedure of choice.
6. Pneumoencephalography.
7. Ventriculography.

SOURCE OF INFECTION

Direct Extension	
Middle ear	20%
Paranasal sinuses	20%
Trauma	10%
Hematogenous	
Lungs	15%

Teeth	7.5%
Osteomyelitis	2%
Miscellaneous	7.5%
Undetermined	10%

REFERENCE

Kern, F. W. Brain abscess. A study of 47 consecutive cases. J.A.M.A., 168:868, 1958.

BRAIN TUMOR

Brain tumors present a diagnostic challenge. It has been stated that more than 2 out of 3 are missed by the average internist. The diagnosis must always be entertained whenever headache or psychic changes or both are present and progress.

DIAGNOSIS

HISTORY AND PHYSICAL

Headache, vertigo, visual changes, diplopia, nausea, vomiting, and fatigue are the most common symptoms. Signs include psychic changes, convulsions, sensory changes, paralysis, aphasia, and unconsciousness in order of decreasing frequency. A carefully performed, detailed, meticulous neurologic examination must be done. This is the most important diagnostic procedure.

LABORATORY

Spinal tap and electroencephalography are each positive in over 90 percent of cases. Angiography and ventriculography are of considerable aid, and skull x-rays show significant changes in about 50 percent of cases.

PATHOLOGY

Gliomas (glioblastoma multiforme, astrocytoma, oligodendroglioma, ependymoma, and spongioblastoma) account for the majority of brain tumors, with meningiomas second. Supratentorial tumors outnumber infratentorial ones by about 2 to 1. Metastatic tumors are very common.

REFERENCE

Netsky, M. G., and Watson, J. M. The natural history of intracranial neoplasms. Ann. Intern. Med., 45:275, 1956.

BRETYLIUM TOSYLATE

This drug, recently introduced, blocks postganglionic sympathetic nerve transmission without depleting catecholamines. Chemically, it produces a state approaching sympathectomy including sensitivity to catecholamines. It is positively inotropic, increases cardiac output, and decreases peripheral resistance while the blood pressure falls or remains unchanged. The drug increases the fibrillation threshold three times, stabilizes ventricular rhythmicity, and is useful in treating ventricular arrhythmias.

DOSE. 2-5 mg/kg I.M. is rapidly absorbed and may be repeated in 8 to 12 hours or sooner. It may be given slowly I.V. diluted in 50 ml 5 percent D/W over a 5-minute period.

REFERENCES

Bucaner, M. B. Prevention and treatment of ventricular arrhythmias and ventricular fibrillation with bretylium tosylate. Univ. Minn. Med. Bull., 38:317, 1967.

____Quantitative comparison of bretylium with other antifibrillatory drugs. Amer. J. Cardiol., 21:504, 1968

CALCIUM

(See also "Parathyroid")

The clinical syndrome of hypercalcemia is most striking and generally is fully developed at a calcium level of 15 mg per 100 ml. Symptoms associated with hypercalcemia include muscular weakness, anorexia, lethargy, nausea, thirst, constipation, insomnia, and restlessness. Delirium, stupor, or coma may develop. The serum calcium can be lowered by correcting the underlying disease (surgery for hyperparathyroidism). Inorganic phosphate (orally), and intravenous sodium sulfate may be effective forms of therapy for hypercalcemia unresponsive to corticosteroids.

DIFFERENTIAL DIAGNOSIS OF HYPERCALCEMIA IN THE ADULT.

1. Laboratory error (most common).
2. Hyperparathyroidism.
3. Neoplasia (with or without bone metastases) especially lung, breast, kidney, ovary, stomach, and multiple myeloma, lymphoma.
4. Sarcoidosis (occurs in approximately 30 percent of cases).
5. Acute osteoporosis of disuse.
6. Milk-alkali syndrome.
7. Vitamin D intoxication.
8. Hyperthyroidism.
9. Acromegaly.
10. Cushing's syndrome.
11. Addisonian crises.

REFERENCES

David, N. J., et al. The diagnostic spectrum of hypercalcemia: Case reports and discussion. Amer. J. Med., 33:88, 1962.

Goldsmith, R. S., and Ingbar, S. H. Inorganic phosphate treatment of hypercalcemia of diverse etiologies. New Eng. J. Med., 274: 1, 1966

Lemann, J., Jr., et al. Calcium intoxication due to primary hyperparathyroidism. Ann. Intern. Med., 60:447, 1964.

CARCINOID SYNDROME

Definition: The symptom complex associated with hyperserotoninemia (5-hydroxytryptamine) produced by metastasizing bronchial and gastrointestinal carcinoid tumors.

DIAGNOSIS

1. Patients with gastric carcinoids have patchy flushes with sharply delineated serpentine borders over face, neck, arms, trunk, and legs. Patients with bronchial carcinoids may have prolonged flushes lasting for 3 to 4 days. Periorbital and facial edema and lacrimation accompany the flush.
2. Chronic or intermittent diarrhea.

3. Respiratory symptoms, especially wheezing and dyspnea.
4. Tricuspid or pulmonic murmurs.
5. X-ray: chest x-ray, bronchography, or barium enema suggestive of tumor.
6. Nodular hepatomegaly.
7. Twenty-four-hour urine – 5-hydroxyindole acetic acid over 25 mg. (Ingestion of bananas, walnuts, or proprietary cough medications containing glycerol guaiacolates) may give false positive results. With gastric carcinoids 5-IAA may be low though 5-hydroxytryptamine or 5-hydroxytroptophan may be elevated.
8. Provocation of flush by intravenous administration of epinephrine.

THERAPY

1. Surgical.
2. Chlorpromazine is effective in abating attacks of flushing and diarrhea in some patients.
3. Alpha-methyldopa may be helpful in relieving symptoms in patients with gastric carcinoid.
4. Corticosteroid therapy may be dramatically effective in ameliorating symptoms in patients with bronchial irritation.

REFERENCES

Grahame-Smith, D. G. The carcinoid syndrome. Amer. J. Cardiol., 21:376, 1968.

Kahil, M. E., et al. The carcinoid crisis. Arch. Intern. Med., 114:26, 1964.

Melmon, K. L., Sjoerdsma, A., and Mason, D. T. Distinctive clinical and therapeutic aspect of the syndrome associated with bronchial carcinoid tumors. Amer. J. Med., 39:568, 1965.

Oates, J. A., and Sjoersma, A. A unique syndrome associated with secretion of 5-hydroxytroptan by metastatic gastric carcinoids, Amer. J. Med., 32:333, 1962.

Roberts, W. C., et al. The cardiac disease associated with the carcinoid syndrome (carcinoid heart disease). Amer. J. Med., 36:5, 1964.

CARDIAC ARRHYTHMIAS TREATMENT

The table (pp. 50-51) outlines the characteristics and treatment of the more frequent cardiac arrhythmias. Congestive heart failure, pulmonary embolus, inadequate pulmonary ventilation, serious electrolyte disturbances and under-oxygenation of the blood all may initiate and help to perpetruate various arrhythmias. These abnormalities should not be overlook and must be treated vigorously. Antiarrhythmic and vasopressor drugs often cause arrhythmias.

ARRHYTHMIA	RATE AND MECHANISM	VAGUS EFFECT	DRUG TREATMENT	ELECTRIC CARDIOVERSION
Sinus tachycardia	SA node rate 100-160; stress	Gradual decrease; returns to previous level	Rest; sedation	Not used
Sinus bradycardia	60 or less	Further slowing	Atropine, isoproterenol	Not used
Paroxysmal atrial tachycardia	150-250; irritable ectopic atrial focus	About 50% have sudden cessation; remainder unaffected	Vagus stimulation; sedation; digitalis in that order. Potassium if due to digitalis in absence of block; propanolol.	Treatment of choice (if not due to digitalis)
Atrial flutter	250-350; ectopic focus or circus	Irregular decrease; gradually returns to original rate	Digitalis first; then quinidine	Treatment of choice

Atrial fibrillation	350-500; ectopic foci	Rate slows; irregularity remains	Digitalis to slow rate; quinidine may convert to NSR	Will convert about 80%
Premature beats	Irritable atrial or ventricular focus	May slow PAC's; no effect on PVC's	If occasional no treatment. If bigemminal APC quinidine. If occasional VPC quinidine or pronestyl. If more than 5 per min, in groups, multifocal, or at apex of T wave, give lidocaine 50 mg I.V. as bolus and repeat if necessary. Bretylium.	Not used
Ventricular tachycardia	150-220; irritable ventricular focus	No effect	Lidocaine 50 mg I.V. as bolus and repeat in 3-5 min if necessary. If effective, follow with I.V. drip 2 g in 500 ml over 24 hr. Bretylium.	Treatment of choice
Ventricular fibrillation	Probable ectopic or circus	No effect	Propanolol	Treatment of choice

CARDIAC CATHETERIZATION

THE NORMAL RANGE OF VALUES USED IN CARDIAC CATHETERIZATION

	NORMAL RANGE
Cardiac output	4 to 8 L/min
Cardiac index	3.1 ± 0.4 L/min/m^2
A–V difference	4.5 ± 0.7 ml/100 ml
O_2 consumption	138 ± 14 ml/m^2/min
Arterial O_2 saturation	94 to 96%

HEART CHAMBER SAMPLES (O_2 CONTENT).

A. Pooled superior vena cava–inferior vena cava: right atrial O_2 diff.	less than 1.0 vol.% ± 2 vol.%. Where sample is greater than 2%, must consider atrial septal defect, anomalous return, ventricular septal defect with tricuspid insufficiency.
B. Right atrium: right ventricular O_2 diff.	less than 0.9 vol.% ± 1 vol.%. If greater than 1 vol.%, consider left-to-right shunt: ventricular septal defect or patent ductus arteriosus with pulmonary insufficiency.
C. Right ventricle: pulmonary arterial O_2 diff.	± 0.5% If greater than 0.5%, consider patent ductus arteriosus, aortic window, or high ventricular septal defect.

PRESSURES.

Right atrium: 0 to 5 mm Hg

Right ventricle: $\frac{18 \text{ to } 30}{0 \text{ to } 5}$

Pulmonary artery: $\frac{18 \text{ to } 30}{6 \text{ to } 12}$ (mean 13 to 17)

Pulmonary capillary: 6 to 12 (Note this is normal in cor pulmonale, high in left ventricular failure and mitral stenosis.)
Left atrium: 4 to 8
Mitral valve area: 4 to 6 cm^2
Pulmonary arteriolar resistance: 47 to 160 dynes sec/cm^{-5}

FORMULAS USED IN CALCULATIONS OF FLOWS IN CONGENITAL HEART DISEASE

CALCULATION OF FLOW.

1. Cardiac output (ml/min):

$$\frac{O_2 \text{ intake (ml/min) } (O_2 \text{ consumption})}{O_2 \text{ content arterial blood (vol. \%)} - O_2 \text{ content mixed venous blood (vol. \%)}} \times 100$$

2. Pulmonary artery flow

$$= \frac{O_2 \text{ intake (ml/min)}}{\text{pulmonary venous } O_2 \text{ content} - \text{pul. art. content (vol. \%)}} \times 100$$

Note: The pulmonary venous blood content value is derived assuming the pulmonary venous blood to be 95 percent saturated.

Example: Pulmonary venous blood

$$= \frac{\text{pul. venous blood content}}{\text{pul. venous blood capacity}}$$

3. Effective blood flow

$$= \frac{O_2 \text{ intake (ml/min)}}{\text{pul. venous } O_2 \text{ content} - \text{mixed venous } O_2 \text{ content}} \times 100$$

CALCULATION OF SHUNTS.

1. Total left-to-right shunt = pulmonary artery flow minus effective pulmonary artery flow.
2. Total right-to-left shunt = systemic flow minus effective pulmonary artery flow.

CALCULATION OF RESISTANCE.

$$\text{Pulmonary arteriolar resistance} = \frac{PA - PC}{CO} \times 1{,}332$$

where: R = pulmonary arteriolar resistance in dynes sec/cm^{-5}
PA = mean pulmonary arterial pressure in mm Hg
PC = mean pulmonary capillary pressure in mm Hg
CO = cardiac output in ml/sec
Normal range: 47 to 160 dynes sec/cm^{-5}

CARDIAC PACING

The major rationale for pacing the heart is to prevent asystole and ventricular tachyarrhythmias. When ventricular asystole complicates heart block, particularly during acute myocardial infarction, the prognosis is grave. Obviously it is much easier to manage asystole occurring after a pacemaker is in place than to attempt bedside placement as an emergency measure during resuscitative maneuvers. Bradycardia may also be complicated by the appearance of rapid ventricular activity which has been well recognized as a cause of Adams-Stokes attacks. The rate below which such attacks occur is referred to as the "critical rate." Although it varies from individual to individual, it is generally in the range of 50 beats or less per minute. Occasionally, the critical rate may be considerably higher, but usually maintaining the ventricular rate at 55 to 60 beats per minute is sufficient to prevent ectopic tachycardia. Depressing agents, such as quinidine and propranolol, are contraindicated in this situation.

Increasing the rate in bradyarrhythmia also has the beneficial effect of producing an increase in cardiac output. Most studies of patients with chronic heart block and slow heart rates show that output is invariably diminished at these rates. Such individuals cannot alter stroke volume because of impaired ventricular function and depend on increasing heart rate for augmentation of cardiac output. Cardiac output usually peaks between 60 and 75 beats per minute. However, there is considerable individual variation and it is difficult to predict the optimal pacing rate. Furthermore, myocardial oxygen demands increase directly with heart rate and, if the coronary vascular bed responds inadequately to these demands, anaerobic metabolism may result. The optimal pacing rate is that at which maximal output is achieved under aerobic conditions. Since it is not possible to predict easily such a rate by current methods, one must be guided by clinical information. If clinical signs of myocardial failure are not present, the primary aim is to prevent asystole and to maintain the ventricular rate above the "critical rate" in order to suppress ventricular tachyarrhythmias. Such goals are achieved by cardiac pacing.

INDICATIONS FOR INSERTION OF A TEMPORARY CARDIAC PACEMAKER

A. Acute myocardial infarction present or suspected
   1. Sinus bradycardia and first degree A-V block with heart rate below 50 resistant to drug therapy (atropine, isoproterenol).
   2. Second degree heart block, complete heart block (regardless of heart rate) or slow junctional rhythm. Others do not consider second degree block of the Wenckeback type an indication for pacing. The Mobitz type is an absolute indication.
   3. Bundle branch block of the bifascicular type. (LBBB or RBBB with LAD or RAD.)
   4. Recurrent ventricular tachyarrhythmia associated with normal heart rate and A–V conduction resistant to drug therapy. Increasing the basic heart rate by "overdriving" the ventricle may suppress the arrhythmia.
   5. Complete heart block.

B. Acute myocardial infarct not present
   1. Prior to insertion of permanent pacemaker (see indications below).
   2. Prophylactic during general anesthesia in patients with incomplete or complete heart block or with a normal ECG and history suggesting Adams-Stokes syndrome.
   3. Unstable heart rhythm with associated bradycardia (any cause).
   4. Refractory ventricular tachyarrhythmia (overdriving).

INDICATIONS FOR INSERTION OF PERMANENT CARDIAC PACEMAKER

A. Chronic bradycardia with or without heart block – symptomatic (Stokes-Adams attacks).

B. Chronic complete heart block with bradycardia – "asymptomatic."

C. Recurrent syncopal episodes due to transient ventricular asystole in individuals with a normal ECG during symptom free periods.

Temporary control of heart rate is best accomplished by transvenous ventricular pacing. The method is relatively safe and, compared to pharmacologic means, is more effective and reliable. Ideally, a No. 6 French bipolar pacing catheter is placed at the right ventricular apex under fluoroscopic vision through a surgical cutdown of the external jugular vein. This vein is preferred for its stability, the low incidence of phlebitis and for convenience of the patient. Veins in either upper extremity, the femoral vein, or the subclavian vein (percutaneous entry) may also be utilized. Apical fixation is chosen, for the catheter may be wedged under a trabeculation for stability. Right atrial pacing may be used if atrioventricular conduction is adequate. The physiologic advantages of synchronous atrioventricular contraction are thus preserved. Blind passage of a "floating" wire or of a stiff catheter to the right atrium is easily achieved using electrocardiographic monitoring. Some clinicians have also effected ventricular pacing by this technique. The major advantage lies in the ability to perform the procedure at the bedside. Although most candidates for temporary pacemakers easily tolerate transfer to a fluoroscopy unit, future availability of a portable image intensifier in the intensive care unit will facilitate insertion of catheters in desperately ill patients. Transthoracic placement of fine pacing wires through a needle into the myocardium is another effective method for bedside pacing.

Once the pacing wire is in place the pacing threshold is determined and a stimulus of 2 to 3 times the threshold is delivered. Pacing may be fixed rate, demand (standby), or synchronous. The last method takes advantage of the benefits of synchronous A-V conduction and avoids the potential problems associated with competition between two pacemakers and the induction of ventricular tachyarrhythmias. Unfortunately, synchronous temporary transvenous pacing has not gained wide acceptance because of the technical difficulties in constructing a reliable pacing system. In contrast, fixed rate pacing is simple and reliable. The pulse generator delivers stimuli at a fixed rate regardless of the intrinsic heart rate. Although cardiac output may not be maximal compared with synchronous pacing, it is usually adequate during the brief periods that artificial pacing is required. A small but definite hazard of induced tachyarrhythmia must be accepted with fixed pacing. At present, demand pacing appears to be the method of choice. The "demand" rate is set at 60 beats per minute. If the ventricular rate is consistently below 60, the instrument will behave as a fixed rate pacemaker. When rate increases above 60 or sinus rhythm recurs, fixed pacing ceases; however, control of heart function is resumed should the rate again fall. Thus, this system avoids competitive pacing.

The most serious complications of transvenous pacing are failure to pace and ventricular tachyarrhythmia. When faced with the first problem it is necessary to examine several possibilities. If a pacing stimulus cannot be seen in the ECG, the problem is most likely caused by battery failure or a faulty connection between catheter and generator. If the stimulus appears adequate, then failure to pace is diagnosed when the stimulus falls between the T wave and subsequent QRS complex but does not capture the ventricle. Merely increasing the amplitude of the stimulus will correct the situation if it is due to increasing threshold of depolarization. In addition, intracardiac ECG or a portable chest x-ray may assist in diagnosing displacement of catheter tip into the atrium. Finally, cardiac fluoroscopy may be necessary to readjust the catheter to an optimal pacing position.

The second problem, ventricular irritability, associated with pacing or the presence of the pacing catheter is managed with intravenous lidocaine by continuous drip. If this fails, quinidine or pronestyl may be tried; eventually the addition of propranolol may be necessary in difficult cases.

REFERENCES

Chardack, W. M. The current status of implantable pacemakers. J. Electrocardiol., 1:135. 1968.

Furman, S., Escher, D., and Solomon, N. Standby pacing for multiple cardiac arrhythmias. Ann. Thorac. Surg., 3:327, 1967.

Gregory, J., and Grace, W. The management of sinus bradycardia, nodal rhythm and heart block for the prevention of cardiac arrest in acute myocardial infarction. Progr. Cardiovasc. Dis., 10:505, 1968.

Jensen, N. K., et al. Intra cavitary cardiac pacing. J.A.M.A., 195:916, 1966.

Johaussau, B. W. Complete heart block, clinical hemodynamic and pharmacological study in patients with and without artificial pacemaker. Acta Med. Scandinav., 180 (Suppl. 451):127, 1966.

Kimball, J. T., and Killip, T. A simple bedside method for transvenous intracardiac pacing. Amer. Heart J., 70:35, 1965.

Lillehei, C. W., Levy, M. J., Bonnabeau, R. C., Long, D. M., and Sellers, R. D. Direct wire electrical stimulation for acute post-surgical and post-infarction complete heart block. Ann. N.Y. Acad. Sci., 111:938, 1964.

McNally, E. M., and Benchimol, A. Medical and physiological considerations in the use of artificial cardiac pacing. Parts I, II. Amer. Heart J., 75:380; 75:679, 1968.

Siddons, H., and Sowton, E. Cardiac Pacemakers. Springfield, Ill., Charles C Thomas, Publisher, 1967.

Sowton, E. Cardiac pacemakers and pacing. Mod. Conc. Cardiovasc. Dis., 36:31, 1967.

CARDIOVERSION

(Electrical Conversion of Cardiac Arrhythmias)

Electrical conversion of cardiac arrhythmias is effective in the restoration of regular sinus rhythm in 94 percent of atrial fibrillation, 97 percent of ventricular tachycardia, and practically 100 percent of atrial flutter and atrial tachycardia. The maintenance of regular sinus rhythm is dependent on the type of the underlying cardiac disease, being about 75 percent in rheumatic heart disease with failure generally in those with giant left atrium, multivalvular disease, or long-standing fibrillation; 80 percent in ischemic heart disease; and 70 percent in hypertensive cardiovascular disease.

The procedure for electrical cardioversion is as follows. Quinidine gluconate, 0.33 g, and 0.1 g pentobarbital are given one hour before cardioversion in nonemergency situations. Light anesthesia with sodium thiopental, 75-150 mg, I.V., is employed in all conscious patients. The DC current cardioverter unit is synchronized to deliver a DC countershock during the downstroke of the R wave so as to avoid the vulnerable period, the first third of the T wave, and the possibility of inducing ventricular fibrillation. Electrodes, 5 inches in diameter, thickly coated with conducting paste, are positioned on the anterior and lateral left chest wall. An initial countershock of 100 watt-seconds, increased by increments of 100 watt-seconds after each unsuccessful attempt at reversion, is employed until restoration of regular sinus rhythm or until a countershock of 400 watt-seconds is unsuccessful. After reversion, maintenance doses of long-acting quinidine, 300-600 mg, q. 8-12 h., are continued. Failure to continue the drug is the most frequent cause of reversion to the arrhythmia, particularly in rheumatic heart disease.

REFERENCES

Ferrer, M. I. The sick sinus syndrome in atrial disease. J.A.M.A., 206:645, 1968.

Futral, A. A., and McGuire, L. B. Reversion of chronic atrial fibrillation. J.A.M.A., 199:12, 135, 1967.

Kuhn, L. A. Electrical conversion of arrhythmias. Amer. Heart J., 67:5, 1964.

Lown, B. Electrical conversion of cardiac arrhythmias. Conference on advances in management of chronic heart disease. N. Y. Heart Assoc., Jan. 21, 1964.

Morris, J. J., et al. Experience with "cardioversion" of atrial fibrillation and flutter. Amer. J. Cardiol., 14:1, 1964.

THE POSTPERICARDIOTOMY SYNDROME

The postpericardiotomy syndrome is a febrile illness with pericardial and at times pleuropulmonary reaction that follows extensive pericardiotomy or nonpenetrating chest trauma. It is strikingly similar to the postinfarction syndrome of Dressler, and a hypersensitivity reaction has been advanced as a reasonable explanation for both conditions. The syndrome has been recorded in all types of cardiac surgery with the one common factor of pericardiotomy. The incidence is about 30 percent following pericardiotomy or nonpenetrating chest trauma. The syndrome is associated with spiking fever of 102°F or higher, persisting or recurring beyond the first postoperative week accompanied with one or more of the following: chest pain, pericardial in type; pericardial friction rub or effusion; pleural effusion; and the serial ECG changes consistent with the diagnosis of pericarditis. The duration is variable and recurrences up to two years have been reported. In postoperative cases it must be differentiated from bacterial endocarditis and the postperfusion syndrome with hepatosplenomegaly and lymphocytosis.

In mild cases treatment is supportive with control of fever and pain by salicylates. In the postinfarction syndrome indomethacin 25 mg 3 to 4 times daily has been effective. In more severe cases with significant pericardial or pleural effusion, a prolonged course, or multiple recurrences corticosteroids are indicated. Large pericardial or pleural effusions may require aspiration.

REFERENCES

Dressler, W. Postmyocardial infarction syndrome. Arch. Intern. Med., 103:28, 1959.

Drusin, L. M., Engle, M. A., Hagstrom, J., and Schwartz, M. S. The postpericardiotomy syndrome. New Eng. J. Med., 272:597, 1965.

Ito, T., Engle, M. A., and Goldberg, H. P. Postpericardiotomy syndrome following surgery for nonrheumatic heart disease. Circulation, 17:549, 1958.

CATHETERS — THEIR MISUSE AND DANGER

THE DRY BED SYNDROME OR FOLEY FOLLY

The dry bed syndrome consisting of a dry bed, a febrile patient, and a dangling Foley catheter is an all too common form of iatrogenic disease born of expediency out of the importuning of the nursing staff. Although at times it is necessary to use a catheter to decompress an acutely distended bladder, the danger of such procedure should never be forgotten even if in such an instance the risk is small and justified. However, the risk of infection and the danger attendant on a Foley catheter left in the bladder over 48 hours are staggering and can never be justified on the grounds of nursing convenience, the dryness of the bed, or accuracy in measuring output. The price to the patient is tremendous compared to the minor advantages that accrue to the nursing and laundry services or the information attained. Far better a wet bed and even excoriated buttocks than an indwelling catheter, a dry bed, repeated kidney infections, chronic pyelonephritis, gram-negative septicemia, and threatened death. The incontinent patient is a challenge to meticulous nursing care, not a problem to be solved by the arrant folly of the indwelling catheter.

REFERENCES

Martin, C. M., and Bookrajian, E. N. Bacteriuria prevention after indwelling urinary catheterization. Arch. Intern. Med., 110:703, 1962.

Vaquer, F., Meyers, M.S., and El-Dadah, A. Prevention of gram-negative rod bacteremia associated with indwelling urinary-tract catheterization. Antimicrob. Agents Chemother., p. 617, 1963.

Waisbren, B. A. Gram negative shock and endotoxic shock. Amer. J. Med., 36:819, 1964.

CEREBROSPINAL FLUID

CONDITION	PROTEIN (mg %)	SUGAR (mg %)	WHITE CELLS	PREDOMINANT CELLS	SEROLOGY
Normal	15-45	45-80	0-5	lymph.	–
Pyogenic meningitis	50-1,500	0-45	25-500	poly.	–
Anterior poliomyelitis	20-350	50-100	10-500	lymph.†	–
TBC meningitis	45-100	0-45	25-500	lymph.	–
Encephalitis lethargica	20-75	50-100	0-100	lymph.	–
Tabes dorsalis	25-100	50-80	10-20	lymph.	may be +
General paresis	50-150	50-80	15-50	lymph.	may be +
Meningovascular syphilis	45-400	20-80	25-2,000	lymph.	+ (in most cases)
Cord tumor	15-100	45-80	0-5	lymph.	–
Brain tumor	50-100	45-80*	0-5	lymph.	–
Guillain-Barré syndrome	over 50	15-45	less than 10	lymph.	–
Viral or aseptic meningitis	45-80	generally normal	10-200	lymph.	–

*Sugar is occasionally quite low.

†Cells may be mostly polys in first few days.

NOTES.

1. There must be about 200 cells/mm before slight turbidity can be seen in the spinal fluid.
2. The lowest CSF sugars are found in bacterial meningitis.
3. A common error is to misidentify red cells and count them as white blood cells.
4. In cases of diabetics and patients who have recently eaten, the sugar may be high. Normally the CSF sugar is approximately one half the blood sugar.

CHOLESTEROL AND ARTERIOSCLEROSIS

The amount of cholesterol in food has practically no effect on the cholesterol level of the blood, for cholesterol is actively metabolized and is in equilibrium with both endogenous and exogenous sources. The primary site of endogenous formation is the liver. Cholesterol is synthesized from acetate and other small molecules derived from the catabolism of carbohydrate and protein as well as fat. About 2 g are manufactured daily with a half-life of about 8 days. Cholesterol and its esters, insoluble in water, are carried in tissue fluids combined in the lipoproteins. Serum cholesterol is determined largely by the nature of dietary fats. These can be divided into three groups.

GROUP I	GROUP II	GROUP III
Highly unsaturated oils: corn and corn oil margarines, cotton, soybean, safflower, sunflower, wheat and rye germ, fish oils	Intermediate oils: olive, peanut, poultry	Saturated oils: butter, hydrogenated shortenings, coconut, cheese, milk, meats, ordinary margarines

Ingestion of foods in the first group tends to lower the serum cholesterol because of the metabolic action of polyunsaturated oils, those in the third group raise the cholesterol level, while those in the second group have little or no effect on serum cholesterol.

There is much debate as to the exact role of cholesterol in the genesis of arteriosclerosis. However, high cholesterol levels are statistically related to the incidence of coronary artery sclerosis, and a heavy consumption of foods containing saturated fatty acids is related to high cholesterol levels.

Practically, the serum cholesterol can be lowered in three ways: 1) By reducing the fat intake to 20 percent of the total calories. This makes for an unpalatable diet. 2) By allowing 30 percent of the total calories in the form of fats made up predominantly of polyunsaturated fatty acids. 3) By the use of various drugs (clofibrate, cholestyramine, d-thyroxine and nicotinic acid).

In following the second course one should be on the alert for the hidden types of fat. Fat constitutes three quarters of the total calories in hamburger, cheese, cakes, and pies, and the fats are of the saturated type. In the production of margarine, hydrogenation changes the liquid oils to hardened saturated fats. Corn oil is highly polyunsaturated. It has an iodine value of 126, which is reduced by hydrogenation to a value of 73 in the formation of margarine. The hypercholesterolemic fats in general have the lowest iodine value.

Dietary prophylaxis of arteriosclerosis means a sweeping reconsideration of the American diet. By the time coronary artery disease is manifest, diet probably does little. Rearrangement of the diet should begin in the early teens or sooner. Butter, milk, ice cream, pastry, and gravies should be replaced in our diets by foods containing predominantly polyunsaturated fatty acids.

DRUG TREATMENT

From among the many lipid-lowering agents the following four are listed in the order of increasing side effects.

1. Clofibrate interferes in the early stage of cholesterol synthesis where acetate is converted to mevalanate. Gastrointestinal upsets are a frequent side effect. It enhances the effect of Warfarin so that the dosage of the anticoagulant must be reduced one third to one half. The daily dose of clofibrate in 500 mg q.i.d.
2. Cholestyramine, the chloride salt of a strongly basic anion exchange resin, binds bile salts and prevents their intestinal absorption. Side effects are mainly gastrointestinal with nausea, diarrhea, or constipation. Mild hyperchloremic acidosis may be produced. The dose is 12-32 g daily in divided doses with meals.
3. D-thyroxine. The main side effects are dose-related and consist of nervousness, palpitation, and diarrhea. With larger doses, 10 percent of patients in the older age groups experience angina. The dose is 2-16 mg daily.
4. Nicotinic acid. The side effects and lipid-lowering property of this drug are dose-related. They are flushing, metallic taste, gastrointestinal disturbances, hyperglycemia, hyperuricemia, and abnormal liver function tests. The dose is 1.0 g daily gradually increased to 3.0 g.

REFERENCES

Chiu, G. Mode of action of cholesterol-lowering agents. Arch. Intern. Med., 108:717, 1961.

Dietary fat and its relation to heart attacks and strokes (special communication). J.A.M.A., 175:389, 1961.

Dole, V., Gordis, E., and Bierman, E. Hyperlipemia and arteriosclerosis. New Eng. J. Med., 269:686, 1963.

Duncan, G. G., et al. Some clinical potentials of chlorophenoxyisobutyrate (clofibrate) therapy (hyperlopidemia-angina pectoris-blood sludging-diabetic neuropathy). Metabolism, 17:457, 1968.

Levy, R. I., and Fredrickson, D. S. Diagnoses and management of hyperlipoproteinemia. Amer. J.. Cardiol., 22:576, 1968.

Sachs, B. A. Appraisal of clofibrate as a hypolipidemic agent. Amer. Heart J., 75:707, 1968.

CIRRHOSIS OF THE LIVER

Hepatic cirrhosis is at present the fifth most common cause of death in this country, accounting for approximately 20,000 deaths per year.

CAUSES

1. Laennec's (alcoholic) cirrhosis	80%
2. Postnecrotic cirrhosis	8%
3. Hemochromatosis	2%
4. Mixed (combinations of the above)	5 to 10%

Rarer causes include cardiac cirrhosis, biliary cirrhosis (each about 2 percent), Wilson's disease, parasitic causes (especially schistosomiasis), and cirrhosis secondary to hepatotoxins (carbon tetrachloride, arsenic, phosphorus, lead, and copper). Malaria and syphilis are said occasionally to cause cirrhosis.

LAENNEC'S CIRRHOSIS. Diagnosis is based upon suggestive historical and clinical findings and is established by liver biopsy.

Liver function tests. BSP is the first test to be abnormal. Later there is a moderate decrease in serum albumin, and elevated globulin. Early, there may be normal bilirubin, alkaline phosphatase, thymol turbidity, and total serum cholesterol. Serum transaminase is elevated in the presence of active necrosis. The prothrombin time may be prolonged and frequently does not respond to vitamin K administration. Urine urobilinogen and bilirubin are increased.

Laboratory tests, in the typical case, show "pure" hepatocellular disease, that is:

1. Reversed A/G ratio with diffuse hypergammaglobulinemia (see "Proteins, Serum").
2. Increase in Bromsulphalein retention.
3. Cephalin flocculation tests, thymol turbidity, and serum transaminase (SGOT, SGPT) levels usually show modest elevation.
4. Cholesterol esterification is decreased.
5. Bilirubin is usually normal except in decompensated, advanced cases.
6. Alkaline phosphatase is normal.
7. Prothrombin time may be elevated; the response to parenteral administration of vitamin K is of diagnostic value. In obstructive states, prothrombin time returns to normal promptly, whereas in primary parenchymal disease, vitamin K does not affect the prothrombin time, or does so very slowly.

POSTNECROTIC CIRRHOSIS. Postnecrotic cirrhosis is better termed "cryptogenic," since a prior history of hepatitis is found in less than 20 percent of American patients and in 33 percent of British patients. In this disease, a more "lumpy" liver is found, and a greater tendency to portal hypertension and varicose bleeding exists, but a lesser tendency to ascites than in Laennec's cirrhosis. Further, the gamma globulin and thymol turbidity are more elevated and serum cholesterol more depressed than in Laennec's cirrhosis.

TREATMENT

The essentials of therapy in cirrhosis of the liver are *diet, rest,* and *abstinence from alcohol.*

DIET. The diet must be high in calories. The relative proportions of carbohydrate fat and protein are of secondary importance. A high caloric diet does not mean that the patient is served two helpings of everything. These patients are often quite ill and are severely anorexic. A heaping plate overloaded with food is not always appealing. The dietician should discuss the diet with the patient. Six feedings are often better than three. If well tolerated the diet may be almost entirely liquid.

The cirrhotic patient needs at least 1 g of protein in his diet per kg of body weight. However, in the face of rapid decompensation, or in the presence of a portacaval shunt, the protein may precipitate coma. Low-protein diet should then be used until better compensation is reached, when the protein can be gradually increased (80-120 g of protein is ideal).

Patients with ascites and edema are frequently placed on low-salt diets. Such diets are frequently unpalatable, and sufficient salt should be allowed to encourage large food intakes.

Frequently patients will state they they are eating well when they are not. It is good practice to have the dietician spotcheck the caloric intake from time to time.

COMPLICATIONS OF CIRRHOSIS

1. Ascites and/or peripheral edema.
2. Hepatic coma.
3. Jaundice.
4. Unexplained febrile disorders. These arise frequently in the cirrhotic. They may be due to viral hepatitis, hemolytic anemia, bacterial infection, or advancing hepatic necrosis.
5. Bleeding esophageal varices.

ASCITES

TREATMENT

Paracentesis accomplishes little or nothing, is often dangerous, and occasionally is fatal. Large amounts of protein are lost, and hypovolemic hypotension and renal failure may ensue. Paracentesis is *rarely* indicated. It may be necessary:

1. As a diagnostic procedure (cytology for malignant cells, culture for bacteria). In this case it is unnecessary to remove more than 1 liter at most.
2. For severe respiratory distress. Here it is desirable to remove no more than 3 liters at one time, or to insert a polyethylene catheter for slower drainage of larger quantities.
3. For enlarging umbilical hernia with danger of perforation and massive decompression. This complication is frequently fatal. Herniorrhaphy under local anesthesia should be contemplated. The procedure listed above in No. 2 should be followed.
4. In unusual situations, such as massive hemorrhoids with or without rectal prolapse or bleeding, and prolapse of the uterus. Again, the procedure under No. 2 should be employed.

OTHER TREATMENT. Assuming an adequate renal blood flow and the absence of hypochloremia, dietary sodium restriction with periodic mercurial or chlorothiazide diuretics is usually successful. If the patient is unresponsive because of low serum Cl^-, priming with l-lysine monohydrochloride, 10 g, q.i.d., until the serum Cl^- reaches 110 mEq/L will then enable the patient to respond to diuretics. If this is unsuccessful, an aldosterone antagonist may be employed in addition to the chloride and mercurials. Aldactone is given in doses of 25 mg, q.i.d. When thiazide diuretics are used alone, potassium supplements (KCl) should be given. No potassium should be used with aldactone, which causes potassium retention.

If all the above fail, prednisone may be added, 10 mg, t.i.d., in a further attempt to suppress endogenous steroid and ACTH production. The majority of patients with even advanced cirrhosis and ascites will respond to the above measures.

The physician must keep in mind that ascites is a symptom of decompensated liver disease. Although it is a great nuisance to the patient, it is not life-threatening, save one exception (perforation of the umbilicus). Heroic procedures associated with high mortality and morbidity (adrenalectomy, portacaval shunt) probably have no sound basis and should not be used to treat ascites. The same applies to the intravenous administration of the patient's own ascitic fluid.

REFERENCE

Reynolds, T. B., Hudson, N. M., Mikkelsen, W. P., Turrill, F. L., and Redeker, A. G. Clinical comparison of end-to-side portacaval shunt. New Eng. J. Med., 274:706, 1966.

HEPATIC COMA

(Hepatic Encephalopathy)

This intoxication is generally attributed to the absorption of nitrogenous products resulting from breakdowns of protein in the intestine which have bypassed the liver (via shunts) and have not been normally metabolized. The precipitating causes are increased dietary protein, gastrointestinal bleeding, or as a terminal episode in far-advanced cirrhosis.

Hepatic coma, arising de novo or following bleeding, is a very grave sign. Recovery from deep coma with jaundice rarely occurs. Lesser states of coma, such as the episodes of confusion, lethargy, and stupor which are seen in patients who have had porto-systemic shunts, are generally reversible. Signs and symptoms include changes in personality, mental confusion progressing to somnolence and coma, clumsiness, ataxia, and hyperreflexia later progressing to flaccidity. Fetor hepaticus is frequently present, as may be the peculiar flapping tremor of the fingers and wrists (asterixis). The latter is not a specific sign, however, and is seen in other diseases, including chronic pulmonary insufficiency with CO_2 retention and uremia.

Electroencephalographic findings are characteristic, showing slow waves of high amplitude, starting bilaterally in the frontal regions, and, in severe cases, becoming generalized.

In hepatic coma, the serum ammonia rises from the normal of 40-70 μcg/100 ml to levels of 150-200 μcg/100 ml.

TREATMENT

1. Discontinue all protein intake. Diet should be composed solely of carbohydrate. Intravenous 10 percent glucose in water may be used.
2. Nitrogenous wastes in the colon are reduced by the use of colonic enemas and antibiotics.
   a. High colonic tap water enemas are given every 4 to 6 hours.
   b. Neomycin, P.O., approximately 1 g, q. 6 h., is of value. If the patient is unable to swallow, intramuscular tetracycline may be given in doses of 100 to 200 mg, q. 6 h.
3. Massive steroid therapy (up to 5 g of cortisone, or equivalent doses of the more potent steroids) has been employed, but is frequently disappointing.
4. Correction of anemia and electrolyte abnormalities. Many electrolyte disturbances occur (respiratory alkalosis, metabolic alkalosis, potassium and magnesium deficiency are common). Metabolic acidosis from administration of chloride ion may occur. Blood is one of the best buffer systems in the body. Correction of anemia helps maintain normal pH.
5. For severe agitation, paraldehyde by rectum or I.M., or chloral hydrate by rectum, may be used. Do not give morphine or Demerol.
6. Glutamates and arginine have been extensively employed but are of doubtful value.

REFERENCE

Trey, C., Burns, D.G., and Saunders, S. J. Treatment of hepatic coma by exchange blood transfusion. New Eng. J. Med., 274:473, 1966.

JAUNDICE

Jaundice occurs in the patient with cirrhosis of the liver for different reasons. Most commonly it represents rapidly advancing deterioration of liver function. It may, however, be a manifestation of a superimposed infection involving the liver (infectious hepatitis). A number of clinical entities can be identified.

1. The cirrhotic patient slowly and gradually becomes jaundiced. The jaundice is usually of mild degree and unassociated with constitutional symptoms or other evidence of rapid liver deterioration. With adequate treatment the jaundice may disappear in 6 to 8 weeks. It represents slowly advancing liver disease.
2. Rapidly advancing liver necrosis may occur in the cirrhotic patient. It is usually associated with jaundice of varying intensity and the occurrence of ascites. Such patients are frequently febrile, and the clinical course is protracted, the mortality rate is high, and 6 to 8 weeks may be required before the recovery to the former state is accomplished.
3. A patient with cirrhosis of liver may develop acute infectious hepatitis.
4. Zieve's syndrome. In this interesting but infrequent complication of cirrhosis of the liver the patient exhibits a protracted febrile course with jaundice, ascites, hemolytic anemia, thrombocytosis, and elevated serum cholesterol. A protracted clinical course is the rule. Most of the patients, however, recover. Liver biopsy generally reveals fatty metamorphosis of the liver.

FEVER

Patients with cirrhosis of the liver frequently run a febrile course with temperature elevations to 102°F to 103°F for many weeks. When the fever is associated with jaundice and ascites there may not be a difficult problem in differential diagnosis. Frequently, however, one sees persistent elevation of temperature without jaundice or ascites. The clinical course is mild, recovery is the rule. The fever may last 4 to 6 weeks.

ESOPHAGEAL VARICES

The incidence of esophageal varices in patients with cirrhosis of the liver is quite high. However, the occurrence of hemorrhage from the varices is only about 25 percent. Although this number is relatively small, a massive hemorrhage from esophageal varices in patients with cirrhosis of the liver is frequently a lethal complication. Whether or not bleeding will occur at some time in the patient's life is difficult to predict. Recent studies indicate that those patients who have high portal pressures are the ones who are prone to bleeding. Those with portal pressures, as measured by splenic pulp manometry, of 300 mm H_2O or higher are those in whom hemorrhage occurs. Hemorrhage does not frequently occur in those with lower pressures (280 mm H_2O or less). Only an occasional patient with esophageal varices will bleed with modestly elevated pressures, e.g., 280-300 mm H_2O.

MANAGEMENT OF ACUTE BLEEDING FROM ESOPHAGEAL VARICES

The presence of cirrhosis of the liver and an elevated portal pressure must be documented. If blood needs to be given it must be fresh to avoid the high ammonia content of stored blood. If bleeding continues after hospitalization, regardless of the amount, the bleeding should be stopped. We feel that the most convenient way to do this is to use local esophageal cooling via a special machine for sustaining the hypothermia. The Sengstaken pressure balloon may also be used, but it is not as simple to operate. The hypothermia device should be used for 24 hours and withdrawn. If the bleeding recurs local hypothermia is restarted, and an emergency portacaval shunt should be done. If the bleeding should cease, then a portacaval shunt should be performed before discharge from the hospital.

PROPHYLACTIC PORTACAVAL SHUNTS. The value of this operation has not been assessed at the present time.

INDICATION FOR PORTACAVAL SHUNT IN PATIENTS WITH CIRRHOSIS OF THE LIVER AND ESOPHAGEAL VARICES

Any patient who has had one previous episode of hemorrhage from esophageal varices, and who has relatively good liver function, should have a portacaval shunt. Before such a procedure is done, however, it should be demonstrated that the portal pressure is elevated and a portogram should be performed to demonstrate the presence of the esophageal varices. By relatively good liver function is meant a patient with a serum albumin of 3.0 g or more, and who is not clinically jaundiced (bilirubin less than 2 mg per 100 ml). The prothrombin time should be less than 22 seconds.

REFERENCES

Conn, H. O., and Lindenbuth, W. W. Prophylactic portacaval anastomosis in patients with esophageal varices. New Eng. J. Med., 279:725, 1968.

Garceau, A. J., et al. Controlled trial of prophylactic shunt surgery. New Eng. J. Med., 270:496, 1964.
—— The natural history of cirrhosis. I and II. New Eng. J. Med., 271:1173, 1964.
Orloff, M. J., et al. The complications of cirrhosis of the liver. Ann. Intern. Med., 66:165, 1967.
Powell, W. J., Jr., and Klatskin, G. Duration of survival in patients with Laennec's cirrhosis. Influence of alcohol withdrawal and possible effects of recent changes in general management of the disease. Amer. J. Med., 44:406, 1968.
Rousselot, L. M., Panke, W. F., and Moreno, A. H. Further evaluation of splenic pulp manometry as a differential diagnostic test of acute upper gastrointestinal bleeding. Amer. J. Gastroenterol. 35:474, 1961.
Schaefer, J. W., Schiff, L., Gall, E. A., and Oikawa, Y. Progression of acute hepatitis to postnecrotic cirrhosis. Amer. J. Med., 42:348, 1967.
Symposium: Liver disease. Medicine, 45:413, 1966
Symposium: Liver disease (continued). Medicine, 46:73, 1967.

BILIARY CIRRHOSIS

(Xanthomatous Biliary Cirrhosis, see also Hyperlipemic States, and the Histiocytoses)

Biliary cirrhosis is a chronic obstructive liver disease of young women. It is rare in males. There are marked elevations of the cholesterol and plasma lipids. When the lipid changes are marked (1,800 mg per 100 ml) and prolonged, striking and grotesque xanthomatous skin lesions appear. Cirrhosis of the liver is present with large nodular areas of regeneration. The fundamental lesion is either biochemical or morphologic, and interferes with excretion of conjugated bilirubin into the biliary radicles. Chronicity is an outstanding feature of the disorder. The patients are more jaundiced than sick. The liver and spleen are enlarged. Pruritus is frequently very troublesome. The tests of liver function suggest an obstructive lesion. The same clinical picture can be produced by chronic mechanical obstruction of the external biliary tree. Any male with this clinical syndrome should be surgically explored, and most of the women probably should be explored.

"COIN LESION"

(See p. 339)

COMA

Definition: Coma is that state of unconsciousness from which the patient cannot be aroused, even by powerful stimuli.

ETIOLOGY

The vowel mnemonic A-E-I-O-U encompasses approximately 99 percent of patients presenting with coma.

A. Alcoholism 60%
 Apoplexy (cerebrovascular accidents) 10%
E. Epilepsy 2%
I. Infection (meningitis, pneumonia, and septicemia) 4%
 Injury (subdural hematoma, etc.) 13%
O. Opiates and other drugs (barbiturates, phenothiazines, etc.) 3%
U. Uremia (1%) and other metabolic causes: diabetic coma (hyperglycemia and hypoglycemia) (2%), hepatic coma (1%)

Also eclampsia, CNS lues, shock secondary to blood loss, myxedema, Addisonian crisis (each less than 1%)

DIAGNOSIS

HISTORY AND PHYSICAL

1. History of drug or alcohol habituation, of hypertension, etc.
2. Examine pockets for cards, medicines, syringes; look inside hat for evidence of dried blood.
3. Odor of breath (acetone, uriniferous, fetor hepaticus).
4. Pupillary and peripheral reflexes.
5. Signs of head injury.
6. Feel skin (cold, clammy or warm, sweaty).
7. Pulse.
8. Character of breathing (Cheyne-Stokes, Kussmaul, Biot).
9. Condition of neck (rigidity).
10. Skin and mucous membranes (icterus, pallor, needle puncture marks).

LABORATORY

1. Urine for sugar and acetone.
2. FBS, BUN, CO_2.

3. Skull x-ray is indicated in every comatose patient presenting with neurologic findings.
4. Gastric aspiration is seldom indicated. The danger of producing aspiration pneumonia is high. If attempted, an endotracheal airway should first be inserted.
5. Spinal fluid examination (when indicated).
6. Serum level of various drugs, e.g., bromide, barbiturate.

TREATMENT

1. See under specific disease or drug.
2. No harm is done by giving 50 ml of 50 percent glucose intravenously.
3. Nalline, 5 mg intravenously, may be used if pinpoint pupils and/or needle puncture marks are seen.

HYPEROSMOLAR NONKETOTIC COMA

This form of coma is associated with hyperglycemia and marked elevation of serum osmolality (normal value = 300 mOsm/L).

The patients are diabetics (usually, but not always of the adult onset type) who develop marked hyperglycemia, while seriously ill, from severe infection, extensive burns, pancreatitis, pancreatic carcinoma, or cerebral disease. The administration of steroids or glucose-containing solutions (intravenously or via peritoneal dialysis) has also been associated with this problem.

Signs and symptoms fall into two categories: 1) hypovolemia and dehydration secondary to osmotic diuresis, and 2) neurologic, i.e., coma, seizures. Diagnosis is made by the finding of marked hyperglycemia (600-3,000 mg/100 ml) and negative serum acetone.

The severity of the hyperosmolality can be estimated by the following equation:

$$2[Na^{+} + K^{+}] + \frac{\text{blood glucose (mg per 100 ml)}}{18} + \frac{\text{BUN (mg per 100 ml)}}{2.8} = \text{mOsm/L}$$

Values over 340 are considered high.

The mainstay of therapy include insulin (usually only in moderate amounts, but occasionally in very large doses) and hypotonic fluids. As an initial fluid, 0.45% NaCl without glucose is probably best used because isotonic sodium chloride may increase the osmotic diuresis and exaggerate the hyperosmolality. In the presence of hypovolemic shock, however, isotonic saline may be used initially for expansion of the severely contracted extracellular fluid volume.

REFERENCES

DiBenedetto, R., Crocco, J., and Soscia, J. Hyperglycemic nonketotic coma. Arch. Intern. Med., 116:74, 1965.

Tyler, F. H. Hyperosomolar coma. Amer. J. Med., 45:485, 1968.

CONGESTIVE HEART FAILURE

Heart failure is due to an inability of the heart to provide oxygen to the tissues, whether through decreased output or failure to keep pace with tissue needs.

In the great proportion of cases of heart failure the cardiac output is low (less than 4.0 liters). The arteriovenous oxygen difference is high. On effort, either the cardiac output does not rise or it falls. This is known as *low output* failure. The most common syndromes associated with congestive heart failure are arteriosclerotic heart disease, hypertension, aortic and mitral valvular lesions, constrictive pericarditis, and the myocardiopathies (acute rheumatic fever, acute nonspecific myocarditis, etc.). The failure of the left ventricle to pump the blood "forward" results in diminished renal blood flow, with consequent retention of salt and water. The edema of heart failure is due to alteration in renal function. Subsequently aldosterone and antidiuretic hormone production are increased, and further salt and water retention occurs.

Congestive heart failure is usually associated with an elevated venous pressure. The mechanism is unknown, but it is probably a compensatory phenomenon to raise ventricular diastolic pressure and force a rise in cardiac output (Starling's law). The combination of elevated venous pressure and increased blood volume contributes to peripheral edema.

Under certain circumstances, congestive heart failure with a similar sequence of events is associated with a high cardiac output. This occurs in Graves' disease, severe anemia, beriberi, arteriovenous fistula, Paget's disease, and patent ductus arteriosus. (The last three are forms of AV fistulae.) In these patients the concept of "forward" failure is not tenable.

In the presence of primary or secondary pulmonary hypertension, thrombosis of the pulmonary artery, pulmonic stenosis, or tricuspid stenosis, the right ventricle fails ("right ventricular failure," "backward failure"). Here the outstanding features are an enlarged, tender liver, ascites, and dependent edema.

From the above it is apparent that the concepts of left ventricular failure, right ventricular failure, forward failure, and backward failure leave much to be desired, because the mechanisms overlap. However, the terms are deeply rooted in medicine and they do serve some purpose in clinical thinking.

DIAGNOSIS

Left heart failure causes acute or chronic passive pulmonary congestion and is usually associated with the following:

1. Dyspnea.
2. Orthopnea.
3. Cough with, rarely, hoarseness.
4. Cyanosis.
5. Hemoptysis.
6. Enlarged heart.
7. Diastolic gallop rhythm.
8. Accentuated pulmonic second sound.
9. Pulmonary rales.
10. Hydrothorax in about one-fourth patients, usually right-sided.
11. Chest x-ray: increased hilar shadows with accentuated pulmonary vessels radiating in a fanlike fashion peripherally.
12. Circulation time is prolonged over 16 seconds.
13. Venous pressure is normal if there is no concomitant right heart failure.

Right heart failure produces congestion in the greater circulation with the following:

1. Weight gain may occur.
2. Easy fatigue.
3. Oliguria and nocturia.
4. Subcutaneous edema.
5. Venous distension.
6. Hepatomegaly with or without tenderness and abnormal parenchymal liver chemistries. Clinical jaundice is occasionally present.
7. Cyanosis.

8. Ascites.
9. Urine with a high specific gravity, low sodium content, and slight to moderate albuminuria.
10. Blood chemistries usually show a low sodium (dilutional) and may show axotemia and hypoproteinemia.
11. The circulation time is prolonged, and the venous pressure is elevated.

Combined left and right failure occurs in most patients. Symptoms and findings then are a composite of those listed above.

TREATMENT

The keystones of successful treatment are rest, sodium restriction, digitalis, and diuretics. On strict bed rest alone a good diuresis usually occurs. Sodium restriction to, initially, 0.5 or 0.25 g of sodium chloride a day is of value.

DIURETICS. Mercuhydrin, 2 ml, I.M., and the thiazide drugs (chlorothiazide, 250-500 mg, b.i.d., or hydrochlorothiazide, 25-50 mg. q.d.) are of value. In long-standing congestive heart failure hypochloremic alkalosis may appear, and in this circumstance the kidney no longer responds to diuretics. The thiazide drugs may cause hypokalemia, and for this reason KCl, 1 g, t.i.d., is employed with the diuretic.

"INTRACTABLE" HEART FAILURE

Intractable or refractory congestive failure connotes a lack of optimal response to full digitalization, adequate sodium restriction, and diuretics in a patient with extravascular accumulations of fluid. When the above therapeutic measures have been employed, conditions poorly responsive to them or not responsive at all, such as masked hyperthyroidism, myxedema, beriberi, constrictive pericarditis, AV fistula, anemia, ventricular aneurysm, and digitalis poisoning, have to be excluded as the cause of the heart failure. The main factor in intractability is usually hypochloremic alkalosis.

SERUM LEVELS (in mEq/L)	NORMAL	HYPO-CHLOREMIC ALKALOSIS
Sodium	138-144	130-135
Chloride	100-110	80-90
HCO_3	23-26	25-30

When the serum chloride drops below 100 mEq/L the kidneys respond poorly to diuretics. To correct the chloride deficit, diuretics are stopped and the blood chlorides elevated by the use of any of the following drugs which increase the concentration of the hydrogen ion and produce a mild hyperchloremic acidosis as outlined above.

1. NH_4Cl, orally, 12 to 14 g daily, in divided doses in enteric coated tablets. The amount of absorption in this form is variable.
2. L-Lysine monohydrochloride, orally in solution, 15 to 40 g daily (1 g = 5 mEq Cl; 40 g = 10 g Cl). This preparation is preferable to the others because of its greater palatability.
3. Dilute HCl, USP (0.1N)(1 L = 100 mEq Cl).
4. NH_4Cl, 2 percent solution slowly intravenously in amounts of 250 ml.

The level of serum chloride is determined every second or third day. When it reaches 110 mEq/L a mercurial, with or without chlorthiazide diuretic, may be given. Satisfactory diuresis then occurs. The acidifying agent is continued. It is most important to withhold the diuretic until the serum chloride reaches a level of 110 mEq/L. Using the diuretic before this point is reached wipes out what has been accomplished in terms of raising serum chlorides.

Ethacrynic acid 50 mg I.V. or 50-100 mg b.i.d. orally or furosemide 40-80 mg orally or I.V. are effective in the presence of hypochloremic alkalosis.

The "low salt syndrome" is mentioned here only to emphasize that in congestive failure a decrease in serum sodium is an expression of dilution due to water retention. The total body sodium is actually *increased.* The proper treatment is as outlined previously with the aim of causing water diuresis. The administration of salt is absolutely contraindicated. In severe refractory failure, limitation of fluid intake to 600 to 800 ml a day is of great value.

The causes of intractable congestive failure other than hypochloremic alkalosis respond only to specific medical or surgical treatment.

DIGITALIS

(See p. 112)

REFERENCES

Akbarian, M., Yankopoulos, A., and Abelmann, W. H. Hemodynamic studies in beriberi heart disease. Amer. J. Med., 41:197, 1966.

Alexander, C. S. Idiopathic heart disease. Amer. J. Med., 41:213, 1966.
Gidekel, L. I., et al. Management of refractory fluid retention with a combination of l-arginine monohydrochloride and mercurials. New Eng. J. Med.. 263:221, 1960.
Skinner, N. S., et al. Hemodynamic consequences of atrial fibrillation at constant ventricular rates. Amer. J. Med., 36:342, 1964.

CONVULSIVE DISORDERS

Definition: This is a group of disorders characterized by paroxysms of muscular convulsions and/or transient episodes of sensory or psychic disturbances. Seizures may be classified in four categories.

1. Grand mal (generalized seizure).
2. Petit mal, with three subtypes:
   a. short stare
   b. myoclonic (bilateral rhythmical jerks)
   c. akinetic, characterized by sudden momentary loss of muscle tone
3. Psychomotor, characterized by loss of contact and some form of irrelevant motor activity.
4. Focal seizures, either sensory or motor.

DIFFERENTIAL DIAGNOSIS

1. *Intracranial causes:*
   a. epilepsy (idiopathic)
   b. epilepsy (symptomatic)
      (1) neoplasms (primary or metastatic)
      (2) inflammation (abscess or meningitis)
      (3) congenital anomalies of the CNS
      (4) trauma
2. *Extracranial causes* (symptomatic epilepsy):
   a. toxic (ethanol, lead, phenothiazines, and other drugs)
   b. hyperpyrexia
   c. anoxia (cardiac, respiratory, or secondary to anemia)
   d. metabolic (hypocalcemia, hypoglycemia, azotemia, and hepatic coma)

Diagnostic procedures:

1. The best single procedure is observation of a seizure.
2. The EEG will show abnormalities in approximately 75 percent of cases.

3. Skull x-rays, lumbar puncture, and appropriate blood and urine chemistries.

TREATMENT

Treatment consists of therapy directed at the underlying cause, wherever possible. Acute attacks of status epilepticus will respond to intravenous sodium amytal, approximately 0.5 g administered slowly. Maintenance therapy usually consists of Dilantin, 100 mg, P.O. or I.M., t.i.d., and phenobarbital, 15-30 mg, t.i.d.

REFERENCE

Andreas, F. D., and O'Doherty, D. S. An analysis of convulsive disorder in a general hospital. Georgetown Med. Bull., 14:172, 1961.

CORONARY ARTERY DISEASE

The spectrum of coronary artery disease extends from angina pectoris to subendocardial infarction to transmural infarction. It varies from transient myocardial oxygen deficit to the death of cardiac muscle cells. Intermediate between the extremes of angina and transmural infarction is the poorly defined entity called, in the past, acute or subacute coronary insufficiency. Anatomically it may be associated with infarction of the subendocardial layers of the myocardium. Its significance and treatment are the same as those of transmural infarction.

ANGINA PECTORIS

Definition: Angina pectoris is a syndrome due to myocardial oxygen deficit. It is manifested by a sense of constriction or pressure behind the sternum with, at times, radiation to the upper extremities, root of the neck, or the jaw. Not uncommonly the pain may start in the volar surface of the wrist as a dull ache, remain there or spread centrally to the chest. Peripheral pain occurs most commonly in the left upper extremity, less frequently in both extremities, and rarely in the right upper alone. The pain pattern is remarkably constant in a given patient and any deviation from the usual pattern in the sense of location of pain, frequency, duration, or intensity should alert one to the possibility of impending or actual myocardial infarction or the onset of an additional disorder. The pain sensation, either tightness, pressure, or fullness, lasts at least 30 seconds and is relieved by rest or appropriate medication.

ETIOLOGY

By far the most common cause of angina pectoris is coronary artery sclerosis producing an obstruction to coronary blood flow. Less common causes are aortic valvular disease, such as aortic insufficiency, either rheumatic or luetic, aortic stenosis, or partial closure of the coronary ostia by luetic aortitis. In aortic insufficiency, angina pectoris is due to low mean aortic pressure with decreased perfusion of the coronary arteries. In aortic stenosis the pain is due to increased oxygen need necessitated by the increased myocardial work necessary to overcome the valvular outlet obstruction. Luetic narrowing of the ostia offers mechanical obstruction to coronary filling. The anginal pain sometimes seen in tight mitral stenosis is due to decreased left ventricular output. Rarer causes of the anginal syndrome are paroxysmal tachycardia, thyrotoxicosis, severe anemia, periarteritis, hypoglycemia, and shock. It is most likely that most of these conditions do not produce the pain of angina unless they are superimposed on a coronary flow already compromised by coronary sclerosis.

Conditions which precipitate attacks of angina pectoris in patients with the underlying causes mentioned are exercise, emotion, eating, and cold.

A certain exercise performed in the morning, such as walking to work, may not produce anginal pain, while the same exertion after a fatiguing day may result in an attack. On the other hand, angina may only occur with the initial exertion in the morning. In reference to exertion as a precipitating factor in angina, a variant form of the syndrome has been recalled to attention by Prinzmetal et al. This variant is not precipitated by exertion or emotional upset. The pain is often cyclic, more severe, and of longer duration than the pain of classic angina. Arrhythmias occur in about 50 percent of these cases when pain is severe. In addition, certain ECG changes to be described later are characteristic of the variant form.

Some patients experience angina after eating. This is probably due to splanchnic diversion of blood. When exercise is added, myocardial work is further increased and accounts for the common complaint of aggravation of angina after eating followed by exercise.

Reflex coronary constriction plays a part in the production of angina after exposure to cold.

DIAGNOSIS

The diagnosis of angina pectoris presents little or no difficulty in classical cases. Typically angina during exertion precedes by some time the appearance of angina at rest. If symptoms in reverse are present the diagnosis is open to question except in the variant form which is rare. The most important element in the diagnosis is a careful history. Physical examination usually adds nothing in those cases due to coronary artery sclerosis but is of value in those due to valvular disease, thyrotoxicosis, and anemia. The standard ECG is usually of no help in the diagnosis of classic angina pectoris. In doubtful cases the exercise ECG may be of value in showing ST depression without reciprocal ST elevation (see "Exercise Tolerance Test," page 177). In the variant form of angina pectoris ST segments are elevated during the attack and reciprocal ST depression may occur. Previously abnormal ST segments and T waves may improve during an attack, and R waves may become taller. In classic angina, if the patient is seen during an attack of chest pain, according to Levine the diagnosis may be established by carotid compression. If the heart rate slows, the patient is then asked, "Is the pain worse?" In angina pectoris the pain may disappear with this maneuver.

TREATMENT

Treatment consists of specific and general measures. Specifically the treatment of the attack consists of the sublingual administration of nitroglycerine, 0.3 to 0.4 mg (1/200 to 1/150 gr). The dosage should be sufficient to produce flushing and transient headache. The patient should be instructed to take the medication when in the sitting or recumbent position until well acquainted with its action. When taken in the erect position syncope and resultant injury have occurred. When the drug is administered and effective relief is obtained in a few moments, residual soreness may persist. Nitroglycerine may be taken as often as necessary to relieve pain. Tolerance to the drug is not acquired, and it relieves the pain of both the classic and variant forms of angina pectoris. Nitroglycerine may also be employed prophylactically. With the knowledge that a certain activity produces pain the patient is instructed to take nitroglycerine before undertaking the activity, but should be made to understand that the use of the drug is not license for unrestricted or violent exercise. Prophylactically it is restricted to the prevention of pain during necessary activity.

The long-acting nitrates, though enjoying a considerable vogue in advertising, have not proved effective in decreasing the number of anginal attacks or the amount of nitroglycerine used by a given patient.

Propranolol, a β-adrenergic blocking agent in conjunction with nitroglycerine or isorbide dinitrate, in some patients strikingly decreases the frequency of anginal attacks. The usual initial dose is 10 mg t.i.d. gradually increased to 20 mg t.i.d. or more if necessary. It should not be used in impending cardiac failure, asthma, or heart block.

Among the general measures in treatment are reduction of weight, avoidance of fatigue, and the dietary measures discussed later.

The surgical treatment of coronary artery disease, such as the Vineberg operation with various modifications, coronary grafting, and endarterectomy, have received an impetus through the technique of coronary arteriography and are being more widely used in the last five years. Their long-range effects can not be assessed at present.

Intractable angina pectoris includes those cases in which the frequency of attacks, their severity or duration is increasing, or in which nitroglycerine is not completely effective. Such a change in the pattern in a given patient should alert one to the possibility of impending myocardial infarction, and the condition should be treated as such with bed rest, relief of pain by morphine or Demerol, and the use of anticoagulants as described under myocardial infarction. If infarction does not occur the patient is allowed up gradually after pains have ceased at rest.

SUBENDOCARDIAL NONTRANSMURAL INFARCTION

Subendocardial infarction is considered by some to be strictly an ECG diagnosis. When symptoms are present, subendocardial infarction differs from angina in that the pain, though similar in distribution, is more prolonged and not relieved by rest or nitroglycerine. Electrocardiographically, ST depression and T wave inversion occur and persist for days or weeks. Q waves do not develop. The ECG pattern is distinguished from that of ischemia in that the abnormalities persist for a greater period of time. Symmetrical inversion of T waves has been considered by some to differentiate this from the ischemic pattern. Slight elevation of temperature, moderate elevation of the ESR, and slight increase in SGOT and later LDH levels may occur. A pericardial rub is never heard.

The treatment of subendocardial infarction is the same as the treatment of transmural infarction except that the period of rest need not be so prolonged. Here the indications for anticoagulation are the same as in transmural infarction.

TRANSMURAL INFARCTION

Infarction of the myocardium results from sclerotic or sclerotic and thrombotic occlusion or critical narrowing of a coronary artery or its branches. Such pathologic processes involve the left coronary artery eight times as often as the right. In over 50 percent of cases the anterior descending branch of the left coronary is involved, and much less often the circumflex and septal branch. Anatomically, anterior apical infarcts are most common, followed by inferior, posterior, and finally combined infarction. Atrial infarction occurs concomitantly with ventricular infarction in about 8.5 percent of cases. Involvement of the right atrium is six times as common as the left. When present, posterior infarction of the right atrium is always associated with posterobasal infarction of the left ventricle.

In 192 patients with transmural infarction the infarct was localized by the ECG as follows:

SITE	INCIDENCE (percent)
Anterior	41.7
Anterolateral	8.9
Anteroseptal	8.8
Inferior	32.9
Posterior	2.9
Combined	4.8

SYMPTOMS AND SIGNS. In the diagnosis of myocardial infarction the history, the ECG and certain laboratory tests are far more important than the initial physical signs. The onset is usually sudden but may be preceded in cases with preexisting angina by an increase in the frequency of the attacks or a change in the pain pattern. The pain distribution is identical with that of angina, but the intensity of the precordial pain usually predominates over the intensity of the pain radiation. The pain varies from an uncomfortable sense of pressure in the chest to excruciating agony but has no relation to the extent of the infarct. In untreated cases the pain lasts with decreasing severity for about 72 hours. In 14 percent of cases showing ECG evidence of previous infarction no history of pain can be elicited. Pain may be the only manifestation of infarction but may be accompanied by weakness, sweating, uneasiness, nausea, vomiting, syncope, and hiccups. In those cases free of pain, shock or syncope may be outstanding.

The appearance of the patient varies from almost normal to that of an obviously ill person, pale, cold, and sweating. The blood pressure is usually initially maintained except in manifest shock. It reaches its lowest level on the third or fourth day and gradually levels off below the preinfarction level. The heart sounds may be faint, and a diastolic gallop is often present.

The incidence of arrhythmias revealed by continuous electrocardiographic monitoring is far greater than the frequency noted on clinical examination. The following table is based on the continuous monitoring of 535 patients with acute myocardial infarction from four coronary care units.

A pericardial rub is heard in from 10 to 15 percent of cases. The frequency with which it is heard depends on the frequency of auscultation, for most of the rubs are fleeting, lasting only a few hours, though they may be present for as long as 14 days. Most commonly heard with anterior infarction they do occur with posterior involvement.

The temperature usually rises at the end of the first day and persists for about a week, not exceeding 101°F. With extensive infarcts hyperpyrexia with levels up to 104° to 105°F is seen, and the elevation may last two to three weeks.

The sedimentation rate increases after the first day, reaches a peak between the first and second week, and remains elevated for from six to eight weeks.

SGOT activity increases earlier than the ESR and is positive only within 1 to 4 days after infarction as a rule. LDH elevation occurs later, reaching a peak at approximately the fifth day, and

ARRHYTHMIAS

SUPRAVENTRICULAR	%	VENTRICULAR	%
S. bradycardia	17.2	VPC	59
S. tachycardia	37.1	Vent. tachycardia	14.6
APC	31.2	Vent. fibrillation	8.0
P.A.T.	8.6	Asystole	8.0
A. fibrillation	14.2		
A. flutter	3.4		
Nodal rhythm	9.2		

CONDUCTION DEFECTS

	%
1° Heart block	8.8
2° Heart block	6.0
3° Heart block	4.7
RBBB	6.7
LBBB	1.5

returning to normal at the eighth to tenth day.

With a typical history and supporting signs of myocardial infarction in the presence of a normal or not diagnostic ECG, one should take serial tracings and obtain precordial leads in the third intercostal space. High anterolateral, direct (true) posterior, and apical infarcts are readily missed in the conventionally taken tracing. Tracings interpreted as subendocardial infarction should also be followed serially, for at times the process evolves into a frank transmural pattern.

COURSE. The overall mortality in general hospitals with an active ambulance service without continuous monitoring had been from 33 to 35 percent. The average mortality in 535 monitored patients which includes experience dating back five years was 22.4 percent. Experience limited to the past five years shows a mortality drop to 18 percent. The decrease has been due to prompt recognition of potentially life-threatening arrhythmias and to prompt treatment in an environment planned to cope with such emergencies.

One out of five suffering a myocardial infarct dies before reaching a hospital. The present mortality statistics are hopelessly confusing, for in many reports no discrimination is made regarding the type of infarct, transmural or nontransmural, age of the patient, or functional status on admission. Some uniformity in reporting must be accepted if a true mortality rate and an accurate evaluation of the worth of coronary care units is to be had.

For these reasons we have been reporting our experience on the basis of functional classification and age. Functional status falls into one of three classes, depending on left ventricular function.

Class I	No. L.V. dysfunction.
Class II	Mild to moderate congestive failure or hypotension (90 mm Hg systolic or less) without clinical shock.
Class III	Shock (pump failure) or acute pulmonary edema.

Age groups considered are 55 years or less, 56 to 65 and over 65.

MORTALITY – ACUTE MYOCARDIAL INFARCTION
(2,174 Patients – USPHS)

Class I	17% (10-22)
Class II	38% (33-55)
Class III	22% (0-100)

MORTALITY ON BASIS OF AGE
AND FUNCTIONAL CLASSIFICATIONS

	55 OR LESS (%)	56-65 (%)	OVER 65 (%)	AVERAGE (%)
Class I	9	23	50	27
Class II	33	50	42	42
Class III	66	91	90	88

Even with this breakdown, associated diseases that influence mortality, such as diabetes, hypertension, and previous infarction, are not considered. If the three classes, three age groups, and three possible complications are considered as variables, 72 possible categories result. In short, when mortality rates from acute myocardial infarction are reported, one should be wary of the nature of the sample.

In 105 patients in a coronary care unit cardiac arrest occurred in 26 percent, and of these 37 percent were discharged living.

In 100 patients on general medical wards cardiac arrest occurred in 32 percent but only 4 percent were discharged living.

Ninety percent of all cardiac arrests took place during the first 72 hours and 75 percent during the first week.

These figures point up the necessity for electronic monitoring of patients with recent infarction and the absolute necessity for the prompt and aggressive treatment of lethal cardiac arrhythmias. External cardiac massage and mouth-to-mouth assisted respiration should be followed as quickly as possible by electric cardioversion. No time should be wasted by attempting to identify the arrhythmia by electrocardiographic means. The salvage rate of patients with actual asystole is extremely low and since most cardiac arrests are due to ventricular tachyarrhythmias nothing is lost and much is gained by electric cardioversion.

TREATMENT OF THE ACUTE PHASE AND COMPLICATIONS

The treatment of uncomplicated infarction is well standardized and essentially consists of the relief of pain and continued rest until healing occurs.

CONSTANT MONITORING. The patient should be placed in an environment, such as an intensive care unit, where emergency resuscitation can be readily attempted. During the first five hospital days he should have constant electronic monitoring of his electrocardiogram and nurse monitoring of other vital signs. After the first five hospital days he can probably be safely transported to an ordinary type of hospital environment, and the monitoring may be discontinued.

Rest is ordinarily continued for from three to six weeks, depending on the clinical and laboratory evaluation of the severity of the case. Rest may be in a bed or in a chair, but the latter type of rest does not seem to have caught on. It should be remembered that in the early hours of an infarct circulatory instability is present and that shock can be precipitated by movement of the patient. Under the heading of rest comes the *bête noire* of most patients – the bedpan and bowel function. Whether the patient has a movement during the first three or four days is of no importance. After this time the initial movement is best accomplished by the aid of a low enema. Such help avoids the necessity of straining (Valsalva maneuver). This mechanism is probably contributory to the so-called bedpan death. After the third or fourth day there is no reason why the average uncomplicated case may not use a commode instead of perching precariously on a bedpan. Mineral oil should not be given to patients on oral anticoagulants, for it interferes with the absorption of the coumarin drugs.

RELIEF OF PAIN. The patient's pain should be relieved as quickly as possible. Meperidine (Demerol) is used in doses of 75-100 mg I.M. and 50-75 mg repeated as necessary. This drug is ordinarily preferable to morphine for it does not have the strong respiratory depressant effect of morphine. However, with severe pain morphine sulfate may be used 15 mg s.c. or 8 mg I.V. combined with atropine sulfate 0.4 mg.

These drugs may be repeated every 3 to 4 hours if necessary. It is better not to leave routine repeat orders for their use but to evaluate the patient's condition at frequent intervals, avoiding oversedation and its attendant complications.

Oxygen should be given in all cases. By raising arterial saturation, the work of the heart is decreased.

The further treatment of myocardial infarction is mainly the treatment of the complications.

CARDIOGENIC SHOCK

Cardiogenic shock is reported to occur in 15 percent of patients with acute myocardial infarction. Despite a variety of treatments the mortality remains about 80 percent. Since the nature of hemodynamic changes associated with cardiogenic shock is widely debated, the concept that vasopressor agents should be used for this condition is not generally accepted.

For the sake of uniformity, shock in acute myocardial infarction is said to be present when the systemic arterial pressure is 80 mm Hg or less (not attributable to arrhythmia or medication), accompanied by clinical signs of shock, cool moist skin, disturbed sensorium, oliguria, and low volume pulse. In shock secondary to myocardial infarction there is almost invariably a reduction in cardiac output; however, the magnitude of the reduction is variable. The usual compensatory reflex increase of peripheral vascular resistance (P.V.R.) *is not* always present; in fact, recent reports demonstrate a normal or reduced P.V.R. in the face of a decreased cardiac output in about 50 percent of patients studied.

With these varying hemodynamic patterns it becomes mandatory that the central venous pressure (CVP), the central aortic pressure (CAP), cardiac output (CO) and peripheral vascular resistance (P.V.R.) be constantly monitored for the intelligent management of cardiogenic shock. The prime object of therapy should be the restoration of cardiac output, adequate coronary and tissue perfusion, correction of hypoxemia and acidosis and prevention of the irreversible state.

PHYSIOLOGIC APPROACH TO MANAGEMENT

1. Correction of hypoxemia and acidosis. Maintenance of arterial pO_2 and saturation in physiologic range may require endotracheal intubation and assisted ventilation. Sodium bicarbonate in large amounts may be required for correction of acidosis in the presence of severe lactic acidosis.
2. Patients with decreased cardiac output, elevated CVP, and normal peripheral vascular resistance will benefit most from the use of agents having both α- and β-stimulating effects. Norepinephrine (Levophed) 4-8 mg in 1,000 ml 5 percent D/W I.V. or metaraminol (Aramine) 100 mg in 500 ml 5 percent D/W I.V. are employed to maintain a mean central aortic pressure of 80 mm Hg. The use of these agents, though maintaining coronary perfusion, may do so at the expense of diminished perfusion to the viscera and kidneys. The increase in coronary perfusion will improve left ventricular function and cardiac output.
3. With high CVP, very low cardiac output, and high peripheral vascular resistance, isoproteronol (Isuprel) infusion 2 mg in 500 ml 5 percent D/W at a rate of 2-6 μg/min may be employed. Systemic resistance falls, cardiac output increases, but if blood pressure does not rise, flow to vital areas will decrease. A disadvantage of the use of isoproteronol is the increased oxygen consumption of the myocardium.
4. Patients with low CVP, decreased cardiac output, and high vascular resistance may respond to volume expansion. Prolonged compensatory vasoconstriction or prolonged use of vasoconstrictor drugs may promote a contracted intravascular volume.

   Low viscosity dextran or plasma may be administered in challenging increments of 100 ml in 10-minute periods, watching for elevation of CVP.
5. Massive steroid therapy has been advocated for its effect in reducing peripheral vascular resistance. This method is not universally accepted.
6. Maintenance of adequate urinary output (greater than 30 ml/hr) is a reliable reflection of tissue perfusion. Mannitol and ethacrynic acid may be of value in achieving the desired urinary flow.

It is important that the treatment of shock not be delayed. The longer it persists the more intractable it becomes.

HEART FAILURE. In myocardial infarction failure may range from a few transient basal rales which rapidly clear to frank congestive failure. In mild cases congestion clears after the second day without treatment. If it is progressive, treatment is that of ordinary failure with salt restriction and diuretics. Digitalis should be withheld because of the infarct and should be used only in rare cases. Pulmonary edema is unusual in the first attack of infarction. When present it may precipitate or aggravate shock. Treatment consists of morphine, oxygen, tourniquets, and digitalis.

DISTURBANCES OF RHYTHM. A definite increase in the mortality occurs with multiple ventricular contractions, atrial flutter and fibrillation, and nodal rhythms.

TREATMENT OF CARDIAC ARRHYTHMIAS IN ACUTE MYOCARDIAL INFARCTION.

Ventricular fibrillation: Electrical defibrillation is the only treatment.

Atrial flutter, ventricular tachycardia, and ventricular flutter: Electric cardioversion is the treatment of choice. Following cardioversion of atrial flutter, long-acting quinidine should be given.

Atrial fibrillation: Initially quinidine should be used. If conversion does not occur in 3 to 4 hours, elective cardioversion should be attempted, followed by maintenance quinidine. Digitalis should be avoided.

Paroxysmal atrial tachycardia: Vasopressor agents are the first choice, followed by quinidine.

The following table outlines the drug treatment of the various arrhythmias.

ARRHYTHMIA	DRUG CHOICE, IN ORDER OF EFFECTIVENESS		
	1	2	3
PAT*	sedation	digitalis	quinidine
Atrial flutter*	*	quinidine	Pronestyl
Atrial fib. (acute)*	*	quinidine	–
Atrial fib. (chronic)	*	–	–
Ventricular PC	Lidocaine	quinidine Pronestyl	–
Ventricular tachycardia*	Lidocaine	Pronestyl quinidine	vasopressors

*The use of direct current synchronized countershock ("cardioversion") is the procedure of choice in most atrial and ventricular arrhythmias at present (see page 194).

For digitalis-induced arrhythmias, potassium administration is indicated.

HEART BLOCK. Complete heart block, complete right and left bundle branch block have a mortality of 70 percent. Complete right bundle branch block in our patients occurred four times more often than left.

In the presence of second-degree heart block, complete AV block, marked sinus bradycardia, or RBBB with right or left axis deviation, we believe that a transvenous pacemaker catheter should be introduced into the right ventricle. With CHB the patient should be paced at a rate of 70-80, until the CHB spontaneously disappears (usually 4 to 7 days). The catheter can then be removed.

ANTICOAGULATION. Anticoagulation theoretically is designed to prevent further extension of a coronary thrombus, to prevent formation of a mural thrombus, and to prevent thrombophlebitis. Anticoagulants are generally employed in the treatment of the acute phase of infarction. Treatment is initiated with intramuscular or intravenous heparin sodium (aqueous) in doses of 7,500 – 10,000 units q. 6 h. Clotting times as generally performed are useless and need not be done. Concomitantly one of the coumarin drugs is administered. There is little to choose between them. The ideal in the acute case is to maintain a prothrombin time between 1½ and 2 times the control level. Heparin prolongs the prothrombin time by about 10 percent. Therefore the prothrombin time should be determined at least 4 hours after heparin administration. Anticoagulants must be used with caution in the presence of pericarditis. An extensive rub precludes their use because of the danger of producing hemopericardium.

There is a rising difference of opinion regarding the value of anticoagulation both in the acute stage of infarction and as a long-term prophylactic measure. Anticoagulation, publicized and popularized by Wright and others, in the past has placed the physician almost under legal compulsion to use the treatment. Lately considerable doubt has been cast on the necessity and effectiveness of long-term postinfarction therapy, and its value even in the acute stage of infarction has been statistically questioned.

THE PERIOD OF CONVALESCENCE FOLLOWING MYOCARDIAL INFARCTION. After four to five weeks of hospitalization the patient may be discharged. During the last weeks of hospitalization he should be ambulatory and able to care for himself (toilet, feeding, dressing). The next two weeks are spent at home, indoors, being up and about. The third and fourth weeks are spent in gradually increased exercise, walking one block at a time, so that at the end of this period he should be able to walk one mile (20 city blocks). The fifth and sixth weeks the patient is allowed to assume full-time activity, and may return to part-time work during the seventh and eighth week. At the beginning of the third month he should resume full work. Sexual activity may be resumed in the second month. This period of rehabilitation must be used by the patient in an attempt to alter his way of life. Weight must be reduced and the diet changed to low fat. The patient must attempt to achieve equanimity. Frequent discussions may be held with the patient, discussing his former way of life and trying to help him to live at a different tempo.

REFERENCES

Gorlin, R. Symposium on the coronary circulation. Amer. J. Cardiol., 9:323, 1962.

Gunnar, R. M., Loeb, H. S., Pietras, R. J., and Tobin, J. R. Hemodynamic measurements in a coronary care unit. Progr. Cardiovasc. Dis., 11:29, 1968.

Halloway, D. H., et al. Systolic murmur developing after myocardial ischemia or infarction. J.A.M.A., 191:888, 1965.

Hultgren, H., Calcino, A., Platt, F., and Abrams, H. A clinical evaluation of coronary arteriography. Amer. J. Med., 42:228, 1967.

Julian, D. G., et al. Disturbances of rate, rhythm and conduction in acute myocardial infarction. Amer. J. Med., 37:915, 1964.

Kuhn, L. A., Eichna, L. W., Dietzmann, R. H., Lillehei, R. C., and Goldberg, L. I. The treatment of cardiogenic shock: Parts I-VI. Amer. Heart J., 74:578,725,848, 1967; 75:136,274,416, 1968.

Pell, S., et al. Immediate mortality and five-year survival of employed men with a first myocardial infarction. New Eng. J. Med., 270:915, 1964.

Prinzmetal, M., et al. Variant form of angina pectoris. J.A.M.A., 174:1794, 1960.

Spann, J. F., Jr., et al. Arrhythmias in acute myocardial infarction. New Eng. J. Med., 271:427, 1964.

CUSHING'S SYNDROME

(See also "Aldosteronism")

Definition: Cushing's syndrome is a symptom complex resulting from adrenocortical hyperfunction.

PATHOLOGY

1. Adrenal hyperplasia	50 to 60% of cases
2. Adrenal adenoma	30 to 40% of cases
3. Adrenal carcinoma	10 to 20% of cases

DIAGNOSIS

HISTORY AND PHYSICAL

1. Weakness and fatigue are the most common presenting complaints.
2. Impotence is common in the male; amenorrhea and hirsutism in the female.
3. Truncal obesity, sparing the extremities.
4. "Buffalo hump" (cervical-dorsal fat pad).
5. Moon facies.
6. Osteoporosis, with back pain and a negative calcium balance.
7. Plethora, ecchymosis and dry skin, acneform rashes, thin skin, and striae are often found together with a moderate hypertrichosis.
8. Diabetes.
9. Hypertension.
10. Mental changes.

LABORATORY

Elevated 17-hydroxysteroids and 17-ketosteroids are usually found. To distinguish the various causes of hyperadrenalism, one should do the following:

1. Obtain baseline 17-hydroxy- and 17-ketosteroids.
2. On days 1 and 2 give 0.5 mg of dexamethasone q.i.d. Collect a 24-hour urine on day 2 and repeat baseline studies.
3. On days 3 and 4, 2 mg of dexamethasone are given q.i.d. On day 4, a 24-hour urine is collected, and again baseline studies are repeated.

INTERPRETATION. In normals or hyperadrenalism secondary to obesity (pseudo-Cushing's) the 17-hydroxysteroids and 17-ketosteroids will be suppressed more than 50 percent of the baseline. If this does not occur on day 2, but on day 4, the patient probably has adrenal hyperplasia. No suppression is strongly suggestive of adrenal tumor.

OTHER SUGGESTED STUDIES.

1. Overnight dexamethasone suppression text. Patient receives 1 mg of dexamethasone by mouth at 11 PM. After adequate sedation with barbiturate a plasma sample is drawn between 8 AM and 9 AM next morning. Levels below 5 mg per 100 ml for plasma cortisol found in

obese patients while patients with Cushing's syndrome have values above 10 mg per 100 ml.

2. Plasma cortisols determined at 8 AM and 5 PM. Normally, there is about 50 percent decrease in late afternoon value. In Cushing's syndrome there is loss of diurnal variation.
3. ACTH stimulation – because of great overlapping of values one must be cautious in interpreting results.
4. Glucose tolerance (diabetic curve).
5. Serum electrolytes (hypernatremia, hypokalemia, azotemia). Patients with hypokalemia should be evaluated for ectopic ACTH source, most commonly due to a bronchogenic carcinoma.
6. Arteriography.

TREATMENT

Bilateral complete adrenalectomy for adrenal hyperplasia and substitution therapy (see page 3). A corticotropin-secreting chromophobe adenoma is seen in about 15 percent of patients post-total adrenalectomy for Cushing's syndrome.

OP-DDD, an adrenal inhibitor, has been used with some success in adrenal malignancy.

REFERENCES

Kuhe, W. J., Jr., and Lipton, M. A. The diagnosis of adrenocortical disorders by laboratory methods. New Eng. J. Med., 263:128, 1960.

Liddle, G. N., Givens, J. R., Nicholson, W. E., and Island, D. P. The ectopic ACTH syndrome. Cancer Res., 25:1057, 1965.

Nelson, D. H., Meakin, J. W., and Thorn, G. W. ACTH-producing pituitary tumors following adrenalectomy for Cushing's syndrome. Ann. Intern. Med., 52:560, 1960.

O'Brien, R. M., et al. Congenital adrenocortical hyperplasia with Cushing's syndrome. J.A.M.A., 187:103, 1964.

Soffer, L. J., et al. Cushing's syndrome. A study of 50 patients. Amer. J. Med., 30:129, 1961.

CYANOSIS

Cyanosis is the bluish color of the skin and mucous membranes due to increased amounts of reduced hemoglobin in the venous plexuses. It is not clinically apparent until 5 g of reduced hemoglobin are present and unless arterial hemoglobin saturation is below 85 percent. *Central cyanosis* results from poor oxygenation of the pulmonary blood flow so that the oxygen saturation of peripheral arterial blood is lower than normal. *Peripheral cyanosis* occurs in the presence of a normal arterial oxygen saturation and results from increased extraction of oxygen in the capillaries, thus producing more than 5 g of reduced hemoglobin in the veins. Due to sluggish peripheral circulation, it is common in shock. *Chemical cyanosis* is due to the ingestion of a reducing agent, such as acetanilid or sulfonamides, which produces an increased amount of reduced hemoglobin. Blue discoloration of the skin of hands and feet with normal blood oxygen may occur on exposure to cold and in an unconscious patient in a cold or air-conditioned room.

DIFFERENTIAL DIAGNOSIS OF CENTRAL CYANOSIS

	ARTERIAL OXYGEN SATURATION			CARBON DIOXIDE
	Resting	Exercise	100% Oxygen	
Hypoventilation Emphysema Pneumonia "Primary"	low	unchanged, lower or higher	saturation usually rises to 100%	high
Alveolar-capillary block	normal	marked	saturation rises to 100%	low due to hyperventilation
Venoarterial shunting Atelectasis Cong. heart dis.	low	unchanged, lower, or higher	saturation rises but less than 100%	normal

NOTE

Cyanosis frequently arises from a mixture of causes. Thus, in acute pulmonary edema, cyanosis may be in part peripheral because of poor peripheral circulation and in part central because of a diffusion block and atelectasis.

DERMATOLOGICAL SURVEY

MACULOPAPULAR DERMATOSES

	COLOR	SCALE	INDURATION	ORAL LESIONS	FACE, PALMS, SOLES	NAILS
Secondary Lues	brown-red	scanty	++++	+	+	+
Psoriasis	dull red	abundant, silvery, with bleeding points	+	0	rare	+++
Pityriasis rosea	rose	adherent on border, fine in center	0	0	rare	0
Tinea versicolor	brown-red	branny	0	0	0	0
Seborrheic dermatitis	dull pink	yellow, greasy	0/+	0	face	0
Parapsoriasis	faded pink	fine opaque	0	0	face	0
Lichen planus	purple	shiny	+	+	0	rare
Lupus erythematosus	purple-red	adherent, "carpet tack"	+	0	face	0

CHRONIC VESICULOBULLOUS DERMATOSES

	AGE	LESIONS	SITES	DURATION	PRURITUS	FEVER	ORAL PAIN
Pemphigus vulgaris	50+	normal skin at periphery	abdomen, scalp, groin, mouth	usually fatal in approx. 1 year	0	0	++++
Erythema multiforme bullosum (Stevens-Johnson)	20-40	iris shaped	eyes, extremities, mouth	6 weeks	0	++	++
Dermatitis herpetiformis	adults	erythema at base	scapulae, trunk, sacrum	several years (without therapy)	++++	0	0
Epidermolysis bullosum	infancy	large bullae	hands, elbows	life	0	0	0

The most common dermatoses, in order of frequency, are as follows:

1. Acne vulgaris.
2. Seborrheic dermatitis.
3. Epidermophytoses.
4. Eczemas.
5. Verrucae and moles.
6. Drug eruptions.
7. Psoriasis.
8. Pityriasis rosea.
9. Lichen simplex.

DIABETES INSIPIDUS

Diabetes insipidus is a syndrome characterized by the passage of large quantities of dilute urine, and polydipsia. The urine specific gravity usually ranges between 1.001 to 1.008, urine volumes of 5 to 10 liters per day are usual, although rarely much greater volumes may be excreted.

There are two mechanisms by which the capacity to form antidiuretic hormone (ADH) is lost: through either a primary or a secondary brain lesion. A rare condition is "nephrogenic" diabetes insipidus in which the renal tubules do not respond to ADH. A condition called "compulsive water drinking," in which there is no disturbance in ADH or the renal tubules, may mimic diabetes insipidus.

ETIOLOGY

1. *Primary diabetes insipidus*
   a. Familial.
   b. Idiopathic.
2. *Secondary diabetes insipidus*
   a. Trauma to brain.
   b. Neoplasm – pituitary, craniopharyngioma, etc.
   c. Metastatic neoplasms.
   d. Infectious disease: granuloma, abscess, encephalitis.
   e. Systemic disease: sarcoid, xanthomas, leukemia, lymphoma.

3. *Nephrogenic*
4. *Compulsive water drinking*

DIAGNOSIS

1. Nicotine stimulation test (2 mg of nicotine base are given I.M.). The nicotine releases ADH from the hypothalamus. Failure to alter the specific gravity of the urine following nicotine indicates that brain damage has resulted in loss of capacity to produce ADH.
2. Hypertonic saline test (10 ml/kg of 3 percent NaCl). The osmoreceptors of the brain respond to the hypertonic fluid normally releasing ADH and forming a more concentrated urine.
3. Aqueous Pitressin, 5 milliunits per minute may be administered by a slow I.V. drip for at least 1 hour, or 5 units of long-acting vasopressin tannate in oil may be given I.M. Patients with diabetes insipidus excrete a more concentrated urine after vasopressin, except with "nephrogenic" diabetes insipidus. In primary diabetes insipidus vasopressin produces more concentrated urine than does dehydration. In compulsive water drinking dehydration usually produces a more concentrated urine than does vasopressin.

TREATMENT

1. Treatment of the primary disease, when feasible.
2. Replacement therapy. Vasopressin may be given by nasal insufflation (dried posterior pituitary powder every 3 to 6 hours).
3. Five tenths to 1 milliliter of Pitressin tannate in oil (5 units in 1 ml), I.M. every 1 to 3 days. Preparation should be warm and the vial thoroughly mixed before administering.
4. Chlorothiazide and hydrochlorothiazide have recently been reported to be of value in reducing polyuria. It has been postulated that the thiazides occupy the same renal receptor sites as ADH.

REFERENCES

Alexander, C. S., et al. Chlorothiazide derivatives for diabetes insipidus. Arch. Intern. Med., 108:218, 1961.

Dies, F., et al. Differential diagnosis between diabetes insipidus and compulsive polydipsia. Ann. Intern. Med., 54:710, 1961.

Randall, R. V., Clark, E. C., and Bahn, R. C. Classification of the causes of diabetes insipidus. Proc. Mayo Clin., 34:299, 1959.

Symposium: Antidiuretic hormones. Amer. J. Med., 42:651-827, 1967.

DIABETES MELLITUS

Diabetes mellitus is a disorder characterized by abnormal carbohydrate metabolism associated with relative or absolute lack of insulin. Recent data suggest that the defect may not be not only in the pancreas but also in lipid metabolic pathways. Nevertheless there is impairment of glucose utilization with subsequent hyperglycemia, and glycosuria occurs as the renal threshold is exceeded. In a normal person, the renal glucose threshold is 140 to 160 mg per 100 ml; however, in diabetics this level may rise to as high as 200 to 250 mg per 100 ml, increasing with the duration of the diabetes and age of the patient.

In the uncontrolled diabetic the elevated glucose in the glomerular filtrate produces an osmotic diuresis, and polyuria and dehydration follow. With polyuria, natruresis also occurs. Potassium is also lost because of glycogenolysis and proteinolysis. The body, unable to utilize effectively glucose, derives more and more energy from fat combustion; ketone bodies (β-hydroxybutyric and acetoacetic acids) are produced, and metabolic acidosis occurs due to excess hydrogen ion formation.

DIAGNOSIS

Polyuria, polydipsia, polyphagia, weight loss, fatigue, pruritus, and frequent infections are the cardinal symptoms. The diabetic is particularly prone to pyelonephritis, tuberculosis and furuncles. A high index of suspicion must be entertained in obese patients and in patients with a positive family history.

LABORATORY FINDINGS

The *sine qua non* for the diagnosis of diabetes mellitus is hyperglycemia. This is established by finding a fasting blood sugar of over 120 mg per 100 ml (Somogyi-Nelson), a two-hour postprandial sugar of over 130 percent, or a characteristic glucose tolerance curve.

In a normal oral glucose tolerance curve the peak blood sugar rarely exceeds 160 at one hour and has returned to the fasting level by two hours. In the diabetic curve, one sees high peaks, with a delay in return to fasting levels.

In the performance of a glucose tolerance test, it is usually unnecessary to prepare patients with a high-carbohydrate diet (250 to 300 g a day) for three days prior to the test. In doubtful or borderline results, however, this procedure should be followed.

Many believe that the intravenous glucose tolerance test is a more reliable index of carbohydrate metabolism, as one of the major variables of the oral test – namely, absorption of glucose – is eliminated.

Other diagnostic tests include cortisone-glucose tolerance tests and tolbutamide tolerance tests; these add little to the oral and intravenous glucose tolerance tests in most cases.

COMPLICATIONS OF DIABETES MELLITUS

1. Ketosis, acidosis and coma.
2. Tuberculosis, pyelonephritis, meningitis, skin and paronychial infections. The diabetic with untreated urinary infection may progress to fulminating and usually fatal renal papillary necrosis. Diabetics are especially prone to staphylococcal infections.
3. Vascular complications:
   a. Arteriosclerosis occurs in diabetics ten times more frequently than in nondiabetics, and is found after 20 years in 80 percent or more of diabetics. Coronary occlusions occur with twice the normal incidence.
   b. Diabetic retinopathy is closely related to nephropathy, but usually precedes the proteinuria.
   c. Diabetic nephropathy. This was formerly referred to as the Kimmelstiel-Wilson syndrome (capillary nodular glomerulosclerosis), and in the full-blown state is manifested by hypertension, edema, albuminuria, and retinopathy with diabetes (remembered by the mnemonic H–E–A–R–D). However, these can occur in the absence of the classical nodular infiltrates, and the general term "diabetic nephropathy" is preferable. Almost 100 percent of patients with diabetes of 20 years' duration or longer will develop nephropathy.
4. Diabetic neuritis, peripheral or autonomic, is manifested by numbness and tingling of the hands and feet with pain, and by "diabetic nocturnal diarrhea," gastric atony, and impotence. Neuropathy is probably unrelated to control. It may begin with the onset of diabetes or may be the presenting symptom of diabetes. Neuropathy is frequently precipitated by stress situations (infections, surgery, etc.). Occasionally it may follow the institution of insulin therapy.
5. Complications of pregnancy include an overweight, edematous baby,

a marked increase in stillbirths and neonatal fatalities, and an increase in congenital abnormalities and hyaline membrane disease.
6. Eye cataracts.

Life-span in diabetes mellitus is 75 percent or less of normal. Good general health habits, including frequent medical supervision and careful control, appear to be associated with fewer complications and a more lengthy survival.

TREATMENT

Treatment consists of dietary restriction and administration of insulin or other euglycemic agents.

DIET. The diabetic diet is normal with the exception that the more rapidly absorbed carbohydrates are eaten sparingly. It is designed to maintain a slightly less than "ideal" weight for age, frame, and height and activity. In general this diet should contain 70-90 g protein, approximately 50-120 g of fat, and about 150-250 g of carbohydrate. The diet, plus the appropriate euglycemic agent, should maintain ideal weight, keep the urine barely free of sugar, and keep the fasting blood sugar at 150 mg per 100 ml wherever possible. A midpath between so-called rigid chemical control and so-called loose clinical control is most acceptable and most desirable for the majority of patients. Complicated calculations and weighing of food are not necessary; good general health measures, frequent testing of urine for sugar, and periodic medical supervision are necessary.

In general, for moderately active adult individuals, the following diet is satisfactory.

	HEIGHT	DAILY CALORIC INTAKE	PROTEIN, grams (1 g = 4 cal.)	FAT, grams (1 g = 9 cal.)	CARBOHYDRATE grams (1 g = 4 cal.)
To reduce weight	short	780	50	20	100
	medium	950	60	30	110
	tall	1120	70	40	120
To maintain weight	short	1720	70	80	180
	medium	2310	80	110	250
	tall	2910	90	150	300
To increase weight	all heights	3130 (or more)	100	170	300

EUGLYCEMIC AGENTS

INSULIN

	ONSET (hours)	PEAK (hours)	DURATION (hours)
Regular or crystalline	1	3-4	6-8
PZI	4-8	12-24	48-72
NPH	2	10-20	28-30
Lente	2	8-14	20-28
Ultralente	8-12	12-24	36-48

These insulins individually, or mixtures of regular insulin with NPH or PZI, will regulate the vast majority of diabetics in any situation.

The mild nonobese diabetic may be empirically started on 15 units NPH a day; and the dose is adjusted according to clinical and chemical response.

Severe diabetics require hospitalization and careful supervision for initial control. They may be started on 20 to 40 units of NPH before breakfast; and then followed by t.i.d., a.c., and h.s. urine for sugar. Five units of regular insulin are given for each plus sugar above one plus. Gradually, the NPH is increased, and "coverage" regular insulin is decreased with continuing response. Mixtures of regular and NPH or PZI insulin can sometimes be tailored to cover postprandial hyperglycemia without producing the hypoglycemic episodes seen with large doses of NPH or PZI. Severe "brittle" diabetes in children and adults is best undertreated, in order to avoid hypoglycemic attacks.

The obese adult diabetic is best treated with diet alone. If the patient will not diet, oral euglycemic agents may be employed.

ORAL EUGLYCEMIC AGENTS

These agents are of value in the age groups over 40 with diabetes of short duration, obesity, and insulin requirements of less than 40 units a day. They are of little or no value in juvenile, ketotic, thin diabetics.

Nausea, vomiting and anorexia are common with doses of phenformin above 200 mg. Chlorpropamide is more likely to cause hypoglycemia than tolbutamide and jaundice has been reported.

NAME	DOSE
1. Tolbutamide (Orinase)	0.5-3.0 g.q.d.
2. Phenformin (DBI)	(0.5 g.b.i.d. or t.i.d.) 50-200 mg q.d.
3. Chlorpropamide (Diabinese)	100-750 mg q.d.
4. Acetohexamide (Dymelor)	250 mg q. 1.5 d.
5. Talazamide (Talinase)	100-500 mg q.d.

MISCELLANEOUS. All diabetics should carry a card indicating their disease. If the patient is on insulin, he should carry a lump of sugar or candy in the event of hypoglycemia. Patients on insulin in large doses do far better with 4 to 6 small meals a day.

DIABETIC ACIDOSIS AND DIABETIC COMA

Mortality from this complication is reported to vary between 2.4 and 43.7 percent.

Acidosis refers to those diabetics with a CO_2 combining power of 15 mEq/L or less. Precipitating factors of acidosis are listed below.

1. Omission of insulin, associated with either emotional upset or neglect 27%
2. Infections of all types: particularly respiratory, urinary, meningeal, and skin infections 18%
3. Acute alcoholism 7%
4. Gastroenteritis 8%

In addition, approximately 30 percent are previously undiagnosed diabetics, presenting in acidosis. In about 10 percent, no definite cause can be determined.

DIAGNOSIS

In addition to the classical symptoms previously mentioned, the commonest symptoms of patients in acidosis are nausea and vomiting, drowsiness or stupor, and abdominal pain.

PHYSICAL FINDINGS

1. Dry skin 90%
2. Flushed face 80%
3. Acetone odor on breath 25%

6. Abdominal tenderness, with or without spasm and rebound 40%

4. Soft eyeballs	25%	7. Hepatomegaly	26%
5. Kussmaul respirations	30%	8. Hyporeflexia	20%
		9. Neck rigidity	rare

LABORATORY FINDINGS

1. Complete blood count: leukocytosis averaging 15,000 is usually found.
2. Hematocrit: this is usually elevated, reflecting the degree of dehydration.
3. Blood sugar: averages 350 mg per 100 ml.
4. Serum CO_2: 15 mEq/L or less.
5. Serum K: initially usually elevated slightly (average 5.5 mEq/L); falls when insulin becomes effective causing glucose to enter the cell as a K-6 glucophosphate compound. Serum K is further lowered by fluid replacement.
6. Serum Na: variable, usually normal or slightly low. Total body sodium low.
7. Serum Cl: usually normal. Total body chloride low.
8. Urinalysis: usually 4 plus sugar and 2 to 4 plus acetone. Pyuria may be present.
9. BUN: usually slightly elevated (25 mg per 100 ml or more).
10. Serum acetone: indicates degree of acidosis, and suggests total insulin requirement.
11. ECG: may reflect hypokalemia, anoxia, etc.
12. Urine culture, blood culture, chest x-ray, and where indicated, sputum culture or lumbar puncture should also be performed.
13. Blood pH falls as low as 7.0.

TREATMENT

Therapy is fourfold: administration of insulin, replacement of fluids and electrolytes, treatment of shock, and treatment of the precipitating cause.

INSULIN. Regular insulin is given: 100 units, I.M. stat., and then 50 units q.h. until urine sugar is less than 4 plus or acetonuria diminishes. Urine sugar and acetone are checked every hour.

1. If glycosuria diminishes but acetonuria persists, administer glucose and continue insulin as above.
2. If glycosuria persists but acetonuria decreases, stop glucose. Subcutaneous insulin is employed, 5 units for each plus sugar above one plus.

Insulin is gradually decreased, according to the glycosuria, to q. 4 h. administration. In moderate acidosis 300 to 400 units of insulin are required for correction.

Fluid and Electrolytes: Physiologic saline with or without Ringer's lactate or 6M bicarbonate should be administered at a rate of approximately 1 liter per hour for 2 hours then ½ liter per hour for 6 hours. The use of lactate or bicarbonate should be based on the blood pH. Total body water deficit in moderate or severe acidosis is about 100 ml/kg (minimum 5 liters). It is better to err on the side of too little fluid until renal function, as measured by urinary output, is established as adequate. An indwelling catheter is inserted only if the patient cannot void; output is measured.

POTASSIUM. In acidosis a deficit of 3 to 7 mEq/kg of potassium exists. However, potassium is never administered until a good urinary flow is established and until several hours of insulin therapy is given. After 3 or 4 hours of treatment, 40 mEq of potassium may be given slowly I.V. over a 2-hour period. In a conscious patient orange juice (1.3 mEq of potassium/ounce), or milk (1.0 mEq/ounce) may be used.

TREATMENT OF SHOCK. In this instance insulin should be given intravenously until the patient responds.

TREATMENT OF PRECIPITATING CAUSE. When the diagnosis of bacterial infection is established, appropriate chemotherapy should be instituted.

SUMMARY OF TREATMENT

1. Urine sugar and acetone, q.h.
2. Insulin. 100 units regular insulin, I.M., stat.; then 50 units, q.h., until acetonuria "breaks" or glycosuria disappears.
3. Fluids. Physiological saline with or without Ringers – 1 L/hr for 2 hours then 0.5 L/hour for 6 hours.
4. Potassium. 40 mEq KCl intravenously over a 2-hour period *after* good urine flow is established and after 200 units of insulin has been given – that is, after 3 to 4 hours of therapy.
5. NPO if the patient is vomiting; if not, attempt 1 liter of fluid/hour, to include orange juice, salty broth, etc.
6. Do not catheterize a conscious patient.
7. Look for the precipitating cause.

NON-KETOACIDATIC COMA AND DIABETES MELLITUS

In diabetes mellitus nonketoacidotic coma may be due to

1. Strokes
2. Drug excess

3. Uremia
4. Liver disease
5. Hypoglycemia
6. Lactic acidosis*
7. Hyperosmolality (hyperglycemia and/or hypernatremia).

REFERENCES

Boshell, B. R. Current concepts in therapy. Hypoglycemic agents for oral administration. New Eng. J. Med., 262:80, 197, 1960.
Brown, J., et al.: Diabetes mellitus: Current concepts and vascular lesions (renal and retinal). Ann. Intern. Med., 68:634, 1968.
Cohen, A. S., et al. Diabetic acidosis. An evaluation of the cause, course and therapy of 73 cases. Ann. Intern. Med., 52:55, 1960.
Danowski, T.S. Diabetes mellitus: Diagnosis and Treatment, pp.145-148, 1967.
Levine, R. (ed.). Symposium on diabetes. Amer. J. Med., 31:837, 1961.
Spurny, O. M., et al. Protracted tolbutamide-induced hypoglycemia, Arch. Intern. Med., 115:53, 1965.
Stenzel, K. H., et al. Diabetic keto acidosis. J.A.M.A., 187:136, 1964.
Symposium: Insulin. Amer. J. Med., 40:651, 1966.
Wruble, L. D., et al. Diabetic steatorrhea: A distinct entity. Amer. J. Med., 37:118, 1964.

DIAGNOSTIC PROBLEMS

The most commonly missed diagnoses are listed below. The diagnosis is missed usually because it is not thought of rather than because of atypical manifestations.

INFECTIONS

Miliary tuberculosis, subacute bacterial endocarditis, and localized abscesses head the list. The last mentioned include brain, hepatic, perinephric, and psoas abscesses. Appendicitis is frequently missed in the elderly patient where fever and localizing signs may be absent.

NEOPLASMS

Multiple myeloma and lymphomas are frequently missed. Brain tumors, hypernephroma, carcinoma of the ampulla of

*Causes 1 through 6 are covered under separate headings. Hyperosmolar coma is usually due to tissue dehydration in markedly debilitated patients. Treatment consists of hydration.

Vater, carcinoma of the pancreas without jaundice, and primary hepatic tumors are usually not correctly diagnosed initially.

MISCELLANEOUS

1. Sarcoid.
2. "Collagen" group of diseases.
3. Cardiovascular: pulmonary infarction, "silent" aortic stenosis; intracardiac myxomas, and coarctation of the aorta.
4. Endocrine: hyperparathyroidism, hyperthyroidism, myxedema and Addison's disease.
5. Porphyria.
6. Amyloidosis.
7. Weber-Christian disease.

DIALYSIS

Compromised renal function produces internal chemical dysequilibrium of varying degrees, from mild azotemia to severe uremia, acidosis, hypocalcemia, and life-threatening hyperkalemia. Dialysis may be used until a diagnosis is made, definitive therapy is employed, or recovery occurs, or to sustain life in cases of irremedial loss of renal function.

INDICATIONS FOR DIALYSIS

1. Acute renal failure: removal of a nephrotoxin, azotemia (a BUN greater than 125 mg per 100 ml), uncontrolled hyperkalemia, severe acidosis, hyper- or hyponatremia, hypercalcemia, severe water retention, pericarditis, progressive somnolence, or uncontrolled convulsions.
2. Chronic renal failure: acute reversible insults to previously compromised kidneys to allow time to establish a diagnosis or to institute therapy, such as preparation for renal transplantation or in irreversible cases chronic repetitive dialysis.
3. Acute poisoning: endogenous or exogenous.
4. Water-retentive states: refractory congestive heart failure, or the nephrotic syndrome.

RELATIVE CONTRAINDICATIONS TO DIALYSIS

HEMODIALYSIS. Hemorrhage, severe hypo- or hypertension, unavailability of vessels for cannulation and pericardial tamponade.

PERITONEAL. Intra-abdominal adhesions or hematoma, gangrenous bowel, recent aortic graft, or abdominal burns.

The choice of method of dialysis is partly determined by availability of equipment and trained personnel. Generally, hemodialysis is utilized in a more urgent situation when rapid lowering of the serum potassium, alleviation of uremic coma, or rapid removal of a nephrotoxin or intoxicating drugs is desired.

Peritoneal dialysis is used in less urgent situations. Both methods have been employed for repetitive dialysis.

Comparison of Clearances of Urea.

1. Kolff twin-coil artificial kidney – 150 to 180 ml per minute.
2. Two-layered modified Kiil, 80 to 100 ml per minute. (At flow rates of 150 to 300 ml per minute.)
3. Peritoneal dialysis: 25 ml per minute (3 liters per hour of 1.8 percent glucose dialysate).

Criteria for judging the applicability of dialysis in the therapy of poisoning.

1. The poison molecules should diffuse through a dialysis membrane, such as cellophane, form plasma water, and have a reasonable removal rate, or "dialysance."
2. The poison must be sufficiently well distributed in accessible body fluid compartments. If substantial fractions of the absorbed poison are bound to protein, concentrated in inaccessible fluid compartments, or attain a significant intracellular concentration, then effective dialysis will be sharply limited. This restriction is diminished, however, if the loculated portion rapidly equibrates with plasma.
3. There should be a relationship between the blood concentration and the duration of the body's exposure to the circulating poison and toxicity.
4. The amount of poison dialysed must constitute a significant addition to the normal body mechanism for dealing with the particular poison under consideration. This should include metabolism, conjugation and elimination of the substance by bowel and kidney.

Specific indications for dialysis.

1. Ingestion of a potentially fatal dose.
   a. 3.0 g of short-acting barbiturate.
   b. 5.0 g of long-acting barbiturate.
   c. 20 g (0.6 g/kg) of acetylsalicylic acid (aspirin).
   d. 10 g (0.15 g/kg) of glutethimide. (Doriden).

The amount of potentially lethal drugs may be obtained from the *Physician's Desk Reference* or by calling poison control centers in most cities.

2. A dangerously high blood level.
   a. 3.5 mg per 100 ml of short-acting barbiturate.
   b. 8 mg per 100 ml of long-acting barbiturate.
   c. 90 mg per 100 ml of acetylsalicylic acid.
   d. 3.0 mg per 100 ml of glutethimide.
3. Removal of a nephrotoxin within 48 hours of exposure.

Nonspecific indications for dialysis.

1. All Reed Class IV coma patients who are suspected of having ingested a dialyzable poison, who remain class IV after initial hydration and aeration.
2. Class III patients who progress to Class IV.
3. Prolonged coma especially in the elderly.
4. Prolonged coma with the development of complications.
   a. Aspiration pneumonia.
   b. Hyperpyrexia.
5. Impairment of the normal routes of excretion.
   a. Refractory hypotension preventing diuresis.
   b. Prior hepatic or renal failure.

CURRENTLY KNOWN DIALYZABLE POISONS

BARBITURATES

Barbital
Phenobarbital
Amobarbital
Pentobarbital
Butabarbital
Secobarbital
Cyclobarbital

OTHER SEDATIVES AND TRANQUILIZERS

Glutethimide
Diphenylhydantoin
Prinidone
Meprobamate
Ethchlorvynol
Ethinamate
Methypyrlon

ANALGESICS

Acetylsalicylic acid
Methylsalicylate
Acetophenetidin
Dextropropoxyphene

HALIDES

Bromide
Chloride
Iodide
Fluoride

ENDOGENOUS TOXINS

Ammonia
Uric acid
Tritium
Bilirubin
Lactic acid
Porphyria
Cystine
Endotoxin

MISC. SUBSTANCES

Thiocyanate
Aniline
Sodium chlorate
Potassium chlorate
Eucalyptus oil
Boric acid

OTHER SEDATIVES AND TRANQUILIZERS

Imipramine
Amitriptyline
Phenelzine
Tranylcypromine
Pargyline
Heroin
Gallamine tetraiodide
Paraldehyde
Chloral hydrate

METALS

Strontium
Calcium
Iron
Lead
Mercury
Arsenic
Sodium
Potassium
Magnesium

ALCOHOLS

Ethanol
Methanol
Ethylene glycol

MISC. SUBSTANCES

Potassium dichromate
Chromic acid
Digoxin
Dextroamphetamine
Sodium citrate
Dinitro-*o*-cresol
Amanita phalloides
Carbon tetrachloride
Ergotamine
Cyclophosphamide
5-Fluorotracil
Methotrexate

REFERENCES

Clark, J. E., and Soricelli, R. R. Indications for dialysis. Med. Clin. N. Amer., 49:1213, 1964.

Linton, A. L., et al. Method of forced diuresis as application to barbiturate poisoning. Lancet, Vol. 2:377, August 19, 1967.

Maher, J. F. Hemodialysis and peritoneal dialysis: A review of their use in renal insufficiency and acute poisoning. Ohio Med. J., 60:235, 1964.

Maher, J. F., and Schreiner, G. E. The dialysis of poisons and drugs. Trans. Amer. Soc. Artif. Intern. Organs, 14:440, 1964.

Randall, R. E., Singh, R., and Fetter, J. G. Increased intracranial pressure from failure to sustain mannitol diuresis during hemodialysis. Clin. Res., 15:51, 1967.

Setter, J. G., Maher, J. F., and Schreiner, G. E. Barbiturate intoxication: Evaluation of therapy including dialysis in a large series selectively referred because of severity. Arch. Intern. Med., 177:224, 1966.

Versaci, A. A. Hemodialysis: Indications and techniques in surgical patients. Surg. Clin. N. Amer., 48:57, 1968.

DIGITALIS

Digitalis, from the time of William Withering, over 175 years ago, up to the present, remains the single most important cardiotonic drug. Although over 30 preparations are available, only about 6 are in common use. Despite drug company claims to the contrary, in clinical practice the therapeutic/toxic ratio is remarkably similar from one preparation to another, approximately 0.6/1. *For this reason, it is best to be thoroughly familiar with one oral and one parenteral preparation.*

Digitalis exerts its therapeutic effect in three areas.

HEART.

1. The major action of digitalis is to increase the force of systolic contraction and thereby raise the cardiac output.
2. Secondary action is depression of the AV node, thus slowing AV conduction.
3. Stimulation of the vagus, thereby slowing the heart rate.

KIDNEY. A lesser effect occurs in the renal tubule by inducing a primary sodium, chloride, and water diuresis.

PERIPHERAL VESSELS. Another minor action of digitalis is a direct effect on arteriolar muscle, thus raising peripheral resistance.

USES

1. Digitalis is the drug of choice in *congestive heart failure.* Here it exerts its primary effect by increasing systolic contraction force. "Low-output" failure responds better than "high-output" failure. Congestive failure unresponsive to average or large doses of digitalis should suggest thyrotoxicosis, myocardiopathy (including that due to active rheumatic fever), or hypochloremic alkalosis. Protracted failure may be a sign of digitalis toxicity (see below).
2. In many *atrial arrhythmias,* digitalis is the drug of choice as a rule. By slowing atrial activity and by slowing AV conduction, digitalis is the first drug to be used in atrial fibrillation, atrial flutter, and paroxysmal atrial tachycardia.

In one atrial arrhythmia digitalis is usually contraindicated. If a previously digitalized patient presents with paroxysmal atrial

PREPARATIONS

	INITIAL DIGITALIZATION				*DAILY MAINTENANCE DOSE*	
	ORAL		INTRAVENOUS		ORAL	
PREPARATION	AVERAGE	RANGE	AVERAGE	RANGE	AVERAGE	RANGE
Digitalis leaf	1.2 g	1-2 g	–	–	0.15 g	0.05-0.3 g
Digitoxin	1.2 mg	1-2 mg	–	–	0.10 mg	0.05-0.3 mg
Acetyldigitoxin	2.0 mg	1.5-2.5 mg	–	–	0.3 mg	0.1-0.6 mg
Gitalin	5.0 mg	4-8 mg	–	–	0.5 mg	0.25-1.0 mg
					ORAL OR PARENTERAL	
Digoxin	2.0 mg	1-3 mg	1,0 mg	0.8-1.6 mg	0.5 mg	0.25-1.0 mg
					PARENTERAL	
Lanatoside C (Cedilanid)	–	–	1.6 mg	1.2-1.6 mg	0.25 mg	0.25-0.75 mg
Ouabain	–	–	1.0 mg	(0.1 mg q.2h.)	–	–

The half-life of Digoxin is 1.65 days. With this knowledge and the patient's B.U.N., appropriate adjustments for the dose in uremic patients can be made according to the level of the B.U.N. as worked out by Jelliffe.

tachycardia (PAT) with block, the usual cause is digitalis toxicity.

A schema for digitalization often found practical in the treatment of acute emergencies is:

1. Cedilanid, 1.0 mg, I.V., stat., then 0.4 mg, I.V. or I.M., four hours later and 0.2 mg, I.V. or I.M., four hours after the second dose.
2. Maintenance dose of digitalis may then be started 24 hours after above digitalization.

In less pressing situations we prefer one of the following:

1. Digoxin, 1.0 mg, P.O., stat.; then 0.5 mg, q. 6 h. for 24 hours (total average dose 2.0 mg in 24 hours). Average maintenance dose is 0.5 mg, q.d., P.O.
2. Equally satisfactory is digitalis leaf. The initial digitalizing dose of 1.2 g may be given over 72 hours. The average maintenance dose is 0.1 g per day.

Slower digitalization may be employed with digitoxin, 0.4 mg, q.d. for three days (total dose 1.2 mg). The maintenance dose is 0.1 mg, q.d.

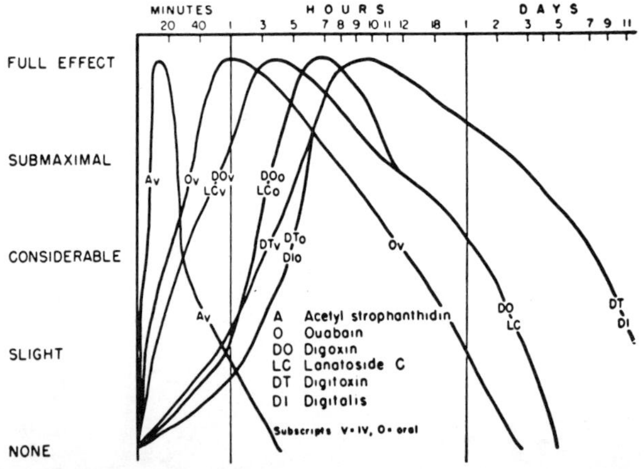

Table and figure adapted from Kay, C. F. Clinical use of digitalis preparations, From *Circulation,* 12:116, 291, 1955. Courtesy of the American Heart Association, Inc.

DIGITALIS TOXICITY

The most common causes of intoxication are:

1. Overdosage
2. Digitalis sensitivity (relative overdosage)
3. Drug-induced diuresis with hypokalemia.

CARDIAC. Any arrhythmia may be induced by digitalis. The most common *atrial* arrhythmia is *paroxysmal atrial tachycardia with block.* The most common *ventricular arrhythmia is premature ventricular contraction(s).*

Other cardiac effects, in decreasing order of frequency, are:

1. First degree AV block (25 percent of conduction defects or arrhythmias due to digitalis toxicity).
2. Second degree AV block, with or without Wenckebach's phenomenon (13.5 percent).
3. Slow atrial fibrillation (ventricular rate less than 60) (11.5 percent).
4. Paroxysmal ventricular tachycardia (11.5 percent).
5. Less frequently, sinus bradycardia, sinus arrest, third-degree AV block, nodal rhythms, and paroxysmal atrial fibrillation occur.

The most frequent ECG change is *ST segment depression.* This, however, merely indicates the action of digitalis as a rule, and *does not indicate toxicity* or even full digitalization. Paroxysmal bidirectional ventricular tachycardia is considered to be pathognomonic of digitoxicity.

The most subtle sign of intoxication is increasing congestive heart failure.

GASTROINTESTINAL. Diarrhea may occur. With the purified glycosides, anorexia, nausea, vomiting, and diarrhea are infrequent and seldom occur before the arrhythmias.

NEUROLOGIC. Headache, vertigo, fatigue, insomnia, depression, confusion, and delirium ("digitalis madness") have been reported. Paresthesias and neuralgias, particularly of the trigeminal nerve, may occur.

VISUAL. Yellow vision, colored halos, scotoma, blurring, and amblyopias occur infrequently. Patients rarely offer the complaint of colored vision. The doctor must ask specifically to elicit this symptom.

MISCELLANEOUS. Urticaria and eosinophilia occasionally occur as an allergic manifestation. Gynecomastia is rare; but very commonly darkening of the mammary areolae is seen.

Arrhythmias, anorexia, and nausea are the most frequent signs of intoxication, each occurring as the initial manifestation in about 30 percent of cases of toxicity. Increasing failure (7.5 percent) is next in frequency; and vomiting is seen in about 4 percent.

TREATMENT OF DIGITALIS TOXICITY

1. Discontinue or decrease the dose of digitalis.
2. Potassium is useful in the arrhythmias but not in AV block, as AV conduction is decreased by potassium. In the face of a ventricular tachycardia, 5 g (67 mEq) of KCl in 100 ml of 5 percent glucose in water is given at the rate of 4 ml a minute until cessation of the arrhythmia. In less dangerous arrhythmias, oral KCl, 3 g (40 mEq), stat. and q. 4 h. for two or three doses is given. If reversion does not occur after 6 g (80 mEq) it is unlikely that more potassium will be effective. Wherever potassium is employed, it is mandatory that adequate renal function be present and that the ECG and serum potassium be followed. Moderate or severe azotemia or oliguria usually contraindicate potassium therapy.
3. Chelating agents, by binding calcium, have been reported of value. EDTA, 600 mg in 250 ml 5 percent glucose in water, may be given slowly with ECG monitoring.
4. Procainamide (Pronestyl) may be of value in the life-threatening ventricular arrhythmias where postassium has failed. Under constant ECG monitoring. 1 mEq per minute injected intravenously may cause prompt disappearance of the arrhythmia.
5. The usefulness of electric conversion for arrhythmia due to digitalis is being evaluated now. In a desperate situation it might be tried after the above have failed.

SUMMARY

Digitalis is the drug of choice in congestive heart failure and in atrial fibrillation with a rapid ventricular rate. It is also of great value in atrial flutter. The best preparations are those with which the physician is most familiar. Doses as outlined represent average ones. Digitalis is best titrated against cardiac response; the physician is thus enjoined to tailor the drug to the patient. Digitoxicity is being seen with increasing frequency, as the drug is being employed more and more in a rapidly enlarging geriatric population. Hypokalemia following mercurial and chlorothiazide diuresis is equally culpable as a contributing factor to toxicity.

The most common signs of toxicity are atrial tachycardia with block, premature ventricular contractions, and anorexia. The last may be most subtle.

The most treacherous sign of digitoxicity is increasing congestive heart failure.

In the face of normal renal function, potassium is the drug of choice in acute toxicity as manifested by the arrhythmias. In AV block, however, potassium is contraindicated.

REFERENCES

Church, G., et al. Deliberate digitalis intoxication, a comparison of the toxic effects of four glycoside preparations. Ann. Intern. Med., 57:946, 1962.

Doherty, J. E., et al. Studies following intramuscular tritiated digoxin in human subject. Amer. J. Cardiol., 15:170, 1965.

Jelliffe, R. W. An improved method of digoxin therapy. Ann. Intern. Med., 69:703, 1968.

Maseri, A., et al. Early effects of digitalis on central hemodynamics in normal subjects. Amer. J. Cardiol., 15:162, 1965.

Mason, D. T., and Braunwald, E. Digitalis: New facts about an old drug. Amer. J. Cardiol. 22:151, 1968.

Mercer, E. N., and Osborne, J. A. The current status of diphenylhydantoin in heart disease. Ann. Intern. Med., 67:1084, 1967.

Weissler, A. M., et al. The effects of deslanoside on the duration of the phases of ventricular systole in man. Amer. J. Cardiol., 15:153, 1965.

DIURETICS

DRUG	ACTION	DOSE	EFFECT ON SERUM Cl^-	EFFECT ON SERUM K^+	TOXICITY	PRIMARY INDICATIONS
Organic mercurials (Mercuhydrin, etc.)	Interferes with proximal Na^+ absorption	1-2 ml, I.M. daily	Decreases; action depends on maintaining Cl^- level over 110 mEq	Suppresses K^+ excretion	Dermatitis	Heart failure
Hydrochlorothiazide derivatives	As above; also interferes with tubular H^+ exchange	250-500 mg, b.i.d. to q.i.d. orally for 3-4 days with rest period of 2 days	None	Decreases	Urate retention; hyperglycemia in diabetes; blood dyscrasias; jaundice; acute pancreatitis; dermatitis	Heart failure
Carbonic anhydrase inhibitor (Diamox)	Interferes with H^+-Na^+ exchange in proximal and distal tubules	250 mg, orally daily, t.i.d.	Elevates	Decreases		Heart failure with pulmonary disease and chronic CO_2 retention

17-Spiro-lactones (aldosterone inhibitors: Aldactone)	Blocks Na^+ retaining and kaliuretic action of endogenous aldosterone	50-400 mg q.i.d. orally		None		Cirrhosis of the liver
Ethacrynic acid	Interferes with proximal and distal Na^+ absorption	50-100 mg b.i.d. orally 0.5 mg/kg b.i.d., I.V.	Decreases	Decreases	Urate retention; hypochloremic alkalosis; GI symptoms; deafness	Refractory states of fluid retention
Furosemide	Interferes with reabsorption of Na^+ in loop of Henle, proximal and distal tubule	40-80 mg orally and repeat same day if necessary. 40 mg b.i.d. I.V.	Decreases	Decreases	Urate retention; dermatitis; paresthias	Refractory states of fluid retention

ETHACRYNIC ACID AND FUROSEMIDE

Ethacrynic acid and furosemide are potent diuretics which are not as dependent on the serum chloride level as the mercurial or thiazide drugs in producing a diuretic effect. Their action is more influenced by the serum sodium than the chloride level. In the presence of hyponatremia the diuretic effect of these drugs is enhanced by elevating the serum sodium in patients with dilutional hyponatremia either by restricting fluids or by liberalizing the dietary salt intake.

When given orally the action of ethacrynic acid or furosemide begins in 1 hour and lasts for 6 to 8 hours. Given intravenously the onset of action is almost immediately with the peak effect within 1 hour.

REFERENCES

Brest, A. N. et al. Clinical selection of diuretic drugs in the management of cardiac edema. Amer. J. Cardiol., 22:168, 1968.

Kirkendall, W. M., and Stein, J. H. Clinical pharmacology of furosemide and ethacrynic acid. Amer. J. Cardiol., 22:162, 1968.

Laragh, J. H. Ethacrynic acid and furosemide. Amer. Heart J., 75:564, 1968.

Muth, R. G. Diuretic properties of furosemide in renal disease. Ann. Intern. Med., 69:249, 1968.

Siegel, W., and Gifford, J. R. W. Efficacy of ethacrynic acid in patients with refractory heart failure resistant to meralluride. Amer. J. Cardiol., 22:260, 1968.

DROWNING

Approximately ten to fifteen percent of the subjects have sufficient laryngeal spasm so that no water enters their lungs and they do not become unconscious from asphyxia. Such patients can generally be resuscitated if they have not been submerged too long. The majority of patients, however, have aspirated into their lungs huge quantities of water. The clinical phenomenon that follows depends on the tonicity of the fluid which is aspirated.

FRESH WATER DROWNING. Rapid absorption of fresh water produces hypervolemia and hemodilution to the point where the circulating blood volume may be doubled. Striking electrolyte abnormalities occur and rapid hemolysis of red cells follows. The hemolysis and the protracted anoxia result in a rapid rise in serum potassium, in spite of the hemodilution. Ventricular fibrillation is common.

SALT WATER DROWNING. The hypertonic fluid draws large quantities of free water into the lungs; there is absorption of electrolytes into the circulating blood volume. Hypovolemia and hemoconcentration appear, with consequent hypotension. Absorption of sodium and potassium raises the concentration of these electrolytes to very high levels. Hemolysis does not occur; death is probably due to hemoconcentration.

PULMONARY EDEMA. Pulmonary edema and hypoxia occur in both fresh and salt water drowning. It may occur 1 to 2 minutes after rescue. It is to be noted, however, that it may occur as late as 48 hours after the onset of spontaneous respiration.

DEATH AFTER APPARENT SURVIVAL. Death may occur after a few days, even though the patient appears to be in good condition during this interval. Pneumonia may develop or recurrent acute pulmonary edema occur. Sudden death after apparent complete recovery may take place as long as 48 hours later, due to apnea or pulmonary edema. After salt water drowning, sudden delayed death appears to be due most often to acute pulmonary edema.

TREATMENT

EMERGENCY

The patient is best treated with mouth-to-mouth respiration and closed chest cardiac massage. Meticulous attention to the control of the airway is mandatory. Postural drainage is of no help. Electrical defibrillation of the patient with ventricular fibrillation, or of the patient with no pulse, may be used.

AFTER CARE

All survivors should be hospitalized. Intermittent positive breathing with oxygen should be instituted and be continued long after the return of spontaneous respiration, and as long as there is x-ray evidence of pulmonary edema. Of major importance is the control of the blood volume and the electrolyte disorders, as indicated above. Phlebotomies may be used or, conversely, transfusions of plasma or hypertonic saline. Perhaps the quickest and simplest way to control the serious electrolyte and fluid disturbance is either renal or peritoneal dialysis particularly in cases of anemia due to hemolysis following fresh water drowning.

REFERENCES

Modell, J. H., Moya, F., Newby, E. J., Ruiz, B. C., and Showers, A. V. The effects of fluid volume in seawater drowning. Ann. Intern. Med., 67:68, 1967.

Wong, F. M., and Grace, W. J. Sudden death after near-drowning. J.A.M.A. 186:202, 1963.

DRUG ADDICTION

True drug addiction with physiologic dependence is considerably rarer in hospitals than one would believe from current publicity. In this institution, which has much experience with the "hippie" society, very little true addiction is encountered. Many young people who take drugs on and off, or even regularly, state they are addicted. However, the "cold turkey" treatment applied to such people is almost uniformly without any ill effect. It is very likely that such people have been taking little or no significant pharmacologic doses of the opiates, even though they pay astonishing prices for whatever they purchase.

The true drug addict is a person with serious psychologic, physiologic, and metabolic disturbances. He is subject to a number of disorders and, when one truly has a convincing history of drug addiction, the possibility of the following must be carefully considered in each of these persons.

1. Endocarditis.
2. Pulmonary complications
   a. Overdose with pulmonary infiltrate
   b. embolic pneumonia
   c. bacterial infection
   d. pulmonary fibrosis or granulomatosis
   e. acute pulmonary edema.
3. Acute hepatitis, subacute hepatitis, and cirrhosis of the liver.
4. Osteomyelitis of various bones, due to repeated injections of bacteria.
5. Tetanus and malaria.
6. Skin lesions, including multiple deep necrotic ulcers.

Consequently, when one approaches a confirmed drug addict one must go through the routine differential diagnosis based on the patient's own complaints and on physical findings. In addition, the physician is obliged to rule out all of the above complications of chronic addiction, even though nothing that the patient states suggests their presence.

Even if the self-asserted drug addict from the youthful and "hippie" population is not addicted to narcotics, this certainly does not mean that such a person is not subject to the disorders listed. These young people injecting almost anything into themselves are subject to pulmonary emboli from poorly dissolved material, malaria, infectious hepatitis, and even tetanus.

REFERENCES

Cherubin, C. E. The medical sequelae of narcotic addiction. Ann. Intern. Med., 67:23, 1967.

Louria, D. B., Hensle, T., and Rose, J. The major medical complications of heroin addiction Ann. Intern. Med., 67:1, 1967.

DIPHENYLHYDANTOIN SODIUM

(Dilantin)

This drug is of limited use in treating cardiac arrhythmias. It is mainly effective in digitalis-induced disturbances of rhythm, such as paroxysmal atrial tachycardia with block, bigeminy and multifocal ventricular premature beats, and ventricular tachycardia. It is ineffective in atrial flutter and fibrillation. The drug has a depressant effect on the sinus and AV node and should not be used in bradycardia or high degrees of AV block.

ADMINISTRATION. Intravenously 250 mg diluted in 5 ml of solvent (3.5-5.0 mg/kg) is given over 3 to 5 minutes. A favorable response if it occurs usually appears in from ½ to 4 minutes. (If the arrhythmia recurs the dose is repeated.) If no ECG changes are noted, the drug is not repeated. The maintenance dose is 200-400 mg I.M. or orally 100-300 mg q.i.d. daily.

REFERENCES

Conn, R. D. Diphenylhydantoin sodium in cardiac arrhythmias. New Eng. J. Med., 272:277, 1965.

Karliner, J. S. Intravenous diphenylhydantoin sodium (Dilantin) in cardiac arrhythmias. Dis. Chest., 51:256, 1967.

DRUG ADMIXTURES

PHYSICAL COMPATIBILITY OF INTRAVENOUS DRUGS

This section is designed to guide physicians and nurses in determining the compatibility or incompatibility of frequently used intravenous additive combinations.

Incompatibilities are generally divided into three classes: 1) physical, 2) chemical, and 3) physiologic.

Physical incompatibilities usually can be seen quite readily by the person combining different drug components. With chemical incompatibilities decomposition may take place without perceptive evidence. Drugs which may be physically and chemically compatible, but with physiologic incompatibility, cannot be detected except by prior knowledge of the actions of each drug in the body.

Changes in pH are probably responsible for the majority of incompatibilities. Medications relatively stable in certain volume solutions at a certain pH may precipitate after the addition of other drugs which result in a pH change. Also, combining two or more injectable drugs with different preservatives, stabilizers, buffers, antioxidants, and vehicles may result in many more combinations unsuitable for intravenous use.

AGENT	INCOMPATIBLE AGENTS
1. Aminophylline	Ascorbic acid, diphenylhydantoin (Dilantin), hydroxyzine (Vistaril), meperidine (Demerol), oxytetracycline (Terramycin), procaine, vancomycin.
2. Amphotericin B (Fungizone)	Penicillin G potassium, tetracyclines.
3. Calcium gluconate	Magnesium sulfate, novobiocin, prochlorperazine (Compazine), streptomycin.
4. Chloramphenicol (Chloromycetin)	Vitamin B complex preparations, hydrocortisone, polymyxin B, tetracyclines, vancomycin.
5. Dextrose	Kanamycin (Kantrex), Vitamin B-12, sodium warfarin (Coumadin), novobiocin sodium (Albamycin).

AGENT	INCOMPATIBLE AGENTS
6. Heparin	Tetracyclines, polymixin B, vancomycin.
7. Hydrocortisone	Vitamin B complex, chloramphenicol, ephedrine, tetracycline, vancomycin.
8. Insulin	Diuril, diphenylhydantoin (Dilantin), sodium bicarbonate, nitrofarantrin (Furadantin), phenobarbital sodium, sodium sulfadiazine, sulfisoxazole (Gantrisin).
9. Kanamycin (Kantrex)	Diphenylhydantoin (Dilantin), hydrocortisone, dextrose, heparin, sulfisoxazole (Gantrisin), phenobarbital sodium.
10. Sodium cephalothin (Keflin)	Oxytetracycline, tetracycline, kanamycin, vitamin B complex with C, erythromycin.
11. Levarterenol (Levophed)	Amobarbital sodium, chlorothiazide (Diuril), diphenylhydantoin (Dilantin), sodium bicarbonate, sodium iodide, streptomycin, sodium sulfadiazine, sulfisoxazole (Gantrisin).
12. Lincomycin (Lincocin)	Diphenylhydantoin (Dilantin), penicillin G, K, or Na.
13. Methicillin (Dimocillin)	Hydrocortisone, meperidine (Demerol), Compazine, metaraminol (Aramine), sodium bicarbonate, vancomycin, tetracyclines.
14. Penicillin G potassium	Amphotericin B, metaraminol, phenylephrine, tetracyclines, vancomycin, ascorbic acid.
15. Procaine hydrochloride	Aminophylline, amobarbital sodium, sodium iodide, chlorothiazide sodium (Diuril Sodium), diphenylhydantoin sodium (Dilantin Sodium), magnesium sulfate, phenobarbital sodium, streptomycin, sulfixoxazole (Gantrisin), tetracycline hydrochloride, nitrofurantoin sodium (Macrodantin), novobiocin sodium (Albamycin).
16. Streptomycin sulfate	Amobarbital sodium, calcium gluconate, heparin sodium, chlorothiazide sodium (Diuril Sodium), diphenylhydantoin sodium (Dilantin Sodium), erythromycin, hyaluronidase (Wydase), phenobarbital sodium, sodium bicarbonate, sodium iodide.
17. Tetracyclines	Amphotericin B, chloramphenicol, heparin, hydrocortisone, methicillin, penicillin G potassium, polymixin B.

Based on material from Amer. J. Hosp. Pharm., 23: 8, 1966.

DRUG POISONING TREATMENT

The choice of treatment depends on the severity of intoxication which is based on the Reed classification after initial hydration and aeration of the patient.

CLASS I. Patient is comatose, but responds to painful stimuli; has all deep tendon reflexes (DTR) and vital signs are stable.

CLASS II. The patient does not respond to painful stimuli, but all DTR are present and vital signs are stable.

CLASS III. No response to painful stimuli, and DTR are absent or almost totally absent; but vital signs are stable and no assistance is required for maintenance of blood pressure or respiration.

CLASS IV. No response to pain, all DTR are absent and support of blood pressure and/or respiration is required.

REGIMEN FOR TREATMENT OF DRUG-INDUCED COMA

1. Maintenance of adequate airway. Intubation if necessary and assisted ventilation via mechanical respirator. Careful attention to removal of bronchial secretions.
2. Support of blood pressure and maintenance of fluid and electrolyte balance. Hypotension associated with clinical evidence of shock or falling urinary output should be treated with vasopressors. Aramine or Levophed is utilized for the hypotension secondary to drug poisoning. Repeated determinations of serum electrolytes is necessary to maintain fluid balance.
3. Frequent change of body position must be employed to prevent the development of hypostatic pneumonia.
4. Prophylactic antibiotics are not indicated.
5. Gastric lavage has been the subject of controversy in recent years. If the patient is alert and awake, removal of the gastric contents may prevent the development of coma. For the patient who is severely intoxicated, the stomach may be lavaged after insertion of a cuffed, endotracheal tube with the cuff inflated. However, lavage fluids are not introduced into the stomach because they may hasten absorption of the intoxicant. Gastric aspiration of a comatose patient may shorten the duration of coma by removing the drug which has not yet been absorbed.

ADJUNCTIVE THERAPY

Forced diuresis has been successfully applied to several types of poisoning. It can be utilized most efficiently in patients who have taken an overdose of barbiturate. Diuresis means a urinary output of approximately 500 ml per hour, if possible.

The contraindications to forced diuresis are

1. Congestive heart failure
2. Renal failure
3. Shock
4. Oliguria and anuria
5. Fluid-overloaded patient.

It is necessary to evaluate carefully the patient's cardiac, pulmonary and renal status before starting diuresis. There are two methods used to create forced diuresis.

1. Diuretic induced.
   a. 500 ml of 5 percent dextrose in water + 50 mEq $NaHCO_3$
   b. 500 ml of 5 percent dextrose in water + 25 mEq KCl.
   c. 500 ml of 0.87 percent sodium chloride.
   d. Rotate the above solutions and administer at a rate of 500 ml per hour.
   e. 40 mg of furosemide are given intravenously and the dose is repeated at intervals when the urinary output falls more than 2,000 ml behind the infusion.
2. Osmotic diuresis.
   a. Twelve and a half grams of mannitol I.V.
   b. 1,000 ml of 5 percent dextrose in water with 12.5 g. of mannitol administered at a rate of 500 ml/hour.
   c. 1,000 ml of normal saline + 12.5 g, of mannitol administered at a rate of 500 ml/hour.
   d. Alternate the following solutions: 1,000 cc of D/W plus 20 mEq of KCl with 1,000 ml of normal saline + 20 mEq of KCl + 12.5 g of mannitol. Administer these solutions at a rate to match the urine output on an hourly basis. A urinary output of 500 ml per hour is desirable. There is no objection to the insertion of a Foley catheter to monitor urinary output in this situation.
   e. Additional doses of 12.5 g of mannitol may be given if the urinary output falls to less than 250 ml per hour. A total dose of 100 g of mannitol should not be exceeded in a given 24-hour period.
   f. Osmotic diuresis should not be stopped abruptly, but rather the patient should be weaned off mannitol. Mannitol diuresis must be continued during peritoneal and renal dialysis or the patient may develop dysequilibrium syndrome.

DIALYSIS

Forced diuresis is an adjunctive form of therapy and does not preclude the use of hemo- or peritoneal dialysis and good conservative management. A current list of dialyzable poisons is published every year in the journal "Transactions of the American Society of Artificial Internal Organs."

EDEMA

Edema is any abnormal increase in interstitial fluid. The mechanisms producing edema are classified as follows.

CARDIAC. Myocardial failure, either primary or associated with valvular lesions or constrictive pericarditis.

HEPATIC.

1. Primary
   a. Portal hypertension.
   b. Hypoproteinemia.
2. Secondary
   a. Renal (with ascites, renal insufficiency may occur).
   b. Adrenal (increased aldosterone secretion).
   c. Pituitary (increased ADH secretion).

RENAL. Two mechanisms play a major role

1. Retention of salt and water from impaired excretion.
2. Hypoalbuminemia.

LOCAL.

1. Obstructive: venous, lymphatic, traumatic, infective. Prolonged sitting (car ride, airplane, etc.) is a notable cause of slight degrees of pedal edema, as are panty girdles and tight garters.
2. Allergic (angioneurotic edema) and toxic.

MISCELLANEOUS.

1. Beriberi: edema is due to hypoproteinemia early in the disease; later cardiac failure also contributes.
2. Endocrine
   a. Myxedematous skin may appear edematous.
   b. Cyclic edema associated with menstruation.
   c. Primary aldosteronism occasionally presents with edema.
   d. Exogenous, secondary to steroid therapy.

THE ELECTROCARDIOGRAM

THE VECTORCARDIOGRAM AND THE VECTOR INTERPRETATION OF THE ELECTROCARDIOGRAM

Mechanical contraction of the heart is preceded by changes in the electrical potential of cardiac muscle. The electrocardiogram and vectorcardiogram are graphic records of such changes in potential, and, although these methods differ in the manner of recording, both mirror the same electrical phenomena arising in the heart (the generator) and transmitted through the body (the conductor) to surface leads.

The vectorcardiogram is a more fundamental approach to the understanding of the sequential electrical changes in cardiac muscle than is the electrocardiogram. In this section, therefore, the characteristics of the vectorcardiogram will be emphasized and the basic principles which they illustrate will be carried over to the interpretation of the electrocardiogram which is more widely used in clinical practice.

The vectorcardiogram displays the electrical activity of the heart in the three orthogonal planes of the body (Fig. 1) as mean instantaneous vectors. The vectors at particular instants of time by their length represent the magnitude of a force, by their direction the relation of the force to the planes of the body, and by their polarity or sense are directed to the positive side of the electromagnetic field set up by cardiac activity. The three characteristics of a vector, magnitude, direction, and polarity, may be displayed in one or all three planes of the body as planar vectors or in the three-dimensional space as a spatial vector (Fig. 2).

When two or more vectors act simultaneously at a particular interval in time, their resultant by vector addition is a mean instantaneous resultant vector (Fig. 2).

The sequence of the generation of the normal electrical forces by the heart depends initially on the distribution of the conduction system and on the spatial relationship of the cardiac chambers.

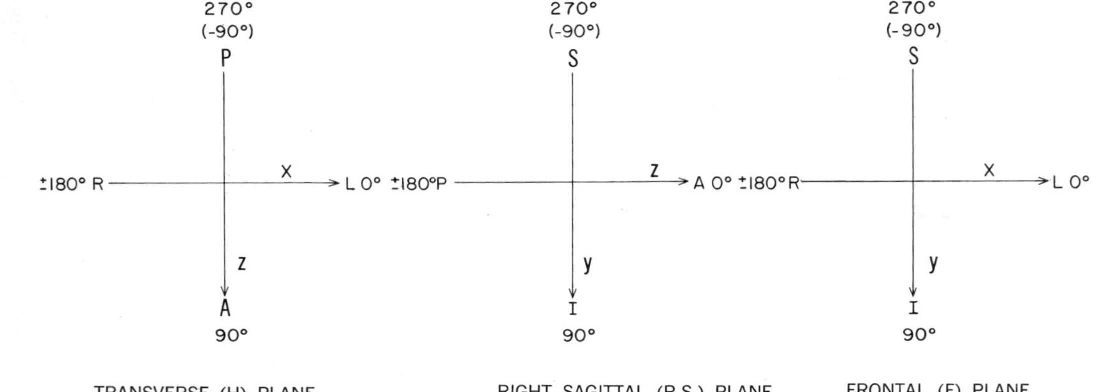

Fig. 1. Orthogonal axes of the planes of the body. Angular notation is indicated with zero degrees to the left in all planes. The positive polarity of the axes is represented by the arrowhead. Note that the sagittal plane is viewed from the right.

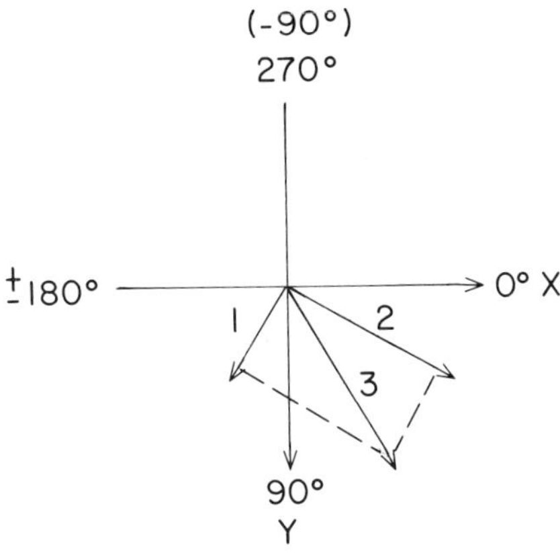

Fig. 2A. Planar vectors in the frontal plane. Vector 1, right and inferior at 120°. Vector 2, left and inferior at 27°. Vector 3, the resultant vector of forces 1 and 2 acting simultaneously, is at 58°. The arrowheads indicate positive polarity.

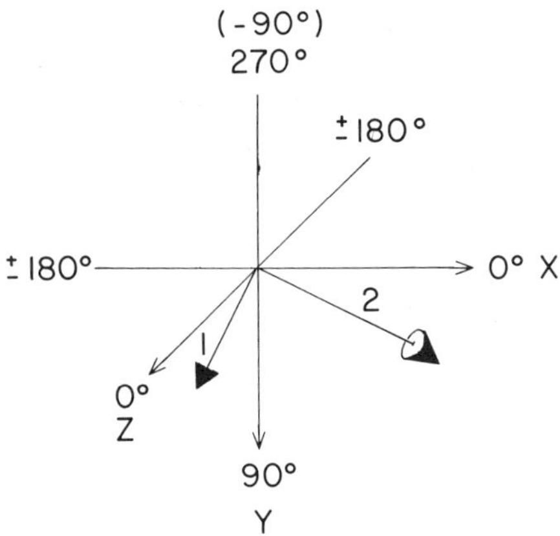

Fig. 2B. Spatial vectors in relation to the X, Y and Z axes. Vector 1 inferior, right and anterior. Vector 2 inferior, left and posterior.

DEPOLARIZATION (ACTIVATION)

ATRIAL. Activation of the atria begins with the rhythmic exit of an impulse from the sinoatrial node (SA) located in the upper lateral right atrial wall. Since the bulk of this chamber is anterior, activation spreads as a wave front in an anterior, leftward and inferior direction. Subsequent spread to the left atrium, a posterior midline structure is posteriorly, inferiorly, and leftward. The vectors of both right and left atrial depolarization are inferior and leftward but those of the right atrium are anterior and those of the left atrium are posterior.

Atrial depolarization is represented in the VCG as the P loop and in the ECG as the P wave.

With the completion of atrial activation the transmitted impulse enters the antrioventricular node (AV) where it undergoes an appreciable delay in the speed of transmission. In the ECG the delay is manifested by the PR segment, the interval between the end of the P wave and the beginning of the QRS complex. From the AV node which straddles the interventricular septum (IV), the impulse passes into the common bundle (bundle of His) which divides into the right and left bundle branches. The right bundle is a long, thin, unbranching filament which, passing along the right side of the septum, reaches the base of the anterior papillary muscle at the apicoanterior portion of the right ventricle where it gives off Purkinje fibers to the inner two-thirds of the right ventricular wall and the apical right septal mass. The structure of the left bundle is more complex. The main left bundle, after leaving the node, divides into two branches. The anterior (superior) division, an extension of the main left bundle, passes along the anterior left ventricular wall to the anterior papillary muscle after giving off fibers to the middle third of the left septal surface and the apicoanterior left ventricle. The posterior (inferior) division of the left bundle consists of fibers from the anterior division and fibers which arise directly from the His bundle. Both groups join to give off fibers to the middle third of the septum, the posterior papillary muscle, and the apical and inferior areas of the left ventricle. Terminally, both divisions of the left bundle arborize into the Purkinje network which carries impulses to the inner two-thirds of the ventricular walls. Purkinje fibers are relatively sparse in the wall of the posterobasal left ventricle and the basal portion of the septum.

VENTRICULAR. The distribution of the conduction system determines the initial area of ventricular activation. The first area to be depolarized is the middle third of the left septal surface in a posterior to anterior direction and from left to right. The interventricular septum, though directed slightly rightward, is mainly colinear with the frontal plane of the body so that the *initial resultant vector of activation is always anterior,* mainly to the right and either slightly superior or inferior. After endocardial activation through the Purkinje system the remainder of ventricular depolarization forces is influenced mainly by the anatomic position and the muscle bulk of the right and left ventricles. The right ventricle facing the anterior chest wall is an anterior chamber. The left ventricle facing posterolaterally is a posterior chamber whose thickness and muscle mass is about three times that of the right ventricle. Because of these anatomic factors the predominant resultant vectors of ventricular depolarization are directed posteriorly, leftward, and usually inferiorly. One should note, however, that early vectors of activation are anterior. Sequential ventricular depolarization takes place in the manner shown in Figure 3, in which the direction, approximate magnitude, and the polarity of the main resultant vectors are shown. Each of the instantaneous vectors represents the resultant of all forces generated in the heart at particular intervals of time. It is apparent that the forces generated by the left ventricle outweigh by far those arising from the right ventricle.

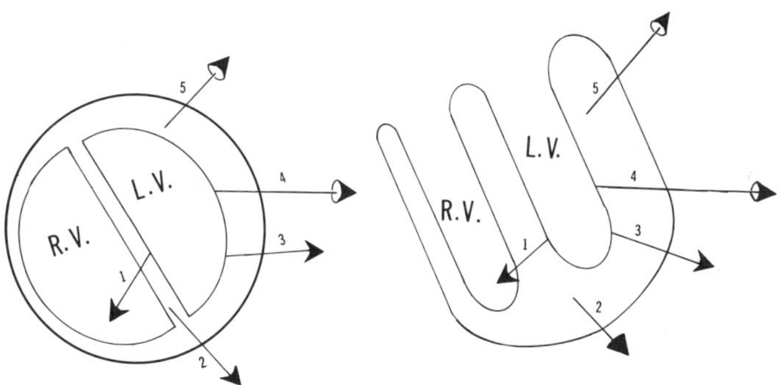

Fig. 3. Sequential resultant ventricular activation vectors in the horizontal and sagittal planes with approximate magnitudes, spatial orientations and polarities.

VECTOR	TIME (sec)	DIRECTION
1. Septal	0.01	Anterior, right, superior or inferior
2. Apicoanterior	0.02	Anterior, left, inferior
3. Anterolateral	0.03	Anterior or posterior, left, inferior
4. Posterolateral (Maximum)	0.04	Posterior, left, inferior
5. Basal	0.05-0.06	Posterior, left, superior*

*In the younger age groups because of the preponderance of the basal right ventricular mass and the right side of the base of the septum the basal vector may be to the right, posterior, and superior.

In the vectorcardiogram the forces of ventricular depolarization are represented by the QRS loop and in the electrocardiogram by the QRS complex.

REPOLARIZATION (RECOVERY)

ATRIAL. The forces of atrial recovery are in the same direction as those of atrial activation, i.e., to the left, inferiorly, initially anteriorly, and terminally posteriorly. Recovery of atrial muscle follows the same sequence as it does in an isolated muscle strip. However, since by convention a vector is directed to the positive side of an electrical field the resultant vector of atrial repolarization is in the opposite direction to the wave of recovery that is to the right, superiorly, and usually posteriorly.

VENTRICULAR. Repolarization of the ventricles begins in those areas of myocardium which were first depolarized, namely, the apical region of the heart. Repolarization forces are directed therefore from apex to base, but as in the case of the atrial muscle the repolarization vector is in the opposite direction, from base to apex. According to rule, ventricular recovery should be also from endocardium, which is first depolarized, to epicardium. The reverse, however, occurs because of the effect of high intracavitary pressure on the endocardium and the cooling effect of intracavitary blood.

The maximum T vector is inferior, anterior, and to the left, usually to the right of a horizontal maximum QRS vector, and to the left of a vertical one. The angle between the QRS and T vectors does not usually exceed 60°.

The forces of repolarization are represented in the VCG as the T loop and in the ECG as the T wave.

The electrical potential of the early phase of ventricular recovery, phase 2 of the membrane action potential, does not vary over time, and as a result the ST vector is often obscured by the origin and termination of the P, QRS, and T loops. When identifiable it is anterior, leftward, and inferior and represented in the ECG as the ST segment between the end of the QRS complex and the beginning of the T wave.

VECTORCARDIOGRAPHIC LEADS AND REFERENCE FRAMES

Vectorcardiographic leads differ from those used in electrocardiography in that 1) the axes of the leads cross each other at right angles through the E point (point of zero potential, null point), 2) the anatomic and electrical axes of the leads correspond as closely as possible, and 3) each lead is equally sensitive to a given electrical force.

To approximate the above ideal characteristics, many lead systems have been devised to correct for the eccentric position of the heart and to compensate for variations in the conductivity of body tissues and body contour. Some lead systems are not adaptable to clinical use because of their complexity. Within the limits of accuracy the most widely used and clinically practicable is the Frank lead system (Fig. 4). This system employs seven electrodes, which, interconnected by suitable resistances, approach the ideal of three equal length or equally sensitive orthogonal axes. The transverse plane of the ventricles is taken as the fourth intercostal space in the recumbent position. Electrode placement is at the anterior midline (E), posterior midline (M), right (I) and left (A) midaxillary lines, and at an angle of 45° (C) between electrodes E and A. Electrodes are also placed on the left leg (F) and on the back or side of the neck (H).

This electrode placement yields three axes at right angles to each other. They are:

1. X axis (right to left) from electrodes I, C, A.
2. Y axis (head to foot) from electrodes H, M, F.
3. Z axis (front to back) from electrodes A, C, E, I, M.

In pairs these axes record the electrical activity of the heart in the three planes of the body. The axes of the transverse or horizontal plane are X and Z, the sagittal plane, Z and Y, and the frontal plane, X and Y.

The vectorcardiographic reference frames are simple. Each plane consists of paired axes as shown in Figure 1.

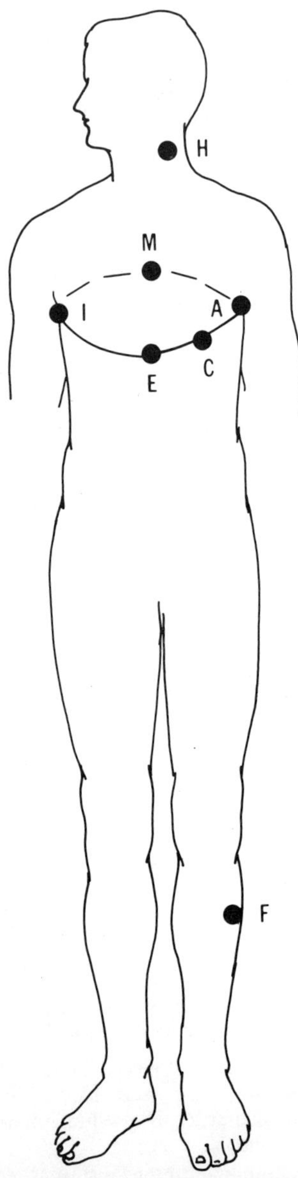

Fig. 4. The Frank system of electrode placement.

ELECTROCARDIOGRAPHIC LEADS AND REFERENCE FRAMES

Electrocardiographic leads differ from vectorcardiographic leads in that they are not orthogonal, their anatomic axes do not correspond to the electrical axes, and the leads are of unequal sensitivity to a given electrical force.

BIPOLAR LIMB LEADS

Bipolar limb leads record the difference in potential of two points on the frontal plane of the body. The arrangement of these leads is represented by the Einthoven triangle (Fig. 5). Arrows indicate the direction of the positive pole.

The midpoint of the triangle theoretically represents the center of the electrical field of the heart in the frontal plane. The

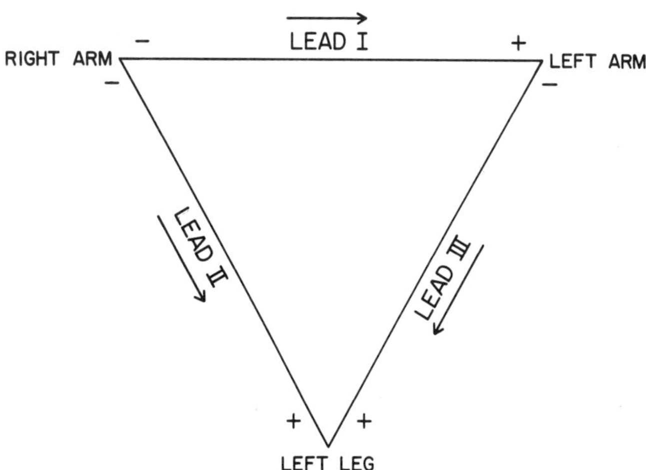

Fig. 5. Lead I. Left arm is connected to the positive pole of the ECG and the right arm to the negative pole.

Lead II. Left leg is connected to the positive pole and the right arm to the negative pole.

Lead III. Left leg is connected to the positive pole and the left arm to the negative pole.

triangle may be rearranged with the original polarity and angular relationship maintained by forming a triaxial reference frame in which the midpoint of each lead passes through the zero point of the original triangle.

UNIPOLAR LIMB LEADS

Unipolar limb leads are obtained by connecting the three extremity leads together at a central terminal so that an approximately zero potential is recorded by the galvanometer. The exploring electrode is attached to the right arm, the left arm, or the left leg and connected to the positive pole of the machine. The central terminal is attached to the negative pole. These leads record small potentials because of their distance from the heart. Goldberger augmented these potentials by disconnecting the lead being taken from the central terminal and recorded a (augmented) VR, aVL, and aVF leads. The potential of the augmented limb leads is about 1.5 times that of the unipolar limb leads.

The relation of the augmented unipolar limb leads to the triaxial reference frame of the unipolar limb leads is shown in Figure 6 as the hexaxial reference frame.

The three bipolar and the three unipolar augmented limb leads represent the electrical forces of the heart in the frontal plane.

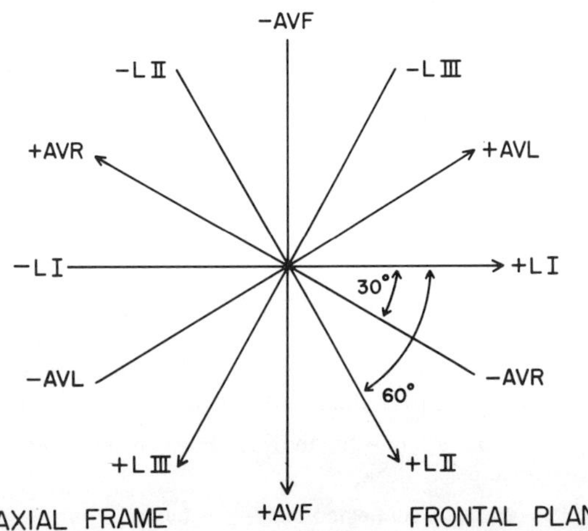

Fig. 6. Uncorrected hexaxial reference frame based on the Einthoven triangle.

The hexaxial reference frame implies that the Einthoven triangle is equilateral in an electrical and anatomic sense. Burger and van Milaan have shown that the axes of the limb leads actually form a scalene triangle with the sides of unequal length or sensitivity, and that the angles between the leads vary with the position of the heart, tissue conductivity, and the contour of the thorax (Fig. 7). Lead I, the shortest axis, is directed upward and backward; Lead III, the longest, is downward and forward; while Lead II is intermediate in length. The plane of the scalene triangle passes behind the cardiac center, and the cephalic end is posterior to the caudal end.

Deriving vectors from the scalar electrocardiogram and projecting them on the scalene reference frame necessitates certain adjustments in the calculation of voltage measured from the different frontal plane leads. Lead III, the longest lead, is more sensitive to a given electrical force than Lead I, the

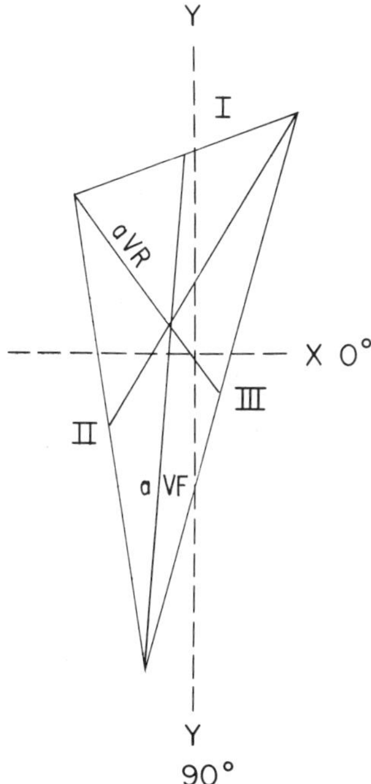

Fig. 7. The scalene triangle of an average normal adult.

shortest lead. In other words, the leads must be equalized by dividing the effective length of Lead I considered as unity by the length of either of the other two sides of the scalene triange. Approximate correction factors for an average position of the heart are:

L I	1.0	VL	1.0
L II	0.56	VR	1.0
L III	0.5	VF	0.8

On the uncorrected triaxial frame a given electrical force will be recorded unequally on L I and L III. The latter lead being of greater sensitivity will record a greater voltage than the former. If L I records 8 mv and L III 4 mv, the actual value on L III using the correction factor 0.5 is 2 mv.

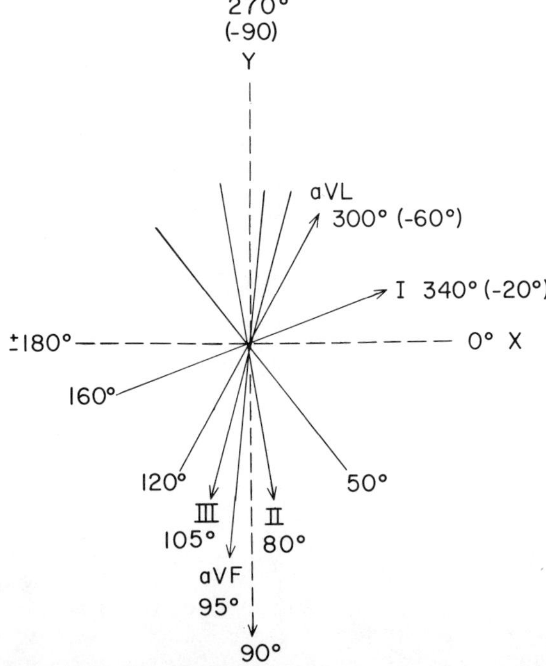

Fig. 8. The scalene triangle rearranged to form an hexaxial reference frame.

A hexaxial reference frame based on the scalene triangle employing the correction factors is a corrected frame. (Fig. 8).

PRECORDIAL LEADS

Records are obtained from the unipolar precordial leads by placing the exploring electrodes in the following positions:

V1 Fourth right intercostal space parasternally.
V2 Fourth left intercostal space parasternally.
V3 Between the fourth and fifth intercostal spaces at a point midway between V2 and V4.
V4 Fifth left intercostal space in the left midclavicular line.
V5 Fifth left intercostal space in the left anterior axillary line.
V6 Fifth left intercostal space in the left midaxillary line.

Occasionally the following leads are of value:

V7 Fifth intercostal space in the left posterior axillary line.
V3R Right side of the chest in the same position as V3 on the left.

Leads taken in these positions represent the electrical forces of the heart in the horizontal plane.

Records from these leads although considered to represent the electrical forces of the heart in the horizontal plane have the same limitations as the uncorrected limb leads. They also are of unequal sensitivity; moreover, they do not lie in the same transverse plane of the body, and their anatomic axes do not coincide with the electrical axes.

The uncorrected and the corrected horizontal reference frame of Helm is shown in Figure 9A-B.

Since most of the terminology used in vectorcardiography has been carried over from electrocardiography, a review is necessary.

In the scalar or conventional ECG the changes in potential were labeled arbitrarily by Einthoven as the P, QRS, and T waves (Fig. 10). These waves are graphically inscribed on electrocardiographic paper in terms of polarity, magnitude, and duration. The polarity of a wave may be positive, negative, biphasic, or isoelectric in relation to the base line. The magnitude of a wave is measured by its relation to the horizontal lines of the ECG paper, which are 1.0 mm apart and represent a potential of 0.1 millivolt (mv). The instrument is standardized so that the induction of 1 mv into the circuit causes a 1 cm deflection of the base line. The duration of a wave or the interval between waves is measured directly from the relation to the vertical lines of the paper, which are 0.04 second apart. Every fifth 0.04-second interval is marked by a heavier line so

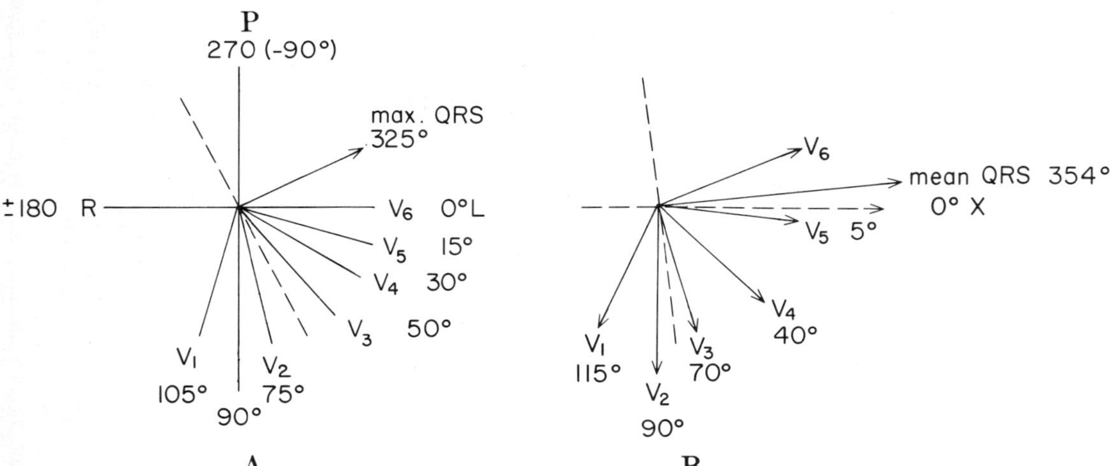

Fig. 9A-B. The uncorrected (A) and corrected (B) horizontal reference frames. The maximum QRS horizontal plane vector derived from the ECG of Figure 11 is at 325° on the uncorrected frame and at 354° on the corrected frame.

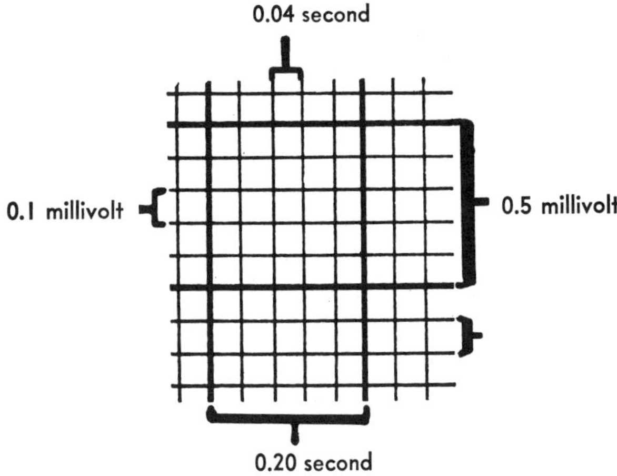

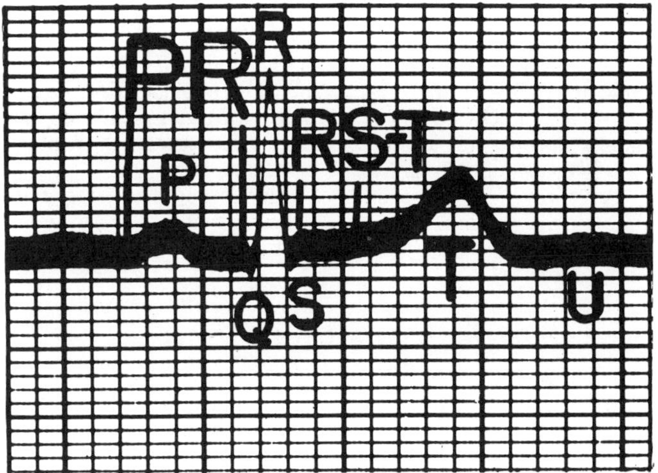

Fig. 10. Illustration of waves on standard ECG paper, identification of time intervals and magnitudes.

that the time interval between the heavier lines represents 0.2 second. There are 1,500 0.04-second lines and 300 0.2-second lines in 1 minute. The heart rate is calculated by counting the number of 0.04-second intervals between the peaks of two adjacent R waves and dividing into 1,500, or the number of 0.2-second intervals and dividing into 300. When the rhythm is irregular, several R-R intervals are counted and the number of 0.2-second intervals over the same distance is counted:

$$\frac{\text{No. R-R intervals} \times 300}{\text{No. 0.2-second intervals}} = \text{heart rate}$$

One QRS complex per five large vertical boxes (0.2 second each) is equal to a heart rate of 60; one complex per four boxes equals a rate of 75; and one per three boxes a rate of 100.

Atrial activation is represented by the time interval necessary to inscribe the P wave. Mechanical contraction of the atria extends through the time interval from the end of the P wave to the end of the R or S wave.

Ventricular activation begins with the onset of the QRS complex and extends to the end of the R wave, or the end of the S wave if present. Mechanical ventricular contraction begins 0.02 second after the peak of the R wave or the nadir of a QS complex and continues for 0.04 second after the end of the T wave.

The QRS complex represents the depolarization forces of the ventricles. The T wave represents the repolarization forces. Normally the QRS complex and the T wave represent predominantly the electrical activity of the left ventricle and the septum, which constitute the main mass of cardiac muscle.

A U wave, the significance of which is not clear, frequently follows the T wave. It is usually best visualized in precordial leads and may occur in healthy patients or reflect electrolyte imbalances.

METHOD OF PLOTTING VECTORS FROM THE ECG

FRONTAL PLANE. By projection of the magnitude and polarity of a complex recorded on two or more of the limb leads in terms of the area enclosed by the complex onto the corresponding limbs of the triaxial reference frame, a mean vector for the complex can be plotted. The area of a complex can be determined by counting the number of small squares enclosed by the wave or by measuring the height of the wave in mv and multiplying by one-half the width of the base in seconds. Each mv/sec is considered a unit. The length of a unit on the axes of the reference frame can be designated arbitrarily for ease in plotting. Perpendiculars are dropped from the determined points on the two limb leads. These will intersect. A line drawn from the zero point to the point of intersection represents the mean vector of the complex in the frontal plane of the body. The mean vector of the QRS complex indicates the mean electrical axis of the heart and not the anatomic position. The direction of the vector was formerly referred to as the "axis deviation." Figure 12 illustrates the method of deriving the mean QRS vector from the accompanying ECG (Fig. 11).

In Figure 13, from the same ECG data the maximum QRS vestor is projected on the scalene reference system. The QRS vector is at 20° compared to 30° on the uncorrected frame. The Einthoven triangle exaggerates vertical forces.

Negative and positive values cancel each other so that the mean deflection on L III is zero. The zero deflection is represented by a line perpendicular to L III drawn from the center of the reference frame.

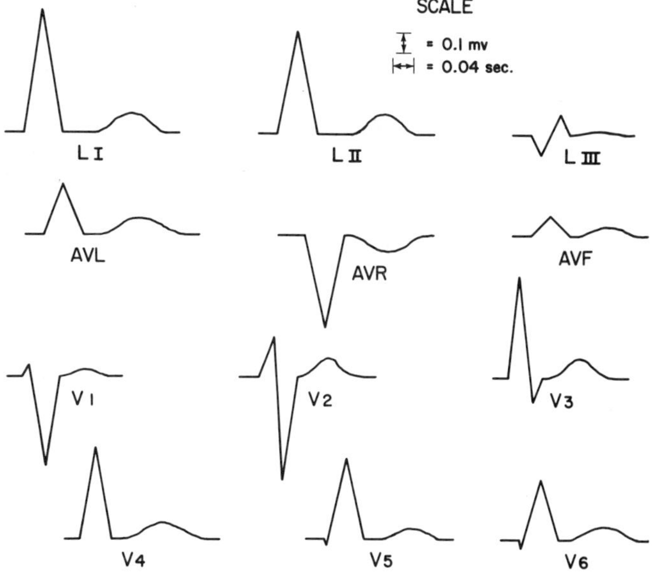

Fig. 11.

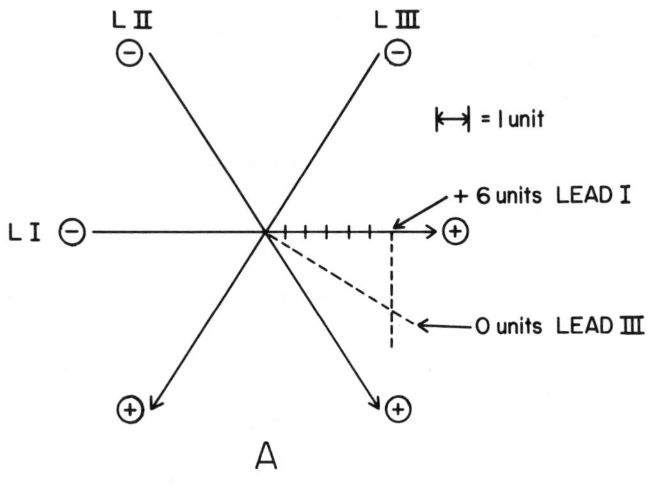

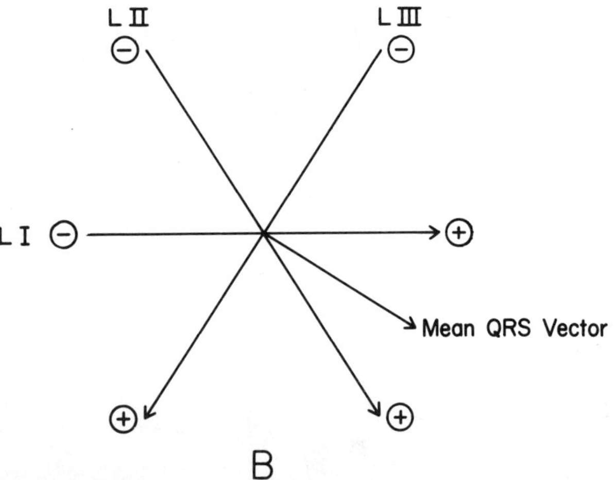

Fig. 12. Lead I. The magnitude of the QRS is +0.6 mv, which can be taken as 6 units for ease in plotting. The size of a unit is decided arbitrarily and measured off on the positive limb of Lead I.

Lead III. The initial limb of the QRS is negative and in magnitude is -0.1 mv, or -1 unit. The terminal limb is positive and the magnitude is +0.1 mv, or 1 unit. The resultant magnitude is zero.

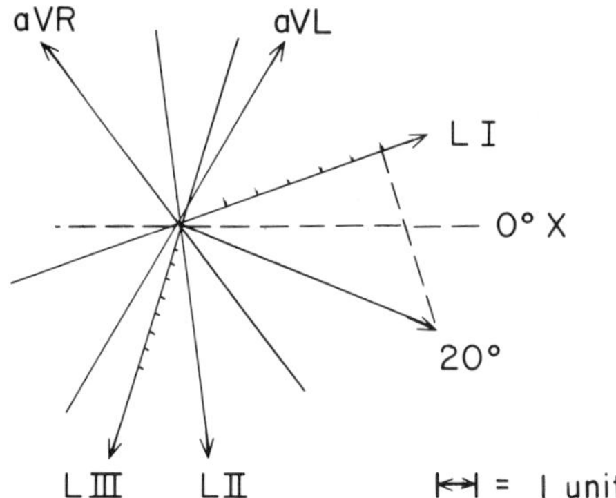

Fig. 13. Method of plotting on the scalene reference frame the maximum QRS vector from the ECG of Figure 11. The QRS voltage is measured on Lead I in arbitrary units. If measured on L III the correction factor 0.5 is used. In this case, the QRS is equiphasic on L III, therefore the maximum QRS vector is at right angles to this lead at 20°. In Figure 12, the maximum vector from the same ECG on the uncorrected reference frame is at 30°.

The mean QRS vector determined from Leads I and III is represented by a line drawn from the zero point of the reference frame to the intersection of the lines dropped from Leads I and III. In Figure 12 the mean QRS vector coincides with the perpendicular of L III. The mean QRS vector has the following characteristics:

1. It points downward and to the left.
2. It is most nearly parallel to L I, and the force of greatest magnitude will be recorded by this lead.
3. It is at right angles to L III, and the mean polarity is zero on this lead.
4. It is in the frontal plane only, because from the data available in the bipolar limb leads one cannot determine whether the vector points anteriorly or posteriorly.

The maximum mean QRS vector in this example is more horizontal than vertical and, if the same arbitrary units are measured on the corrected scalene system, the vector would be even more horizontal in position.

HORIZONTAL PLANE. The maximum horizontal QRS vector is determined by inspection of the precordial leads. That lead which is of equally negative and positive polarity, the transitional lead is identified. If none of the five leads is of algebraic zero potential, the zone between the predominantly positive and negative adjacent leads is considered transitional. The vector is at right angles to the axis of the transitional lead or zone. In the ECG of Figure 11 the transitional zone is between V2 and V3. A line drawn between the axes of these leads marks off the null or zero plane which divides the electrical field in the transverse plane into two parts. On one side of the plane are predominantly positive deflections and on the other negative deflections. The maximum QRS vector at right angles to the null plane points in the direction of the positive half of the field and away from the negative half, and as a result the vector is rotated a certain number of degrees anteriorly or posteriorly. When positive complexes are to the left and negative ones to the right, the vector is directed leftward. The maximum QRS horizontal plane vector is projected on the corrected and uncorrected reference frames in Figure 9A-B.

If the complexes are predominantly positive in all five leads, the vector is an indeterminable number of degrees anteriorly. If all complexes are predominantly negative, the vector is an unknown number of degrees posteriorly.

Some rules of thumb are useful in roughly estimating by inspection the direction of a vector from the ECG. A vector is at right angles to the axis of a lead on which an equiphasic complex is present. If the QRS complex of L I is equiphasic, the vector may be at 270° (−90°) or at 90°. If the complex is positive on aVF, the vector is along the positive half of the axis of aVF, i.e., at 90°, an equiphasic complex on aVL is represented by a vector at right angles to aVL which coincides with the axis of L II. If the complex is positive on L II, the vector is along the positive half of the L II axis at 60°.

A vector is directed along the axis of the lead on which the complex is of greatest magnitude. If the complex is predominantly positive, the vector is along the positive half of the axis of the lead; if negative, along the negative half.

The calculation of a vector from the ECG is only approximate unless two or more leads are taken simultaneously so that identical time intervals of the complexes are selected. The beginning or the end of one or the other complex may be isoelectric because of phase differences across the leads and as a result different time intervals may be measured. Practically this is of little importance for vectors derived from the ECG are only approximate.

THE VECTORCARDIOGRAM

The electrical activity of the heart produces a myriad of forces. The vectorcardiogram (VCG) by electronic selection displays them as resultant vectors which represent all the activity taking place at particular intervals of time.

The basic parts of the vectorcardiograph are a cathode ray tube with a contained cathode and anode metal plate. The anode is at high positive potential so that a strong electrical field exists between it and the cathode. Electrons emitted by the cathode pass at high velocity through a hole in the anode as a fine beam of cathode rays, which in turn passes between pairs of deflection plates set at right angles to each other and strikes the inner surface of the viewing screen of the tube. The deflection plates are connected to the patient by lead wires. If the plates are uncharged or equally charged, the beam remains at a fixed point on the screen. When a potential difference is present between the plates, the beam is deflected toward the positively charged plates and away from the negative ones. A potential difference across the horizontal plates in the X axis displaces the beam from side to side, and a difference between the vertical plates in the Y axis displaces the beam upward or downward. The magnitude and direction of the movement of the beam is the resultant of the potential differences across the X and Y plates. The magnitude of the movement of the beam can be regulated by a selector switch. The beam can be projected on the transverse (horizontal), sagittal, and frontal planes. A timer is used to increase or decrease the intensity of the beam so that portions of the continuous loops made up by joining the termini of many resultant vectors are blanked out at predetermined time intervals. The usual time interval selected is 0.0025 second (2.5 msec). For permanent records the loops are photographed directly from the oscilloscopic screen.

THE NORMAL VECTORCARDIOGRAM

The normal vectorcardiogram (VCG) consists of three loops. The P loop is usually the smallest, the T loop is intermediate, and the QRS loop is the largest. All three loops appear to begin and end at the E point (null or isoelectric point) which at the usual amplification also consists of an isoelectric ST vector of very small magnitude (Fig. 14).

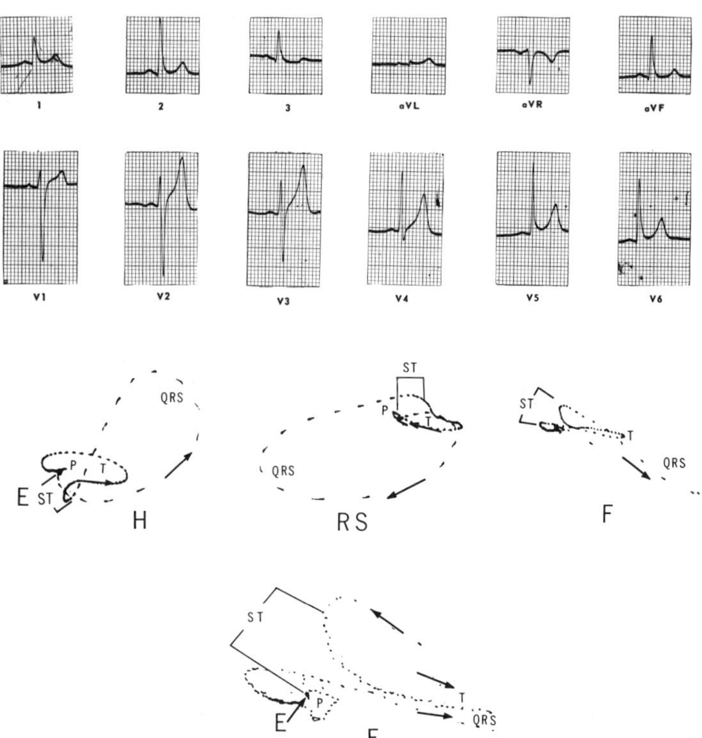

Fig. 14. The ECG and VCG of a normal young man. The P, T and QRS loops are shown with the ST vector and the E point.

P LOOP. The loop is the largest on the sagittal and frontal planes, and its length normally exceeds its width. In the transverse (H) and right sagittal (RS) planes the initial vectors of the loop are anterior from the right atrium, and the terminal vectors are posterior from the left atrium. The mean direction of the loop is inferior and leftward. Inscription is counterclockwise (C-CW) in the transverse (H) and frontal (F) planes and clockwise (CW) in the right sagittal (RS) plane. The magnitude does not exceed 0.18 mv in any plane. The angular range of the maximum P vector is shown in Figure 15.

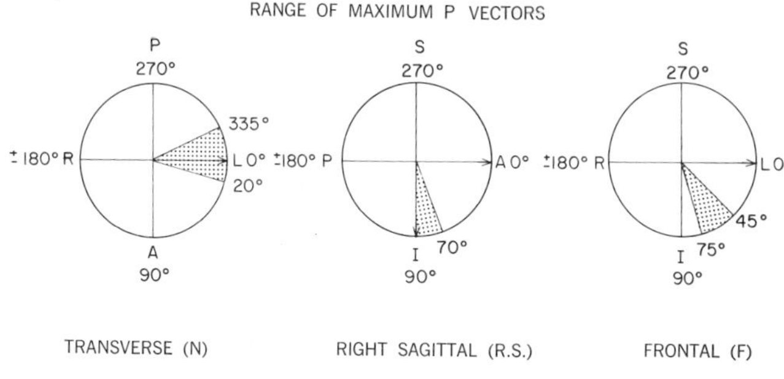

Fig. 15.

ELECTROCARDIOGRAPHIC APPLICATION

When the mean inferior and leftward P vector is projected on the uncorrected frontal reference frame the P wave is upright on L I-II-aV-L but may be positive or negative on L III. In the latter case the vector is not more leftward than 330° (–30) so that the normal P wave remains upright on L II. The normal P wave is always negative on L aVR.

In the horizontal plane the P wave is diphasic (±) in V1 corresponding to the sequential anterior and posterior direction of the initial and terminal P vectors. It is upright on the other precordial leads.

The P wave of the ECG is 0.08 second in duration and the amplitude does not exceed 2.5 mv in the limb leads. The PR interval, from the beginning of the P wave to the onset of the QRS complex or the time for excitation to spread from the SA node to ventricular muscles, does not exceed 0.20 second in the adult. Measuring this interval on the planar VCG is impracticable.

The Ta segment corresponding to the atrial repolarization vector to the right and posteriorly is represented in the ECG in a direction opposite to the direction of the P wave. If these forces are prolonged through ventricular depolarization, they may produce apparent depression of the ST segment.

QRS LOOP. This, the largest of the three loops formed by connecting the termini of successive instantaneous vectors of ventricular depolarization, is oval, elliptical, or triangular and smoothly inscribed without notching. The early and late portions of the loop are slowly inscribed (close spacing of the time dashes) (Fig. 14). The maximum duration of the loop in any of the three planes is 0.1 second (100 msec). The maximum magnitude of the loop (maximum QRS vector) is the distance from the E point to the most distal portion of the loop if the loop is oval or elliptical. The maximum vector of triangular or irregular loops is taken as a half area vector, which by estimation divides the loop into two equal areas. The angular range of the maximum planar QRS vectors is shown in Figure 15.

The term "S loop" refers to terminal forces in the right superior posterior quadrant. A Q loop represents initial forces in the right, anterior, and either superior or inferior quadrant.

The QRS loop has different characteristics in the three planes.

HORIZONTAL. The loop is smooth in contour and C-CW in direction. The maximum vector is 1.5 to 3 times the width of the loop. One-third or less of the area of the loop is anterior to the X axis in the adult with the early initial forces always anterior and in 95 percent of cases rightward. The loop may extend into the right posterior quadrant as an S loop. (Fig. 16A.)

RIGHT SAGITTAL. The loop in this plane is elongated or a figure eight with the initial forces always anterior and either superior or inferior. The maximum vector is inferior and posterior. The terminal portion may form a S loop. In 95 percent of the cases the loop is CW with the remainder either C-CW or figure eight. (Fig. 16B.)

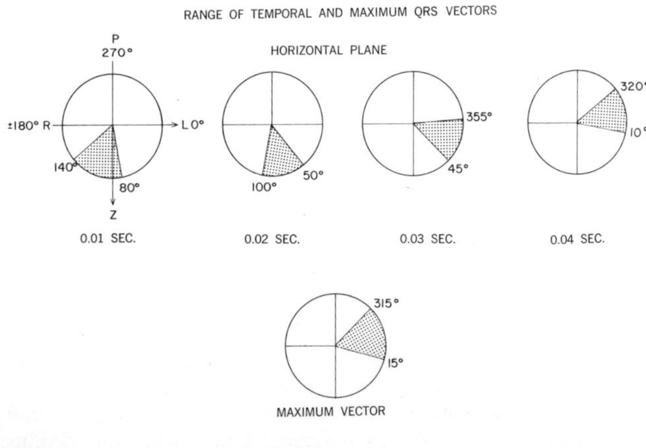

Fig. 16A.

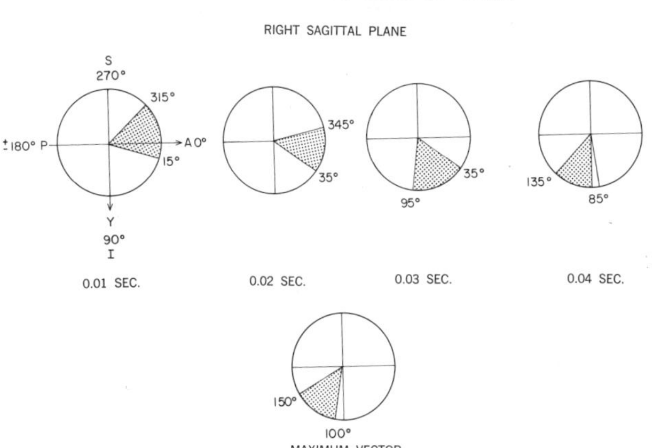

Fig. 16B.

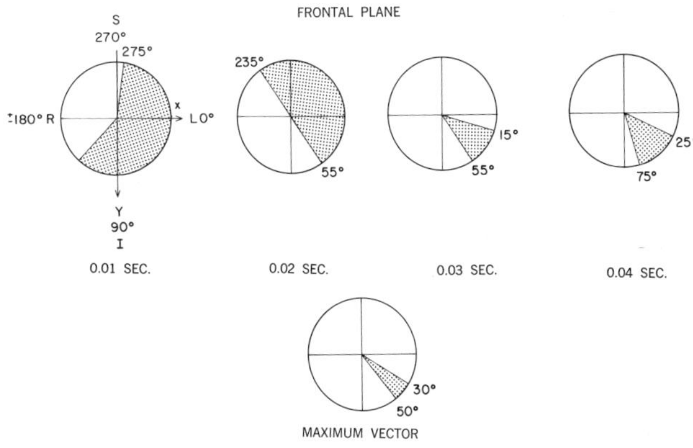

Fig. 16C.

FRONTAL. Contour and inscription vary in this plane from vertical loops which are CW (60 percent), figure eight (25 percent) to horizontal C-CW loops (15 percent). The maximum vector is in the left inferior quadrant. If it is at less than 0°, left axis deviation (LAD) is present; if more than 90°, right axis deviation (RAD). (Fig. 16C.)

ELECTROCARDIOGRAPHIC APPLICATION

The QRS interval in the normal adult does not exceed 0.10 second. In the precordial leads the early anterior forces always record an initial R wave over the right precordium. Absence of the R wave is always abnormal. Since the magnitude of successive vectors increases from right to left as they move from anterior to posterior, the initial R wave gives way to a developing Q wave and the magnitude of the R wave increases. The transitional zone is usually between V3 and V4.

The contour of the bipolar and unipolar QRS complexes depends on the electrical position of the heart. The direction of the maximum vector in the frontal plane reflects the direction of the electrical forces about an anteroposterior axis. When the vector is upward toward the positive half of the axis of L I, the electrical axis is horizontal with the tallest R wave in L I. The more leftward the vector, the less is the amplitude of the R wave on aVF. When the vector is inferior and to the right toward the positive half of the axis of aVF the heart is electrically vertical. In the frontal plane the normal maximum QRS vector is between 330° (–30) and 90°.

The axis of aVR is toward the ventricular cavities. The contour of QRS on this lead depends on the relation of the axis to the septum. If it is toward the right side of the septum, an rS or an rSr′ complex results. The r′ is due to late depolarization of the posterior basal portion of the right ventricle and the right basal septum. When the axis is toward the left septal surface, a QS or Qr complex results.

The contour of aVL and aVF also varies with the electrical position of the heart. In the horizontal position aVF records an rS complex, the r wave being due to septal and apicoanterior depolarization in an anterior, inferior direction and the S wave to posterolateral and basal activation in a superior, leftward, and posterior direction. The activation forces are recorded on aVL as a qS complex. In the vertical position an rS is inscribed on aVL and a qR on a VF.

The electrical position of the heart described by Wilson included the concept of rotation about a longitudinal axis extending from apex to base. With CW rotation the right ventricle rotated anteriorly and leftward and the left ventricle posteriorly and rightward. This moved the transitional zone to the left so that V1-2 resembled aVL and V5-6 resembled aVF, for more of the positive portion of the electrical field generated by the right ventricle was directed toward the aVL electrode. With C-CW rotation the left ventricle moved to the right and anteriorly, and the right ventricle moved to the left and posteriorly. The transitional zone of the field moved rightward so that V5-6 resembled aVL and V1-2 resembled aVF.

It is emphasized that rotation in this sense applies to the electrical field and not to the anatomic position of the heart. Grant using autopsy material and Prinzmetal experimentally have shown that, despite the presence of CW or C-CW rotation in an electrical sense, the septum remained relatively parallel to the frontal plane so that anatomic, longitudinal rotation cannot account for the contour of the QRS complex on the different leads.

In the ECG the term "intrinsicoid deflection" refers to the time interval from the onset of the QRS to the peak of the R wave. It is the measure of the ventricular activation time. In the right precordial leads it ranges from 0.015 to 0.035 second; in the left leads from 0.035 to 0.05 second. The shorter interval over the right or the early R peak is due to the initial septal and apicoanterior vectors; the longer interval on the left, to the completion of later activation of the left ventricular free wall and base. A delay in the intrinsicoid deflection is characteristic of block in the conduction system.

ST VECTOR. At the usual amplification of the VCG an ST vector is not apparent. With increased magnification the E point is actually the beginning of the P loop. None of the loops is closed. An ST vector extends from the beginning of the QRS loop to the beginning of the T loop. Spatially it is downward, leftward, and anterior.

ST SEGMENT. This in the ECG corresponds to the ST vector which normally is anterior to the frontal plane so that in the limb leads the segment from the end of the QRS complex to the beginning of the T wave is usually isoelectric. In youth early repolarization forces may be increased in magnitude and be more anteriorly directed so as to produce upward displacement of the ST segment, particularly in leads V3-4. This normal variant may be recognized by the narrow angle formed by the vectors of the QRS and T wave and by the ST vector being approximately parallel to an increased mean T vector.

T LOOP. The latter phase of repolarization is responsible for the successive instantaneous vectors of recovery represented by the T loop which consists of a slowly inscribed efferent limb and a more rapidly inscribed afferent limb. The loop, open or elliptical in one plane, may be linear in the others. The length:width ratio is 2.5:1 or greater. The direction of inscription usually follows that of the QRS loop. The angle of the maximum T vector is best considered in relation to the angle of the maximum QRS vector. The enclosed angles do not exceed 40° in the frontal plane or 80° in the horizontal. In infancy the T vector points posteriorly away from the predominant right ventricle. This direction may persist into adult life. In the adult successive T vectors are directed leftward and downward. The range of the maximum T vector is shown in Figure 17.

ELECTROCARDIOGRAPHIC APPLICATION. The contour of the T wave mirrors the normal velocity differential of the T loop. The ascending limb is slowly inscribed and slurred; the descending limb is more rapidly inscribed so that the wave is normally asymmetrical. Because of the leftward and downward direction of the maximum T vector the T waves are upright in the limb leads except aVR and upright in the precordial leads from V2 to V6. In V1 the T wave may be positive or negative. As a rule they are in the same direction as the QRS complex. Persistence of the infantile, posteriorly-directed T vector may invert the T wave in some adults from V1 to V4.

RANGE OF MAXIMUM T VECTORS

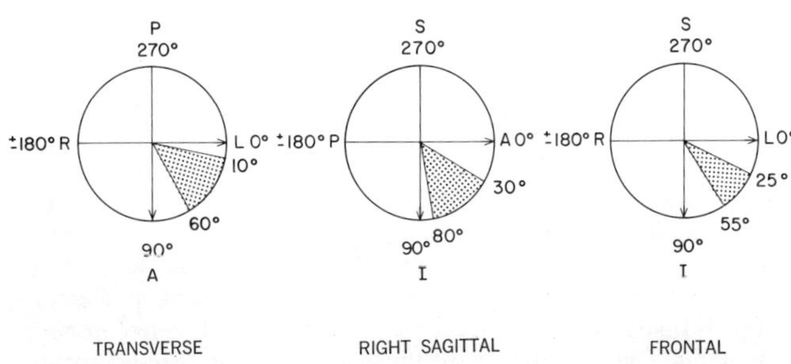

Fig. 17.

QT INTERVAL. Measurement of this interval is most easily done from the ECG. It extends from the beginning of the Q to the end of the T wave. The range in men is 0.24 to 0.48 second; in women 0.22 to 0.42 second depending on the heart rate. The interval is decreased with increased heart rate and digitalis, and increased by quinidine, procainamide and hypocalcemia. In the last instance prolongation is due to the increased duration of the ST segment.

The QT interval, corrected for heart rate may be calculated by Bazett's formula:

$$\frac{QT}{\sqrt{R\text{-}R}} = 0.42 \text{ sec or less}$$

CHAMBER ENLARGEMENT

RIGHT ATRIUM

VCG. The spatial vector in right atrial enlargement (RAE) is increased in magnitude and directed anteriorly, leftward, and inferiorly. The maximum P vector is more vertical than normal and approaches 90°. The duration of the loop is not increased. In the H plane the magnitude of the maximum vector is greater than 0.1 mv and inscription is C-CW; in the RS plane magnitude exceeds 0.18 mv and inscription is CW; in the F plane the loop is C-CW and the magnitude is more than 0.18 mv.

ECG. The voltage of the P wave is increased but not the duration. The wave is peaked on L II-III-aVF because of the more vertical direction of the mean P vector and is predominantly upright in V1-2 due to increased anterior forces. These features are characteristic of P pulmonale.

LEFT ATRIUM

VCG. The spatial vector is mainly posterior, inferior, and leftward. The magnitude may not be increased but posterior forces are especially prominent. The loop is increased in duration and less vertical than normally. In enlargement due to mitral disease, irregular, bifid and mitten-shaped loops are common. The direction of inscription usually follows the normal.

ECG. In V1 the dominant posterior forces project a diphasic P wave (+ –) with the negative portion prolonged and slurred. In the F plane the increased leftward forces and the increased duration of the loop project as a broad, notched P wave greater in duration than 0.10 second on L I-II-aVL-V5-6. The above contour and distribution constitutes P mitrale.

COMBINED ATRIAL ENLARGEMENT

VCG. Both the early anterior forces from the right atrium and the later posterior left atrial forces are increased in magnitude especially in the H and RS planes. In the latter plane the loop is often broad and triangular. Inscription is normal in all planes.

ECG. In V1 the P wave is diphasic (+ –), initially tall and peaked, and terminally broad and slurred. In L II-III-aVF the P wave is not only tall but increased in duration.

In general the magnitude of the P wave in relation to that of the QRS complex is important. If the magnitude of the P wave in the limb leads is greater than one-third of the QRS amplitude, atrial hypertrophy should be considered.

LEFT VENTRICULAR HYPERTROPHY (LVH)

VCG. The normal electrical preponderance of the left ventricle is reflected in the major forces of the VCG. In LVH such forces are exaggerated and rotate more posteriorly toward the effective electrical site of the left ventricle. The main feature of LVH is an abnormally posterior maximum QRS vector of increased magnitude directed leftward, posteriorly, and inferiorly. The initial forces tend to move leftward from their usual rightward position. The terminal forces are posterior, superior, and always leftward. The increased magnitude exceeds 2.0 mv in the H and F planes and 1.6 mv in the RS plane. LVH is one of the few VCG entities that require accurate measurement of the maximum vector for diagnosis.

The H plane QRS loop is narrower than normally and usually C-CW with initial forces rightward and anterior. One fifth of cases are figure eight loops with the initial vectors to the left and anterior. In rare instances the loop may be CW. Figure eight and CW loops are related to left ventricular conduction defects and resemble the sequence of activation in left bundle branch block (LBBB) without prolongation.

In the RS plane initial vectors remain anterior but are inferior. Terminal vectors are superior. The inscription is CW.

The maximum F plane vector is more superior than normally, but contrary to some proposed criteria LAD is not present unless there is a conduction defect in the anterior (superior) division of the left bundle. The initial vectors are often leftward and inferior rather than rightward. The terminal vectors remain to the left. Inscription is C-CW.

ECG. The increased voltage and the abnormally posterior direction of the maximum forces in LVH are manifested in the ECG by increased S wave amplitude in the right and R wave amplitude in the left precordial leads. The following precordial voltage criteria have been proposed:

1. R V5 or R V6 > 26 mm
2. R V5 or 6 S V1 or 2 > 35 mm
3. R V6 > R V5

In the limb leads the leftward and inferior direction of the initial forces produces a diminished or absent Q wave in LI-aVL-V5-6 which resembles the contour of LBBB. The more posterior and superior the maximum vector, the less will be the forces projected on the frontal plane, and for this reason, evidence of hypertrophy may be absent in the limb leads. However, the accepted voltage criteria in the limb leads are:

1. Lewis index (R1+S3) – (R3+S1) > 17 mm
2. R1 + S3 > 26 mm
3. RaVL > 15 mm
4. RaVF > 20 mm

The voltage criteria of LVH are not reliable in individuals below the age of 35.

The T loop and the ST vector are to the right, anterior, and superior. The T loop, either CW or C-CW, is inscribed with normal conduction differential. The QRS-T angle often approaches 180° so that the T wave in the left precordial leads decreases in magnitude to the point that T V1 > TV5-6. The ST segment tends to be opposite the QRS complex and in the same direction as the T wave.

RIGHT VENTRICULAR HYPERTROPHY (RVH)

Considerable hypertrophy of the relatively thin right ventricular wall must be present to overcome the preponderant forces of the left ventricle. The degree of hypertrophy may produce changes ranging from isolated RAD to VCG loops which are oriented entirely anteriorly due to resultant vectors directed toward the anatomic site of the right ventricle anteriorly to the right, superiorly, or inferiorly. The net effect of increasing degrees of RVH is to increase the magnitude of early anteriorly-directed vectors so that the initial portion of the loop is more anterior than normally; to affect the mid and terminal vectors so that the afferent limb of the loop moves anterior to the efferent though the loop is mainly leftward, or to affect all vectors so that the entire loop is displaced to the right and anterior.

The QRS loops of RVH are more varied than those of LVH and are influenced not only by the degree of hypertrophy but also by selective anatomic hypertrophy and the effects of diastolic or systolic overload of the RV. In general RVH may affect early vectors, mid and terminal vectors, or all vectorial forces; sometimes, the only clue to the presence of RVH may be RAD in individuals over 35 provided that they are not tall and linear and that chest deformity is not present.

DISPLACEMENT OF EARLY VECTORS

The effect of increased magnitude of early vectors is most apparent in the H and RS planes. The loop remains normally inscribed but the vectors up to 0.03 second are anterior to the normal 320° to 10° range due to exaggerated forces from the apicoanterior and lower anterior RV wall. More than one-third of the loop is anterior to the X axis in the adult and more than one-half after the age of three. In the F plane the loop is more vertical than normally. If the maximum vector is more than 90°, the initial forces are leftward and inferior.

This type corresponds to the normal right ventricular preponderance in infancy.

The T loop is leftward and posterior. An ST vector is not present.

The anterior loop type of RVH may be present in early pulmonary hypertension secondary to mitral stenosis.

ECG. In the precordial leads a relatively tall R wave (>6 mm) and an R/S ratio > 1 is present in V1. An S wave projects on L I-V5-6. The T wave is inverted in V1-2. A relatively vertical frontal axis is present.

DISPLACEMENT OF THE MID AND TERMINAL VECTORS

In this situation two types of loop are found. Both have these common characteristics in the H plane: 1) initial anterior forces are leftward or less to the right than usual, 2) the larger area of the loop is rightward, 3) the main portion of the loop is anterior, 4) a significant terminal conduction delay is not present, and 5) the maximum F plane vector is $\overset{=}{>} 90^\circ$.

The first type in this group is a figure-eight loop with the afferent limb either anterior or posterior to the efferent limb. The second type is an anterior, open, mainly CW loop to the right.

The T loop is posterior and leftward with CW inscription in the H and F planes and C-CW in the RS plane. An ST vector if present is superior, rightward and posterior opposite the QRS loop.

Loops in this group are found with selective hypertrophy of the basal RV such as occurs in moderate mitral stenosis and increased diastolic overload in atrial septal defect.

ECG. The vectors project on the right precordial leads as R, Rs, RsR′, rSr′ or RS complexes with significant S waves in L I-V5-6. Asymmetric inversion of the T wave is present in the right precordial leads. The frontal axis is vertical and diphasic QRS complexes may be present in all the unipolar limb leads with a tall late R wave in aVr.

DISPLACEMENT OF ALL VECTORS OF THE QRS LOOP

In this group inscription of the H plane QRS loop is CW. The larger area of the loop is rightward and entirely anterior. The T loop is posterior and leftward with inscription reversed to CW in the H and F planes and C-CW in the RS plane. The ST vector is posterior and leftward, either inferior or superior.

This type of loop occurs with generalized RV hypertrophy, as seen in pulmonary stenosis, tetralogy of Fallot, and marked pulmonary artery hypertension due to mitral stenosis or cor pulmonale.

ECG. An Rs, RsR′ or qR complex is present in the right precordial leads. On the left an RS or rS complex is present. In the limb leads increased rightward forces diminish the R wave and increase the S wave in L I. The inferior direction of the loop increases the amplitude of the R wave in L III-aVF-II. The T wave may be inverted across the precordium and in the inferior limb leads.

In all groups of RVH the diagnosis is reinforced by ancillary findings of P. mitrale or P. pulmonale.

BIVENTRICULAR HYPERTROPHY (BVH)

The VCG findings in hypertrophy of both ventricles may be dominated by either right or left ventricular forces; the forces may balance each other producing in effect a normal loop, or the individual characteristics of right or left hypertrophy may present separately. This last possibility is responsible for increased anterior and posterior forces which are greater than the lateral extension of the H plane loop. Such a loop, common in BVH in infants and children, is also common in congenital heart disease in adults with ventricular septal defect or patent ductus arteriosus. In the ECG this QRS loop produces the Katz-Wachtel complex with large diphasic deflections in the midprecordial leads.

In two-thirds of adult patients with BVH another QRS loop type can be identified by the following characteristics in the H plane.

1. The QRS loop is C-CW.
2. Initial forces are anterior, either to the right or left.
3. The half area vector approximates the Z axis.
4. An S loop constitutes 45 percent of the time duration of the QRS loop.
5. The maximum S vector is 70 percent of the magnitude of the maximum QRS vector.
6. Conduction time is not increased.
7. RAD is present in the F plane CW loop.

In the precordial leads the magnitude of the S wave increases markedly between V1 and V2 and an S wave is present in V6. RAD is present.

COMPLETE LEFT BUNDLE BRANCH BLOCK (CLBBB)

A block in the left bundle alters the normal sequence of ventricular activation. Septal depolarization instead of being from left to right and posterior to anterior is reversed. Initial activation is from right to left and anterior to posterior in the lower one-third of the right septal surface and to the right and anterior over the right ventricular anterior wall. The resultant vector of these two forces is usually leftward, anterior and inferior. A variation in the direction of the resultant vector is possible if the forces of the anterior RV wall are dominant. In this case the resultant vector will be to the right, anterior, and inferior.

The second vector of activation represents forces arising from the left septal mass and the adjacent free wall of the LV. It is directed to the left, inferiorly, and posteriorly. The resultant vector of the last area to be activated, the lateral wall of the LV, is leftward and posterior, either superior or inferior.

The VCG characteristics of CLBBB are:

1. Narrow QRS loops of increased magnitude and duration (> 0.12 sec), mainly CW in the H and RS planes and C-CW in the F plane.
2. An abnormal initial vector usually leftward and anterior.
3. The afferent limb of the QRS loop is to the left of the efferent limb.
4. A conduction delay in at least two planes involves the mid- and afferent portions of the loops.

The ST vector and the T loop are anterior and rightward, either superior or inferior, almost 180° away from the axis of the QRS loop. The position of the T loop is secondary to abnormal depolarization, for normal inscription velocity is maintained. In the H and F planes the T loop is CW, and C-CW in the RS.

ECG. The duration of the QRS complex is > 0.12 second. The intrinsicoid deflection exceeds 0.5 second.

The leftward direction of the initial vectors is mirrored by an absent Q wave in L I-aVL-V5-6. The peak of the R is slurred or notched and the terminal limb of the wave is thickened in the same leads. The magnitude of the R wave is small and practically constant in V1-2-3 and suddenly increases in V4. An absent R in V1-2-3 is uncommon without complicating myocardial infarction.

Depression of the ST segment and T wave negativity are present in leads with a predominant R wave (L I-aVL-V5-6). The ST segment is elevated and the T wave upright in leads with predominantly negative QRS complexes (V1-2-3).

INCOMPLETE LEFT BUNDLE BRANCH BLOCK (ILBBB)

This type of block is due to incomplete interruption of the LB so that conduction is at a slower than normal rate. The QRS duration is less than 0.12 second. Activation follows the same pathways as in CLBBB. The QRS loop in magnitude and orientation is the same as in CLBBB but mid- and terminal conduction delays are absent.

ECG. The Q wave is diminutive or absent in L I-V5-6. Tall R waves are present in these leads and deep S waves in the right precordial leads. The ST segments and T waves are opposite the QRS complexes.

The abnormal direction of initial vectors in LBBB obscure the Q wave, the hallmark of myocardial infarction. The diagnosis is difficult except in septal infarct which directs initial forces to the right and produces a Q wave in LI-aVL-V5-6 in the presence of LBBB. If the rightward vector is also posterior QS complexes appear in the precordial leads. The ST vector and the maximum T vector of infarction in LBBB are directed respectively toward and away from the infarcted area so that ST segment elevation and T wave inversion are present in LI-aVL and the precordial leads.

COMPLETE RIGHT BUNDLE BRANCH BLOCK (CRBBB)

In this conduction defect the early sequence of activation through the intact LB is normal so that initial and midtemporal vectors are in their usual position. Late and terminal vectors, however, are displaced anteriorly and rightward, either superiorly or inferiorly toward the position of the right ventricle which is the last chamber to be activated. Activation time is prolonged to at least 0.12 second.

The QRS loop of RBBB consists of two parts; the first, normally oriented in the usual type, consists of the initial efferent and early afferent limbs; the second is a slowly inscribed, fingerlike appendage due to delayed activation of the right side of the septum and the RV wall. This second part of the loop as a distinct terminal conduction delay in at least two planes is anterior and rightward, inferior or superior and is the most distinctive feature of RBBB.

The characteristics of RBBB, most apparent in the H plane, are:

1. The major portion of the QRS loop is C-CW.
2. The terminal conduction delay is CW or C-CW to the right and anterior at approximately 150°.

With this type loop an ST vector is not present. T The loop is directed 180° away from the maximum vector of the terminal conduction delay.

Such a loop may or may not be associated with clinical heart disease.

Some variations in the inscription and the position of the QRS loop may be found in RBBB.

1. The midtemporal vectors may be anterior to the E point with the loop C-CW and the conduction delay CW. This variety may be associated with atrial septal defect, pulmonic stenosis, or pulmonary disease with or without cor pulmonale.
2. The entire loop may be anterior to the X axis with the main portion CW and the conduction delay C-CW. This form may be present in RVH with either systolic or diastolic overload.
3. The entire QRS loop and the conduction delay may be CW. This is commonly associated with marked RVH.

The RS plane has essentially the same features as the H plane. The direction of inscription varies when the loop is inferior but is usually C-CW with superior loops.

In the F plane the conduction delay is less apparent. It may be inferior, horizontal along the X axis or superior. When inferior it is inscribed more commonly CW; when superior, C-CW. In the latter case LAD is present representing a block in the superior division of the left bundle in addition to RBBB.

In the advanced forms of RBBB an ST vector is present to the left and posterior paralleling the maximum T vector. The T loop is inscribed with normal conduction differential.

ECG. The QRS complex is 0.12 second in CRBBB. The intrinsicoid deflection is greater than 0.035 second. An rsR′ or rSR′ complex is present in V1. The initial r is due to the initial rightward and anterior forces. The S wave varies in depth. Posterior midtemporal vectors project deep S waves. With anterior vectors the S wave may be small, absent or represented by a notch on the R wave. The R′ is slurred and corresponds to the anterior rightward conduction delay. The magnitude of the R wave is decreased in V5-6 and terminal, slurred S waves are present.

In the limb leads the conduction delay may project inferiorly, horizontally or superiorly. In the last instance in addition to the S wave in L I there will be S waves in LII-III-aVF and LAD will be present.

INCOMPLETE RIGHT BUNDLE BRANCH BLOCK (IRBBB)

This is a debatable diagnosis. Some consider it warranted when the features of CRBBB are present but the QRS duration is less than 0.12 second and as short as 0.09 second. Others make the diagnosis on the basis of a QRS loop which is C-CW with a terminal conduction delay of more than normal duration in the right posterior quadrant of the H plane.

In the ECG an rsR′ complex is present in V1 if the terminal vectors are anterior or the terminal R′ is of greater magnitude than the initial R wave. IRBBB may also include the S1-S2-S3 pattern.

When confronted with an rSr complex in V1, one must be certain that the electrodes have not been placed in the third interspace for, with terminal vectors superior and rightward, this interspace will record an R wave in V1.

MASQUERADING BUNDLE BRANCH BLOCK

In this entity the F plane shows the features of LBBB with marked LAD, and the precordial leads resemble RBBB with predominantly upright complexes in V1-2. Higher than normal electrode placement may produce such precordial patterns.

LEFT VENTRICULAR PARIETAL BLOCK

This type of block, which is true LAD, is manifested in the VCG by a maximum vector more superior or leftward than 0° in the frontal plane. The maximum QRS vector approaches the X axis with increasing age, i.e., the heart assumes a more horizontal electrical position, but the leftward direction does not become superior. Maximum forces more leftward or superior than 0° are common in coronary artery disease with myocardial fibrosis which impairs conduction in the superior, anterior division of the LB. Contrary to some criteria LAD is not a necessary feature of LVH.

ECG. In the uncorrected lead system a maximum QRS vector superior to 330° (–30°) constitutes parietal block (LAD) and is recorded on L III-II-aVf as predominantly negative QRS complexes.

PREEXCITATION

Wolf-Parkinson-White Syndrome (W-P-W),
Anomalous AV Conduction,
Accelerated Conduction,
Bundle of Kent Syndrome

Preexcitation is generally considered to be due to a functioning accessory bundle of Kent bridging the atrioventricular groove between the right atrium and right ventricle, the right atrium and the left ventricle, or the left atrium and the left ventricle. The effect of this accessory pathway is to permit the atrial impulse to by-pass the normal delay in the AV node and to shorten transmission time between the atrium and the ventricle. The PR interval is shortened and the QRS interval is lengthened by the extent of the PR shortening. The P-QRS interval remains unchanged. The spread of the anomalous impulse in ventricular muscle is slow in accord with the decreased rate of muscle transmission and produces slowly inscribed forces as the initial and early vectors of the QRS loop. The impulse eventually enters the conduction system, and the rate and direction of further spread are normal for that part of the conduction system that the impulse enters. At the same time the atrial impulse after undergoing normal delay in the AV node enters the conduction system so that ventricular activation is the result of the fusion of two impulses.

Prinzmetal believes that preexcitation results from injury to certain fiber tracts in the AV node so that the atrial impulse passes more rapidly than normally to the ventricles.

The characteristics of preexcitation are most completely displayed in the ECG, for the PR shortening is difficult to identify in the VCG. It should be mentioned however that W-P-W may occur with heart block. In the VCG the anomalous conduction is represented by the delta segment of the QRS loop. This is an initial conduction delay of up to 0.08 second which in one or more planes abruptly changes direction when the impulse enters the conduction system. The delta segment of the QRS loop may be either anterior or posterior; anterior when there is early activation of the basal septal and posterobasal LV; posterior when there is early activation of the anterolateral and basal septal areas of the RV.

ECG. Two main types of preexcitation are described. In both the PR interval is classically less than 0.12 second and the QRS interval is between 0.11 to 0.18 second.

Type A has predominantly upright QRS complexes and upright delta waves as a slur or notch on the upstroke in all precordial leads. In this type RV activation follows LV and the QRS has the contour of RBBB.

Type B shows predominantly negative QRS complexes in the right precordial leads and a negative delta wave due to posteriorly directed delta vectors. Preexcitation in this instance may normalize an existent RBBB if activation is distal to the block.

The ST segments and the T wave are opposite in direction to the QRS complex.

In the F plane preexcitation forces may be markedly superior and leftward and produce significant Q waves in L III-II-aVF which simulate inferior infarction. When the forces are anterior they may obscure the initial Q wave of anterior infarction.

CLINICAL IMPLICATIONS OF W-P-W

Preexcitation may cause no symptoms. In the ECG it should not be confused with bundle branch block. Alternating normal and preexcitation beats must be differentiated from atrial, premature beats with aberrant conduction and fusion beats with bundle branch block. In atrial fibrillation the ventricular rate may not be controlled by digitalis when a functioning bundle of Kent is present. Digitalis lengthens conduction time through the AV node and predisposes to conduction through the accessory bundle.

Paroxysmal atrial tachycardia is the most common complication of preexcitation. During the paroxysm the QRS complexes are of normal configuration due to normally directed transmission through the AV node and retrograde conduction through the bundle of Kent. When the tachycardia ceases, the QRS complexes again manifest a delta wave. Quinidine is the drug of choice in paroxysmal tachycardia associated with the Wolff-Parkinson-White syndrome.

MYOCARDIAL INFARCTION

Myocardial infarction is due to a critical decrease in the blood supply which may affect the entire thickness of the myocardial wall, the endocardium alone or scattered intramural areas. Depending on the extent of the decrease in the blood supply, infarction may be transmural, subendocardial, or intramural (nontransmural).

The following changes occur in transmural infarction:

1. Ischemia and injury to muscle cells manifested by abnormal ST vectors.
2. Ischemia manifested by changes in the T vectors.
3. The above changes plus death of the involved areas of the myocardium manifested mainly by changes in the resultant 0.025 to 0.04 second vectors of the QRS loop.

ST VECTOR. An abnormal ST vector is the earliest change to appear in transmural infarction. At the end of depolarization the area of injury continues to exert positive polarity so that the ST vector is directed toward the site of injury which is the positive side of the electrical field. With aging of an infarct, usually in a matter of days, the ST vector returns to the normal position. Persistence of an abnormal vector beyond 6 weeks may be due to a ventricular aneurysm.

T VECTOR. The first area to depolarize is the first to repolarize. The necrotic area of an infarct does not depolarize so the T vectors representing unopposed repolarization forces are directed away from the infarct in the direction of intact muscle.

Q VECTOR. Dead tissue in the infarcted area does not contribute to the electrical activity of the heart at particular time intervals. Depending on the location and the extent of the necrotic area, resultant vectors are displaced, in general, away from the infarcted area at that particular time interval at which depolarization would ordinarily occur. The vectors affected are those usually between 0.025 to 0.04 second.

As a rule anterior wall infarcts displace resultant QRS vectors posteriorly and leftward and are best displayed in the H and RS planes. Inferior infarcts (formerly called "posterior") displace resultant vectors superiorly in the F and RS planes. True posterior infarcts allow the resultant vectors to shift anteriorly in the H and RS planes. In each case all resultant vectors are displaced to a greater or lesser degree for the normal electrical balance of the heart has been disturbed.

In general, the electrical effects of infarction coincide with the area involved anatomically. Lack of correlation is usually due to the effects of multiple infarcts.

It has also been proposed that the effects of myocardial infarction are due to disturbances in the conduction system due to impairment of the blood supply. This theory proposes that the adequacy of the blood supply to the conduction system determines the resultant vectorial forces and attributes the QRS-T changes to an altered sequence of intraventricular activation.

The anterior (superior) division of the left bundle is supplied by the anterior descending branch of the left coronary artery. If blood flow through this vessel is compromised, conduction along the anterior division is delayed and is transmitted initially posteriorly and inferiorly along the unaffected posterior (inferior) division. This results in the initial forces in the VCG being posterior and inferior and records in the ECG Q waves in V1-4 and, depending on the extent of involvement, also in L I-aVL. Terminal activation of the superior lateral left ventricle then occurs anteriorly and to the left through the superior division in which conduction has been delayed. These forces are recorded in the ECG as terminal R waves in the leads noted above.

According to the conduction theory the T loop changes of infarction are secondary to altered intraventricular conduction. The inferior, posterior left ventricle being the first area to be depolarized is the first to repolarize and in the same direction. These forces are recorded as inverted T waves in those leads with initial Q waves.

Impaired blood supply through the right coronary artery delays conduction through the posterior (inferior) division of the left bundle and the AV node. This delay results in initial activation of the superior left ventricle in a superior, leftward and anterior direction and terminally downward through the intact inferior division. With this sequence in conduction initial forces are registered in the ECG as Q waves in L III-II-aVF and R waves of increased amplitude in V1-2. Repolarization forces, superior and anterior, project as inverted T waves in the leads with significant Q waves.

ANTERIOR MYOCARDIAL INFARCTION

ANTEROSEPTAL INFARCTS

Anteroseptal infarcts involve the anterior part of the IV septum and the paraseptal anterior left ventricular wall resulting in a loss of normal anterior, rightward and superior forces. As a result early vectors up to 0.02 second are directed posteriorly and leftward and the early efferent limb loses its normal anterior convexity. Both of these features are apparent in the H plane which is inscribed C-CW.

In the RS plane the loop is CW and initially posterior and inferior. The F plane is not characteristic for the abnormal forces are perpendicular to the plane.

In all types of anterior infarction the ST vector is to a variable degree rightward, anterior, and inferior. The T loop is uniformly inscribed and directed posteriorly and to the left.

ECG. The initial leftward and posterior direction of the QRS loop is responsible for a QS complex in V1-2 and the loss of the normal Q wave in V5-6. The limb leads are normal.

MIDANTERIOR INFARCTS

Midanterior infarcts affect forces arising from the anterior wall of the LV. The normal initial anterior and rightward forces are not affected. In the H plane the loop is C-CW. The 0.02 to 0.03 second vectors are posterior and leftward. Part of the efferent limb tends to be concave anteriorly.

In the RS plane initial forces are also preserved, but the early efferent limb is posterior. Inscription is generally CW. Since the abnormal vectors are displaced anteroposteriorly, no changes are present in the F plane.

ECG. Abnormal Q waves are present in V3-4 with qR or QS complexes. The normal r wave is preserved in V1-2 and a small q wave in V5-6 because of intact initial forces. The limb leads are normal.

ANTEROLATERAL INFARCTS

Forces generated by the normal anterolateral wall are anterior and leftward. Infarction of this area does not affect initial forces but displaces later resultant vectors posteriorly and rightward, changes which are most apparent in the H plane. The initial forces are exaggerated rightward and anterior. The efferent limb is posterior and to the right of the afferent so that the loop is CW.

The RS plane is not diagnostic. The F plane records the left to right displacement. The loop is C-CW. Initial forces are normal but the efferent limb is to the right and inferior. The maximum vector is rightward.

ECG. V1-2 record normal rS complexes. Prominent Q waves are present in V5-6 because of the rightward displacement of the efferent forces. Depending on the degree of the rightward displacement QS or QR complexes may be present in V3-4. Q waves of 0.04 second are present in LI-aVL, but the magnitude of the R wave is reduced in these leads because of the vertical position of the maximum vector.

EXTENSIVE ANTERIOR INFARCTS

These present with the combined features of anteroseptal, midanterior and anterolateral infarction. The QRS loop is CW or a figure eight. Anterior forces are completely absent and the loop is entirely posterior in the H and RS planes.

ECG. QS or QR complexes are present across the precordium with significant Q waves in LI-II-aVL.

INFERIOR INFARCTS

The inferior wall of the LV, formerly called the "posterior wall" is supplied by the right coronary artery. Infarction of this area which is, in fact, the lower third of the posterior wall results in dominant superior and leftward forces opposite the involved area. The abnormal forces are vertical and are apparent mainly in the F and RS planes.

The F plane is characteristic with:

1. Superior forces either to the right or left for at least 0.025 second with magnitude greater than 0.16 mv.
2. A QRS loop either entirely CW or with the proximal portion CW. The entire loop may be superior to the X axis and concave inferiorly.

In the RS plane the QRS is CW, superior the Z axis for 0.025 second and anterior.

A conduction defect to the right but superior is common in inferior infarction.

The ST vector is left and anterior. The T loop is superior and leftward and opposite the QRS in inscription.

ECG. Because of the superior direction of the initial forces abnormal Q waves are present in L III-II-aVF.

INFEROLATERAL INFARCTS

In this type normal inferior and leftward forces are unbalanced. The early portion of the QRS is displaced superiorly and to the right; features of this are best displayed in the F plane. The loop is CW. The initial forces are to the right, superior, and of greater than normal magnitude.

ECG. In addition to the abnormal Q wave of inferior infarction in L III-II-aVF, abnormal Q waves are also present in L I-V5-6 due to the abnormal rightward forces.

POSTERIOR INFARCTS

This type primarily involves the posterobasal (dorsal) area of the LV, the last portion of the chamber to be activated. Normally, forces from this area are posteriorly directed, but with infarction unopposed anterior forces predominate and resultant vectors are displaced anteriorly. This shift of forces is best displayed in the H and RS planes. In typical cases, at least two thirds of the QRS loop is anterior to the X axis. Displacement affects mainly the afferent limb which may show an anterior convexity. Normal C-CW inscription may persist but if the afferent limb is anterior to the efferent CW rotation or a figure-eight loop may result.

In the RS plane the QRS is mainly anterior and usually CW.

The ST vector is posterior, superior, and leftward. The T loop is prominent and its position is important. It is at least 70° anterior and even more to the right if the lateral wall is also involved. The location of the T loop is of importance in differentiating the anterior QRS loop of posterior infarction from that of RVH. In the latter instance, the T loop is posterior. The more commonly vertical F plane axis in RVH is also a differential point as is the presence of right or left atrial enlargement.

ECG. The voltage and the duration of the R wave is increased in V1-2 and that of the S wave decreased. The RS ratio is often greater than unity. The T waves are prominent and upright in the right precordial leads.

POSTINFARCTION BLOCK

This type of conduction defect may appear in the acute stage of infarction or develop later in the course. It may be transient or permanent. Two types of postinfarction block exist:

1. Intrainfarction block which is a delay of conduction through the infarcted area.
2. Peri-infarction block or a delay of conduction around the infarcted area.

In the VCG intrainfarction block is present if there is an initial conduction delay of 20 msec or more or if there is a delay of 10 msec within an abnormal Q loop. In the ECG the frequently present slurring of all or part of the Q wave of infarction is the counterpart of this conduction delay.

Peri-infarction block in the VCG is manifested by a terminal delay greater than 30 msec which is located opposite the abnormal vectors of infarction. The QRS duration may or may not exceed the normal. The delay is never anterior and to the right as it is in RBBB; it is not a midconduction delay, as is present in LBBB. Moreover, in LBBB the angle between initial and terminal vectors is rarely greater than 45°. When this angle is more than 100° in the presence of infarction, the cause is peri-infarction block and not LBBB.

Two types of peri-infarction block can be identified, anterolateral and inferior. In both types of peri-infarction block the angle between the initial and terminal vectors is greater than 100°.

ANTEROLATERAL PERI-INFARCTION BLOCK

The initial vectors are rightward, posterior, and inferior away from the infarct. They project Q waves on L I-aVL-V5-6 and R wave on L III-aVF. The terminal vectors, directed toward the infarct, project terminal R waves on complexes with an initial Q wave, and S waves on those with an initial R wave.

INFERIOR PERI-INFARCTION BLOCK

The initial vectors away from the infarct are leftward, superior, and anterior and project as Q waves on L III-II-aVF and as R waves on L I-aVL-V5-6. The terminal vectors rightward, inferior, and posterior inscribe R waves on leads with initial Q waves and S waves on those with initial R waves.

MYOCARDIAL INFARCTION WITH BUNDLE BRANCH BLOCK

WITH RBBB. In RBBB terminal vectors are affected but initial ones are normally positioned. Since infarction primarily involves the initial vectors, the usual evidence of infarction is not masked.

WITH LBBB. Here the problem is difficult since LBBB affects the initial vectors diagnostic of infarction. However, four sites of infarction can be identified in the presence of LBBB.

1. Infarction of the lower two-thirds of the IV septum reverses the initial right-to-left septal activation of LBBB so that forces from the apicoanterior RV wall are dominant. The resultant vectors are to the right and anterior, in contrast to the left and anterior forces of uncomplicated LBBB. The remainder of the QRS loop is typical of the block.

ECG. In this and all the following types the QRS interval is prolonged with mid- and terminal slurring of the R wave, and in this type a Q wave is present in L I-aVL-V5-6.

2. Infarction of the lower third of the septum also involves the paraseptal areas of the right and left ventricles. This abolishes all initial anterior forces so that the initial vectors are to the left and posterior and the usual CW inscription of the H plane QRS loop in LBBB is reversed to C-CW.

In this type QS complexes are present from V_1 to V_4. In uncomplicated LBBB, QS complexes may be present from V_1 to V_3. In forty-five percent R waves are present in right precordial leads; 35 percent have absent R V1; 15 percent absent R V1-2; 5 percent absent R V1-2-3.

3. Infarction of the free wall of the LV in the presence of LBBB displaces late vectorial forces away from the site of the infarct so that the afferent limb of the QRS loop in the H plane is posterior and rightward. The loop is C-CW or a figure eight with the afferent limb

to the right of the efferent. Terminal forces to the right are usually present in the F plane.

ECG. S waves are prominent in V 5-6 and less so in L I-aVL.

4. Inferior infarction with LBBB presents no problem. There is markedly superior displacement of the entire QRS loop and an absence of initial inferior forces.

ECG. Diagnostic Q waves are present in L III-II-aVF.

SUBENDOCARDIAL INFARCTION

The diagnosis of subendocardial infarction is rarely made in the ECG unless the anterior wall of the LV is involved. There is considerable evidence that the endocardium does not contribute to the positive potential of cardiac activity so the absence of QRS changes in this type of infarct is not surprising even though necrosis is present. It is a common clinical experience to see tracings without significant Q waves, but with ST depression and symmetrical T wave inversion, which occur suddenly in a setting of chest pain indistinguishable in location and duration from the symptoms of transmural infarction. These changes persist over weeks with increasing negativity of the T waves and moderate alterations in the serum enzymes. The prolonged T wave changes cannot be explained on the basis of continuing ischemia and injury and in the clinical setting represent subendocardial infarction. It is probable that many cases of this type of infarct are missed, for circumferential infarctions of the left ventricular endocardium from the apex to the base have been reported with absent or minimal ST and T wave changes.

VENTRICULAR ISCHEMIA

A discussion of ventricular ischemia necessarily centers around the characteristics of the normal T loop and the T wave. The former has already been, described, and, since changes in the T wave are studied more commonly in clinical practice, emphasis will be mainly on the ECG features rather than on the T loop.

Normally, the T wave in L I-II must be positive or upright. In all other limb leads it may be negative or diphasic. There is a normal relation between the maximum QRS vector and the T vector. In the uncorrected frontal plane the angle between them does not exceed 45°. If the maximum QRS vector is vertical (about 70°) the T vector which is to the left must be sufficiently parallel to produce a positive T wave on L III-aVF. If the maximum QRS vector is horizontal the T vector which is to the right may project either an isoelectric or negative T wave on L III-aVF. The normal T voltage in all limb leads exceeds 0.2 mv.

In the precordial leads the T wave may be positive or negative in V_1, but it is always positive from V_2 to V_6.

T wave abnormalities beyond the age of 40 should be considered, after the elimination of other causes, to be due to left or right ventricular ischemia. However T wave changes also occur in

1. Postprandial state.
2. Obesity.
3. Orthostasis.
4. Pericarditis.
5. Pericardial calcification.
6. C.N.S. damage.
7. Pneumothorax.
8. Malposition of the heart.
9. Isolated T wave negativity.
10. Conduction defects.
11. Myocardial infarcts.
12. Electrolyte disturbances.

When it is not possible on clinical and other grounds to identify the cause of abnormal T waves they should be classified as nonspecific T wave changes.

In left ventricular ischemia the direction of the maximum QRS vector often is not altered. The position of the T vector is determined by the uninvolved areas of the heart so the vector points away from the ischemic area and is more anterior and rightward than normally. This widens the QRS-T angle to more than 45° in the F plane and more than 60° in the H plane uncorrected reference frames. The T waves in Leads I-aVL and V6 decrease in magnitude and finally become negative, and the increasing anterior direction of the vector produces a tall T wave at V1.

When the mean QRS vector is horizontally directed, the T vector of ischemia also rotates to the right and anteriorly, so that in the frontal plane the T waves become smaller but not inverted while the T wave at V1 becomes taller.

With a vertically directed mean QRS vector the T vector of ischemia rotates to the left and anteriorly, so that the T wave in Lead III-aVF gradually becomes inverted and the T wave in V1 becomes taller.

In right ventricular ischemia when the mean QRS vector is directed downward, to the right, and anteriorly, the T vector points to the left away from the right ventricle and posteriorly so that the magnitude of the T wave decreases in V1 and increases in V6-LI.

ANGINA PECTORIS

The ST vector in this syndrome points away from the injured area so that the ST segment may be depressed more than 0.5 mm in Leads I and II and the left precordial leads. The T wave may or may not be inverted. The changes are transient. On the other hand, the only manifestations may be frequent ventricular extrasystoles or transient T wave inversion in Leads I-II and the left precordial leads. In 50 percent of cases the ECG is within normal limits.

A variant of the usual ECG of angina pectoris has been reemphasized by Prinzmetal. The ST segment is elevated in Leads I and II and some of the precordial leads with inversion of the T wave. The R wave is increased in amplitude. This represents subepicardial injury and is attributed to diminution in the blood supply through the larger superficial branches of the coronary vessels. Symptomatically this form of angina differs from the classical type in that pain occurs at rest, is relieved by exercise, and is cyclical in character.

THE EXERCISE TOLERANCE TEST. The test is based on the observations published by Scherf and Goldhammer in 1932 that the ECG obtained after exercise could be used to diagnose coronary artery disease. The test has been popularized by Master, who in 1942 introduced tables of standard exercise according to the sex, weight, and age of the patient. The tables are a carry-over from an old examination still widely used by insurance companies and government agencies. They set criteria for the amount of work that could be performed by the normal individual whose pulse and blood pressure would return to the resting level within two minutes after standardized exercise. Though it appears to be here to stay, Master's exercise tolerance test (so far as standardization goes) has lost all semblance of validity by the introduction of the double two-step test in which the amount of exercise for the normal individual has been doubled. The double two-step test also contains the false assumption that one can quantitate the degree of coronary artery disease. It implies that a normal standard test means less coronary artery disease than an abnormal double two-step test. Using the tables advocated by Master we prefer to follow the criteria of Scherf for a positive test. They are:

1. ST depression of 1.5 mm in the unipolar or bipolar leads
2. ST depression of 2.0 mm in one or more of the precordial leads

Depression is measured from the beginning of the QRS complex and not from the level of the PQ segment.

More recent criteria have been devised in an effort to increase the validity of the test. These include RS-T depression of 2 mm or more, QX-QT fraction of 50 percent or more, QT ratio of 1.08 or more, inverted U waves, and many others. They await the test of time.

The test should not be performed after a meal or after an infectious disease, for T wave inversion may occur in normal individuals in these settings. Obviously with an abnormal resting ECG there is no necessity for the test. It is of no value in the digitalized patient, for the drug itself in the normal individual will cause ST depression during exercise and even T wave inversion.

REFERENCE

Scherf, D. The electrocardiographic exercise test. J. Electrocardiog., 1:141, 1968.

PULMONARY EMPHYSEMA

In addition to producing overinflation and decreasing the conductivity of the lungs, pulmonary emphysema also results in lowering of the diaphragm so that the heart assumes a more vertical position in the frontal plane. The electrical center of the heart is displaced downward. The magnitude of the electrical forces is increased along the vertical axis (Y axis) and decreased along the horizontal axes (X-Z axes). In 90 percent of cases vertical forces are increased inferiorly. In the remainder the axis is superior and leftward, and left axis deviation occurs (left axis illusion).

In the F plane the loop is narrow with the maximum vector not beyond 90°.

There is no satisfactory explanation for the posterior QRS loop which is narrow and decreased in magnitude in the H plane.

ECG. The magnitude of the R wave is greater in L III-II-aVF than in L I-aVL due to the increased vertical forces. Left axis deviation (axis illusion) may be present. Because of the posterior direction of the QRS loop and the position of the electrodes above the electrical center of the heart, QS complexes may be recorded in V1-2 and must be differentiated from anteroseptal infarction. The T wave in emphysema, however, is upright.

ACUTE COR PULMONALE

Acute cor pulmonale is usually due to acute pulmonary embolization. Such a catastrophic episode usually does not permit direct VCG recording so the following features are based on the analysis of vectors derived from the ECG.

1. One-third of the patients or more may show no ECG changes. If changes are present they are transient, lasting no more than a few days.
2. The mean QRS vector may be directed downward and to the right in the frontal plane and posteriorly in the horizontal plane, producing a SI-QIII pattern (the McGinn-White pattern). The ST segment is depressed in Lead I and ascends in stepwise fashion to the upright T wave. QIII is less than 0.03 second in duration. QII does not occur as it does in inferior infarction.
3. If marked right axis deviation occurs, an SI-II-III pattern appears in the bipolar leads with the mean QRS rotated posteriorly in the horizontal plane as evidenced by marked "clockwise rotation" in the V leads. The SI-II-III pattern may be normal in young individuals or it may appear following myocardial infarction.
4. Transient RBBB believed to be due to right ventricular dilation may occur.
5. P pulmonale attributed to right atrial dilation occurs rarely. This is seen much more frequently in chronic cor pulmonale.
6. Previous arrhythmias may revert to sinus rhythm, or various atrial arrhythmias may appear.
7. In patients with underlying coronary artery disease, the fall in cardiac output following pulmonary embolization may produce an ischemic pattern of depressed ST segments and upright T waves in V5 and V6 together with ST elevation and at times T wave inversion in V1 and V2.

CHRONIC COR PULMONALE

The most important cause of chronic cor pulmonale is diffuse obstructive pulmonary emphysema which results in increased mean pulmonary arterial pressure and hypertrophy of the RV, the extent of which depends on the degree and duration of the hemodynamic changes.

The VCG characteristics depend on the anatomic site of RV hypertrophy. In the early stages, which involve mainly the crista and the basal right septum, the H plane QRS loop is C-CW and posterior with initial forces anterior and either to the right or left. The afferent limb extends into the right posterior quadrant. The T loop is anterior.

Further involvement of the RV includes hypertrophy of the free wall. This produces a figure of eight loop proximally C-CW with the distal loop mainly in the right posterior quadrant. The initial forces are anterior and leftward.

In severe degrees of cor pulmonale the QRS loop may be completely CW and mainly anterior with the initial forces to the left either anteriorly or posteriorly.

In the F plane the main loop is CW with the maximum vector to the right of 70°. If axis illusion is present as a manifestation of emphysema, the loop is C-CW.

The P loop is narrow with increased magnitude in the F and RS planes. It is directed anteriorly and inferiorly either to the right or left.

ECG. The following criteria for the diagnosis of chronic cor pulmonale in the presence of pulmonary emphysema are in the main conclusive:

1. R/S ratio in the right precordial leads greater than unity.
2. Predominant R waves in the right precordial leads.
3. rSR′ pattern of incomplete RBBB in these leads.
4. An enlarged heart with right axis deviation of the QRS.
5. Together with P pulmonale.

Less conclusive features are:

1. Right axis deviation greater than 110°.
2. Wide S waves in Leads I, II, III, V5, V6.
3. QS, Qr, or qr waves in Leads V1-3 but with upright T waves to distinguish the contour from that of anteroseptal infarction.
4. R/S ratio in V6 less than one.

DIGITALIS

Digitalis effects an early onset of repolarization, particularly of the endocardial layer, so that recovery is in the same direction as depolarization; from endocardium to epicardium. Early repolarization produces an ST vector directed away from the maximum QRS vector. It is directed superiorly, anteriorly, and rightward from the end of the QRS loop to the beginning of the T loop. When the ST vector is about 210° (−150°) the greatest depression of the ST segment in the ECG is in L II and the left precordial leads and the greatest elevation is in aVR. The typical ST segment of digitalis effect is a straight segment, convex, neither upward or downward. The Q-T interval is shortened by early repolarization.

The T loop is also affected by digitalis in that the loop is inscribed with uniform velocity and the maximum T vector, though normal in position, is decreased in magnitude. The QRS-T angle is widened. In the ECG normal T asymmetry is lost and the amplitude of the T wave is decreased.

QUINIDINE

In therapeutic doses quinidine prolongs the Q-T interval by increasing the duration of the T complex. With increasing dosage the T wave becomes broader, decreases in magnitude, and may be inverted. Quinidine may prolong all parts of the QRS complex equally, and in toxic doses produce right or left BBB, AV block, VPC's, or ventricular tachycardia.

POTASSIUM

HYPERPOTASSEMIA	*HYPOPOTASSEMIA*
T WAVE CHANGES	
When plasma K exceeds 6.5 mEq/L the T wave increases in magnitude, becoming sharp and peaked, particularly in right precordial leads. Inverted T waves (aVR) become deeper. Abnormally inverted T waves become less inverted and at times upright.	T waves decrease in magnitude and finally invert. A U wave, if present, fuses with the T wave producing a double contour.
QRS CHANGES	
These succeed T wave alteration. With a K level of 8 mEq/L, S waves increase in magnitude and R waves decrease in left precordial leads. At 9-11 mEq/L, RBBB develops. With further increase QRS and T fuse into a biphasic complex.	Usually no change.
P WAVE CHANGES	
The P wave decreases in magnitude. SA block occurs. A ventricular pacemaker takes over, and ventricular fibrillation may occur.	Ectopic atrial rhythms may develop.

CARDIAC RHYTHMS

REGULAR SINUS RHYTHM. Normally the impulse for cardiac activation arises in the sinoatrial node (SA) at rates from 60 to 100 per minute. The P-P intervals do not vary more than 0.16 second. The P-R intervals are more than 0.12 second and within upper limits for age and heart rate. The upper limit in adults is 0.21 second and average 0.03 second less in children.

SINUS BRADYCARDIA. The basic mechanism is sinoatrial with rates below 60/min. The P axis is nearly parallel to Lead I. Rarely is the rate below 40/min. The P-R intervals are normal. It occurs particularly in athletes and in conditions of increased vagal tone. Sinus arrhythmia usually accompanies sinus bradycardia.

SINUS TACHYCARDIA. This is an SA mechanism with rates of 100 to 140/min. Rarely rates as high as 180 in the adult and 220 in children may occur. The axis of the P wave is nearly parallel to Lead II. The T-P interval is shortened so that with very rapid rates the P wave may be superimposed on the preceding T wave. If the R-R interval is less than 0.58 second, the P merges with the preceding T wave. Sinus tachycardia is a normal response to exercise, fever emotion, etc.

SINUS ARRHYTHMIA. This SA mechanism is due to periodic fluctuations in the discharge of the sinus node. Variations in the P-P intervals exceed 0.16 second. Two types are distinguished:

1. Respiratory or phasic, in which cycle lengths become shorter with inspiration and longer with expiration. P-R intervals are normal, but the P waves may show some variation in contour due to respiratory shift in the heart position.
2. Nonrespiratory or nonphasic, in which variations in the P-P intervals are not related to respiration. P-R intervals are 0.12 second or longer.

Any factor which increases the heart rate tends to abolish sinus arrhythmia. Slower rates accentuate it. It is prominent from childhood through adolescence.

Sinus arrhythmia may be accompanied by:

1. Wandering of the pacemaker in the SA node. Since the node is 2.5 cm long and the site of exit of the impulse from the node to the atrial muscle alters the direction of the atrial vector there may be a change in the contour of the P wave and the P-R interval which, however, does not become less than 0.12 second. The taller P waves and longer P-R intervals are associated with faster beats (Fig. 18).
2. Wandering of the pacemaker to the AV node is a normal variant of cardiac rhythm. The shift may or may not be phasic with respiration.

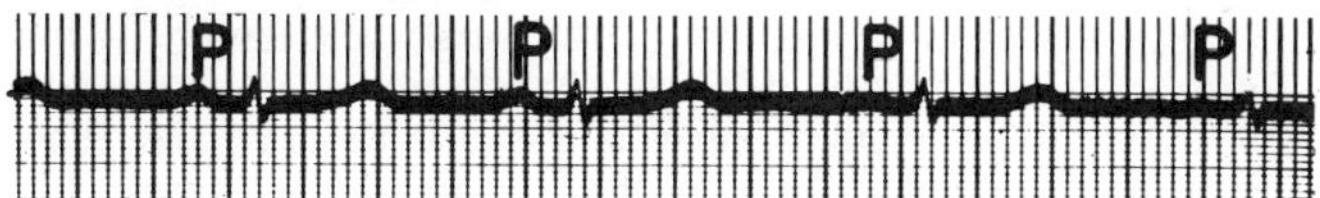

Fig. 18. Sinus arrhythmia with wandering of the pacemaker in the SA node.

Increased vagal tone suppresses the faster pacemakers earlier than the slow ones. The T-P interval may be so prolonged that the pacemaker shifts to the AV node. The diagnosis is made when the P wave in a given lead undergoes changes in size, shape, and direction of its vector concurrently with slowing of the rate and a decrease in the P-R interval to less than 0.12 sec (Fig. 19).

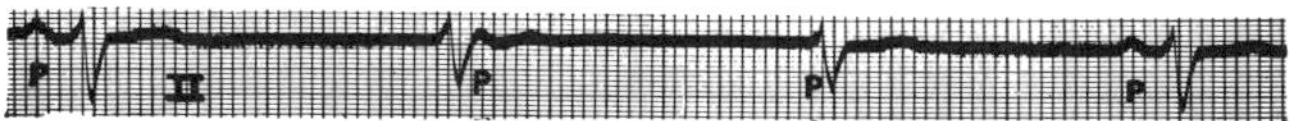

Fig. 19. Shift of the pacemaker to the AV node in nonphasic sinus arrhythmia.

SINOATRIAL BLOCK. In this arrhythmia a normal impulse is formed in the SA node but is not conducted to the atria. For a definite diagnosis regular sinus rhythm must be present, followed by a pause which does not contain a P-QRST complex. Pauses may occur after every second, third, or fourth beat. The duration of the pause is an exact double or any other multiple of the R-R intervals of normal sinus rhythm (Fig. 20).

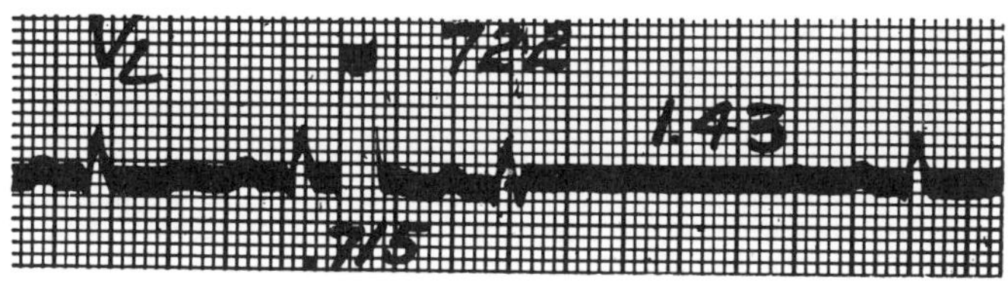

Fig. 20. Sinoatrial block. The pause is twice the duration of the P-P interval.

SINUS ARREST. This is due to the transient absence of impulse formation in the SA node. There is a complete suspension of atrial and ventricular activity for varying intervals. The duration of the pause is not a multiple of the usual cycle length. If the pause is prolonged, the AV node or a ventricular pacemaker takes over as the rhythm center, and escape beats appear. This arrhythmia is rare and may be due to carotid sinus sensitivity, digitalis, quinidine, or coronary artery disease.

Following pauses in SA block or sinus arrest there may be:

1. Resumption of regular sinus rhythm.
2. Nodal escape manifested by retrograde P wave (positive in aVR and negative in aVF) and a normal QRS complex, or the P wave may be buried in the QRS complex.
3. Ventricular escape in which the QRS complex does not resemble that of regular rhythm.

HEART BLOCK

INTRA-ATRIAL BLOCK. This is manifested by a P wave of more than 0.11-second duration, usually notched, which resembles the contour associated with mitral disease. The diagnosis is justified only in the absence of a mitral lesion and any other cause of atrial hypertrophy.

ATRIOVENTRICULAR BLOCK. Disturbances of cardiac conduction through the AV node may be of three degrees.

First-Degree AV Block (Delayed AV Conduction). The PR interval is prolonged beyond 0.21 second in the adult. The prolongation is slight when up to 0.28 second, moderate between 0.28 and 0.5 second, and extreme when up to 0.88 second. A QRS complex follows every P wave. No beats are dropped.

Second-Degree AV Block (Partial AV Block). Here the ventricular rate is slower than the atrial because some atrial impulses are prevented from passing through the AV node. The ratio of atrial to ventricular complexes may be constant or may fluctuate due to vagal tone in ratios of 2:1, 3:1, 4:1, etc.

Two types of partial AV block occur:

1. Wenckebach type is due to a progressive increase in the duration of the PR interval in successive cycles until an atrial impulse fails to activate the ventricles. Dropping of a QRS complex usually occurs when the PR interval reaches 0.34 second or more. When the phenomena is vagal in origin the degree of block or the frequency of dropped beats may be decreased by exercise, atropine, or the erect posture (Fig. 21). Characteristically Wenckebach periods consist of a) progressively shorter cycles separated by a long one, b) the sum of the duration of any two consecutive short cycles is greater than the duration of the long cycle, and c) the cycle immediately preceding the pause is shorter than the first following it. On the basis of these characteristics, Wenckebach periods can be identified in SA block and nodal rhythm.

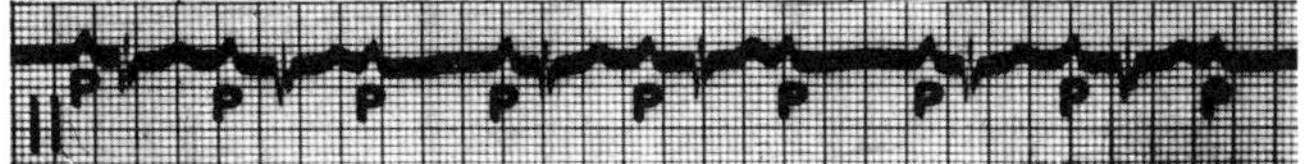

Fig. 21 Wenckebach phenomenon.

2. Moebitz type is rare and manifested by a normal or prolonged but constant P-R interval with a regular sinus P wave not being followed by a QRS complex.

Third-Degree Heart Block (Complete Heart Block). In complete heart block the atria and the ventricles each are controlled by independent pacemakers. Not only are atrial impulses not conducted to the ventricles, but there is also total absence of retrograde conduction from the ventricles to the atria. When the atrial rhythm is sinus, regular P-P intervals are present.

The ventricular rate is usually between 30 and 40 per minute, but may be more rapid when the block is digitalis induced (Fig. 22). When there is a single ventricular pacemaker the ventricular rhythm is regular and the QRS complexes are similar. With more than one ventricular pacemaker, the rhythm is irregular, and the QRS complexes differ. A pacemaker above the bifurcation of the bundle of His produces QRS complexes of normal contour. A pacemaker in the left bundle produces QRS complexes characteristic of RBBB, in the right bundle those of LBBB. When the pacemaker is in the ventricular muscle, the QRS complexes are broad and bizarre, and change in contour.

The mortality rate in patients with complete heart block, with or without Adams-Stokes attacks, is 40 percent within the first year. Permanent cardiac pacing reduces this to 17 percent.

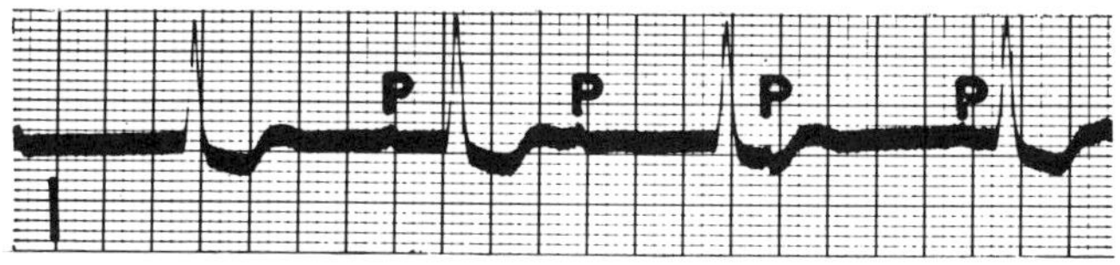

Fig. 22. Complete AV block due to digitalis. (From Barker. *The Unipolar Electrocardiogram.* Courtesy of Appleton-Century-Crofts.)

PREMATURE BEATS

Premature beats may be single, paired, or occur in runs. If they occur after each sinus beat, the rhythm is coupled or bigeminal; if after each pair of sinus beats, it is trigeminal.

Premature beats may be supraventricular (atrial or nodal) or ventricular in origin. Premature beats with basic sinus rhythm have one characteristic in common: they occur earlier than expected in the rhythm cycle.

1. Atrial premature beats have a shortened P-P interval between the sinus P wave and the succeeding premature ectopic P wave. If, as is usually the case, the ectopic atrial pacemaker discharges the SA node, the pause following the premature atrial systole is longer than a regular sinus interval, but the duration of the cycle preceding and the duration of the pause are less than two normal sinus cycles. The pause is usually not fully compensatory. The ectopic P wave of an atrial premature beat differs in contour from the sinus P wave. If its prematurity is great, it may be hidden in the T wave of the preceding complex. In such cases, however, inspection of the T contours and comparison with those of regular sinus beats will reveal a difference varying from subtle to marked. The P-R interval of the ectopic beat varies with the location of the ectopic focus, the prematurity of the beat, and the conduction through the AV node. If the beat arises in the right atrium, the P wave is inverted in aVR; if from the left atrium, the P wave is upright in aVR. The ventricular complex following a premature atrial beat may show varying degrees of aberrancy and at times be mistaken for ventricular premature beats unless a premature P wave is diligently sought (Fig. 23).

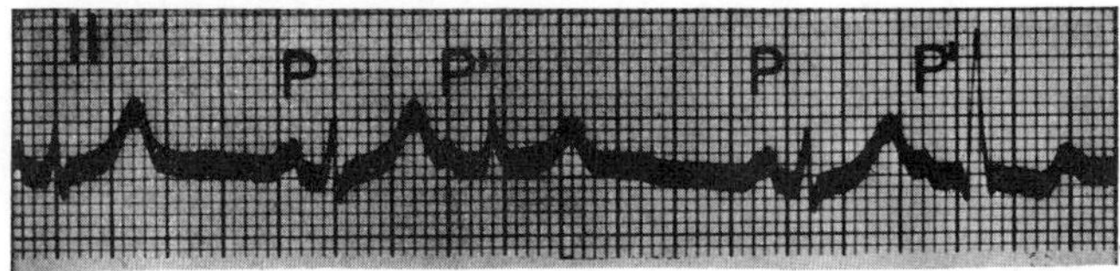

Fig. 23. Atrial premature beats with and without aberrant ventricular conduction. (From Barker. *The Unipolar Electrocardiogram.* Courtesy of Appleton-Century-Crofts.)

2. Nodal premature beats manifest inverted P waves in Leads II, III, and aVF and upright ones in Leads I, aVR, and aVL. The pause after a nodal premature is usually compensatory, and the duration of the P-P interval of two sinus beats enclosing the ectopic beat is equal to the duration of the interval between three sinus beats. The P wave of a nodal premature beat may precede, be buried in, or follow the QRS complex which initiates it, depending on whether it is "upper" (Fig. 24), "middle," or "lower" nodal in origin.

   When the nodal P wave precedes the QRS, the P-R interval is less than 0.12 second. "Middle" nodal P waves are buried in the QRS,

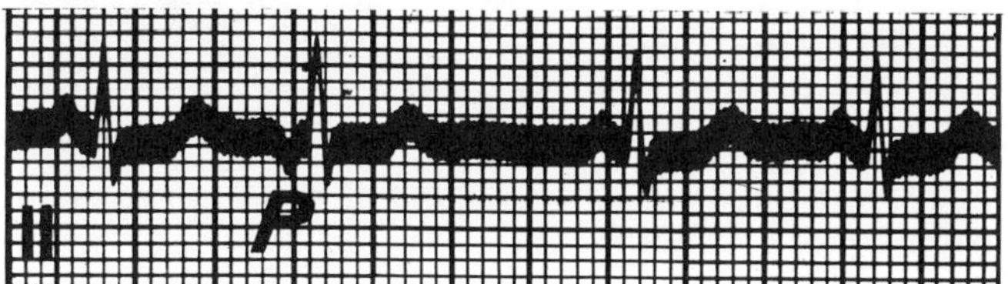

Fig. 24. "Upper" nodal premature beat.

while in "lower" nodal premature systoles, the retrograde P wave follows the QRS by 0.01 to 0.20 second. The ventricular response varies with the prematurity of the ectopic nodal impulse. The QRS may be identical with that of sinus activation, but the more premature the nodal P wave, the more aberrant will be the resulting QRS, because the ventricles will not have recovered from the previous activation.

3. Ventricular premature beats are manifested by premature QRS complexes of an unusual configuration not preceded by a P wave. They may be followed by a P wave due to retrograde stimulation of the atria. If the ectopic beats arise from a single ventricular focus, the premature QRS complexes in a given lead will have the same contour and will occur at the same interval after the preceding sinus-induced QRS, i.e., their coupling will be fixed. When the contour of the premature QRS complexes differ in the same lead, more than one focus is active. Ectopic ventricular beats usually occur early in diastole, but they may occur late, superimposed on the sinus P wave or shortly after it. The latter instance may produce a fusion beat in which the initial bizarre portion of the QRS is due to the ectopic focus, and the terminal portion, supraventricular in contour, is due to normal activation throughout the bundle of His (Fig. 25).

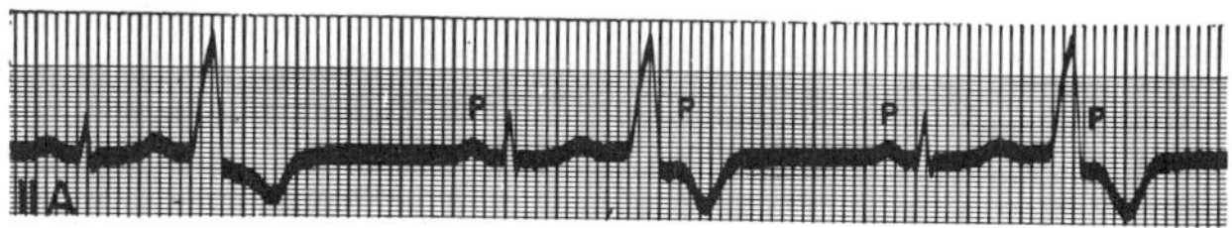

Fig. 25. Ventricular premature beats, unifocal with fixed coupling producing bigeminy. (From Barker. *The Unipolar Electrocardiogram*. Courtesy of Appleton-Century-Crofts.)

In sinoatrial rhythm, the pause following a ventricular ectopic beat is compensatory. Ectopic ventricular beats interpolated between two sinus beats without affecting the regularity of the sinus rhythm are the only true extrasystoles (Fig. 26).

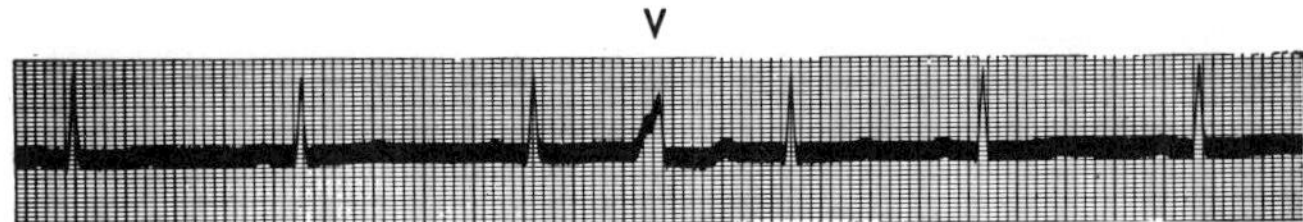

Fig. 26. Sinus rhythm, interpolated ventricular extrasystole. (From Barker. *The Unipolar Electrocardiogram*. Courtesy of Appleton-Century-Crofts.)

The pause following a ventricular ectopic beat may be terminated by a supraventricular beat and the resumption of normal sinus rhythm. Long pauses are usually terminated by an AV nodal escape beat or a succession of them.

4. Parasystolic ventricular premature beats may or may not have identical contours, but characteristically the premature beat occurs at different times in the cardiac cycle (variable coupling to the preceding beat), and intervals between successive premature beats are equal or multiples of a common denominator, the least common of which represents the basic rate of the parasystolic pacemaker, which ranges between 20 and 70 per minute, though rates as high as 400 per minute have been reported. Because of variable coupling, fusion beats are common, i.e., the ventricle may be activated by both a supraventricular and ventricular impulse. Parasystolic rhythms may be atrial, nodal, or more commonly ventricular in origin.

ATRIOVENTRICULAR DISSOCIATION

Atrioventricular dissociation is due to independent pacemakers in the atria and in the ventricles. When the rate of an atrial pacemaker is slower than that of a pacemaker located in the AV node, the bundle, or the ventricular muscle, the control of rhythm becomes dissociated, and two independent pacemakers control, respectively, the atria and the ventricles. The two pacemakers are separated by a barrier in the AV junction.

AV dissociation may be complete or incomplete. Complete dissociation may be due to equalization of the rates of the atrial and ventricular pacemakers without antegrade or retrograde conduction. More commonly, incomplete AV dissociation occurs when the ectopic ventricular rate is faster than that of the sinus node (Fig. 27). QRS complexes occur at shorter intervals than P-P intervals. Succeeding P-R intervals become shorter and shorter (reversed Wenckeback phenomena), and, finally, atrial impulses occur late enough so that the AV node is responsive, and a transmitted atrial impulse reaches the ventricle as a "ventricular" capture for one or several beats. The P-R interval of such beats is greater than 0.12 second.

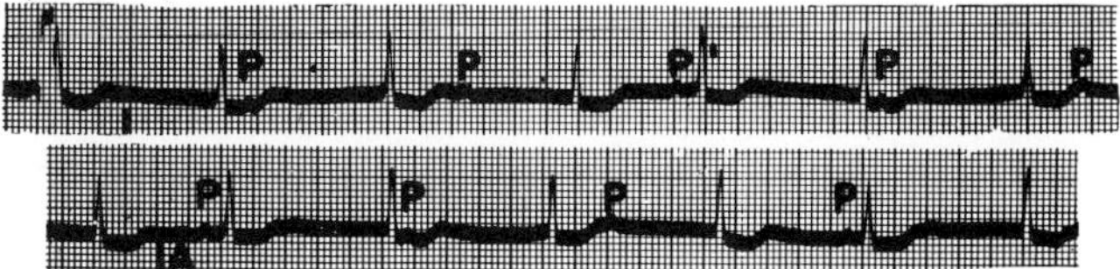

Fig. 27. Incomplete AV dissociation. Complex P′ QRS is a capture beat occurring early in R-R cycle.

NODAL RHYTHM

Nodal rhythm occurs when the ventricles are activated by antegrade impulses and the atria by retrograde impulses from the AV node. Nodal rhythm may be either passive or active.

1. Passive nodal rhythm occurs when the SA node is depressed. P waves are nodal in origin and regularly spaced (upright in aVR and aVL, downward in aVF). The rate is usually below 100. QRS complexes are normal in uncomplicated cases. It is customary to designate the rhythm center as being in the upper, middle, or lower portion of the AV node. This classification assumes that antegrade conduction to the ventricles and retrograde conduction to the atria occur at the same rate. Scherf and Shookhoff first pointed out that the position of the P wave, preceding, buried in, or following the QRS complex, might be due to a conduction disturbance of the impulses from the AV node retrogradely to the atria or down to the ventricles or in both directions and not depend on the anatomic site of impulse formation in the node.
   According to their concept there are:
   a. AV rhythm with preceding activation of the atria due to antegrade delay to the ventricles ("upper" nodal rhythm). The P wave precedes the QRS by less than 0.12 sec, upright in Leads I, aVL, aVR, downward in Leads III and aVF (Fig. 28).

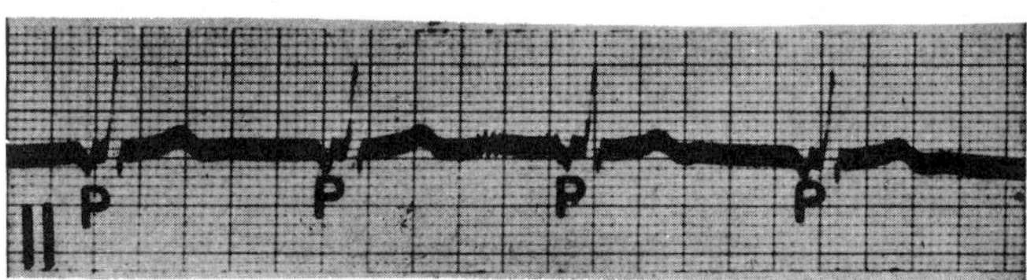

Fig. 28. "Upper" nodal rhythm. (From Barker. *The Unipolar Electrocardiogram.* Courtesy of Appleton-Century-Crofts.)

b. AV rhythm with simultaneous activation of atria and ventricles ("middle" nodal rhythm). The P wave is buried in the QRS complex (Fig. 29).

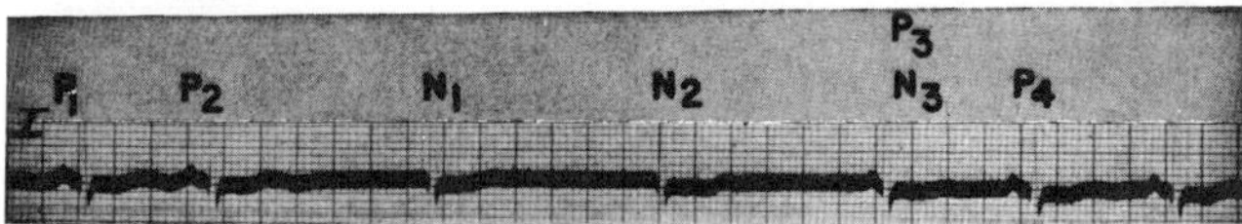

Fig. 29. "Middle" nodal rhythm at N_1, N_2.

c. AV rhythm with preceding ventricular activation due to retrograde conduction delay to the atria ("lower" nodal rhythm). The P wave follows the QRS complex from 0.02 to 0.20 sec (Fig. 30). Reciprocal rhythm is apt to occur in this type especially when retrograde atrial transmission is appreciably delayed. The retrograde atrial impulse reverses its direction, reenters the AV node, and moves antegrade to activate the ventricles a second time. The interval between the R wave of the nodal beat enclosing a retrograde P wave and the R of the reciprocal beat is less than 0.5 second. Reciprocal beats are also called "echo beats" (Fig. 31).

2. Active nodal rhythm arises from an irritable focus in the AV node. The rate exceeds 100 and usually is over 150. It is a form of supraventricular tachycardia with P waves like those of passive nodal rhythm.

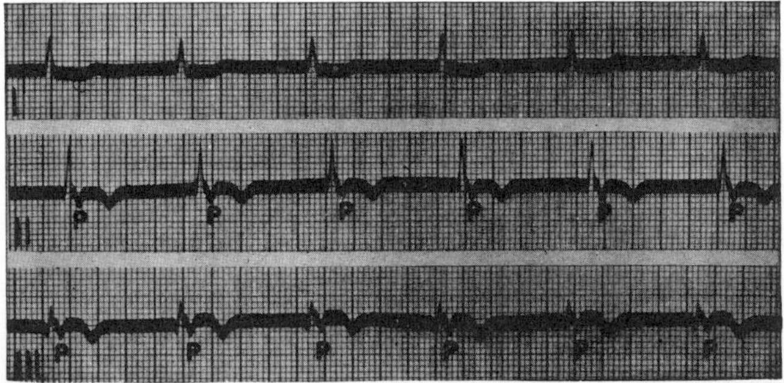

Fig. 30. "Lower" nodal rhythm.

CORONARY NODAL RHYTHM

In this type, the P-R interval is between 0.02 and 0.10 second, with upright P waves in Leads I and II. The direction of the P

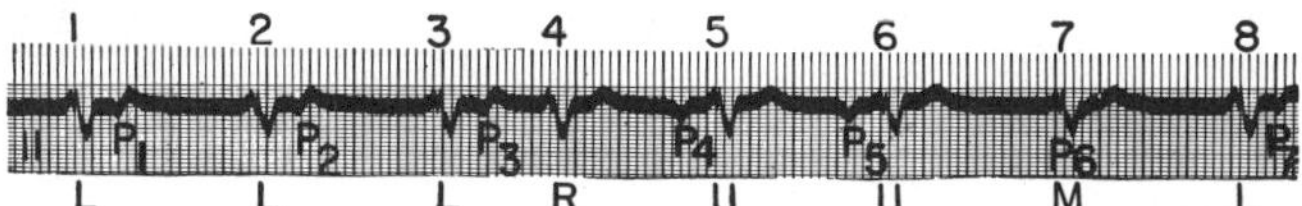

Fig. 31. Reciprocal beat following P3 with transition from "lower" nodal to "upper" and "middle" rhythms. Reciprocal beating may initiate supraventricular tachycardia. (From Barker. *The Unipolar Electrocardiogram.* Courtesy of Appleton-Century-Crofts.)

vector is normal, for the impulse arising close to the tail of the SA node is directed from right to left and from the back to the front of the atria. An alternate explanation is that a normally generated sinus impulse may pass along an accessory rapid conduction pathway, joining the atria and the ventricles above the bifurcation of the bundle. Coronary nodal rhythm may occur in isolated beats or as a form of coronary nodal tachycardia.

ECTOPIC ATRIAL RHYTHMS

These are due to replacement of the sinus node by an ectopic atrial focus or foci which assume pacemaker function.

ATRIAL TACHYCARDIA. The P waves are similar to the P waves of sinus rhythm, but with very rapid rates may be fused with the T wave. The atrial rate is between 150 and 220 per minute. With difficulty in clearly identifying the P waves and differentiating them from retrograde waves from the AV node one classifies this arrhythmia as supraventricular. The ventricular response may be in a 1 to 1 or 2 to 1 ratio, or may be irregular in the presence of variable block. It is stated that atrial tachycardia differs from atrial flutter on the basis of a slower atrial rate an[illegible] the presence of an isoelectric interval between the P waves in t[illegible] former. The isoelectric interval is a function of the atrial [illegible]te and [illegible] [illegible]ntricular resp[illegible]. The shorter the T-Q interval [illegible]nd the more rapid the atrial rate, the [illegible] time is available f[illegible] the inscription of an isoelectric interval. Lown an[illegible] [illegible]vine c[illegible]nsider atrial tachycardia with variable degrees of block to be the most common manifestation of digitalis toxicity. Atrial flutter is considered to be an uncommon manifestation of digitalis poisoning. The difference between these two arrhythmias seems to be mainly a difference of definition which assigns a more rapid rate to flutter. Variable block may occur in each, and whether there is continuous undulation of the base line, as in flutter, or isoelectric intervals, as in atrial tachycardia, depends on the atrial rate and the ventricular response rather than on a basically different mechanism. Atrial flutter with varying AV block and atrial tachycardia with varying block are identical, save for a confusion in terminology which exists in the literature at present.

ATRIAL FLUTTER. The atrial rhythm is regular and manifested by flutter (F) waves which are continuous undulations of the base line without isoelectric intervals between them, and conventionally are described as having a "sawtooth" configuration. Flutter waves are usually best seen in the aVF or the right precordial leads. The atrial rate is usually between 250 and 300 per minute. The atrial-ventricular ratio may be 2 to 1, 3 to 1, 4 to 1, or more, or it may vary in different cycles (Fig. 32).

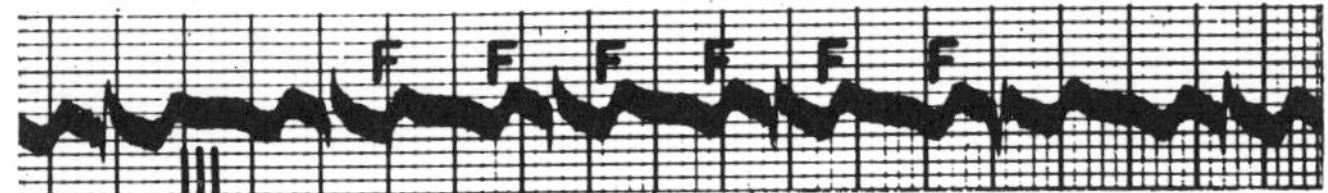

Fig. 32. Atrial flutter.

ATRIAL FIBRILLATION. The atrial rhythm is totally irregular and is manifested by f waves which vary in spacing and contour. The atrial rate is usually between 400 and 600 per minute. The ventricular response is also totally irregular, depending on the degree of AV block, so that the ventricular rate may vary from 50 to 200 per minute (Fig. 33).

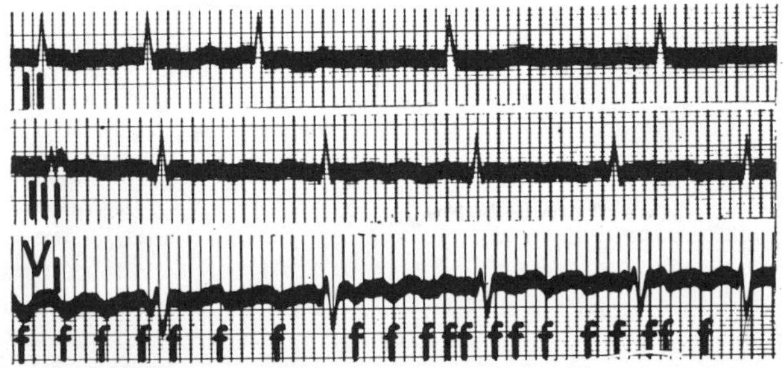

Fig. 33. Atrial fibrillation.

ECTOPIC VENTRICULAR RHYTHMS

VENTRICULAR TACHYCARDIA. This consists of a rapid, regular, or irregular succession of three or more bizarre ventricular complexes with the QRS prolonged to more than 0.12 second and oppositely directed T waves continuing into the QRS. Antegrade atrial conduction is blocked, and identifiable P waves have no relation to the QRS complexes. The rate is from 120 to 250 per minute (Fig. 34).

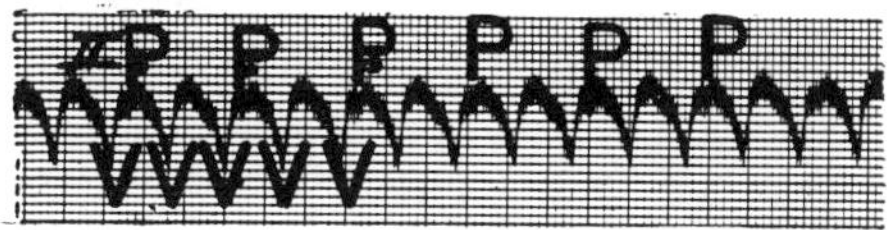

Fig. 34. Ventricular tachycardia.

This arrhythmia is frequently confused with atrial tachycardia with aberrant ventricular conduction. Whenever the ventricular complexes have the contour of RBBB, one should be suspicious of atrial tachycardia with aberration.

VENTRICULAR FLUTTER. This extremely rare arrhythmia is characterized by regularly spaced QRS complexes at a rate of over 250 per minute. All complexes are strikingly alike with the QRS and T waves fused.

VENTRICULAR FIBRILLATION. Ventricular fibrillation shows irregular, bizarre complexes which differ from each other in contour and spacing. There is fusion of the QRS and T waves (Fig. 35).

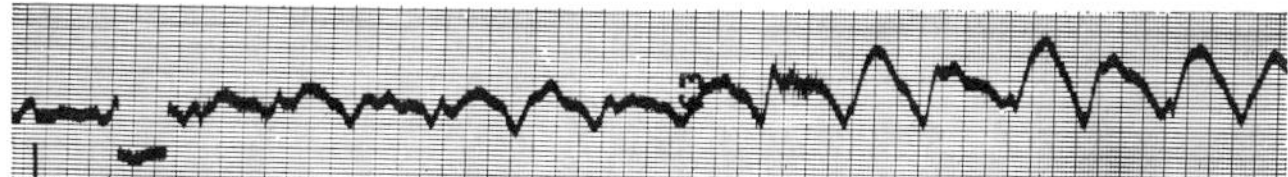

Fig. 35. Ventricular fibrillation.

The following table (page 194) outlines the more frequent cardiac arrhythmias.

ARRHYTHMIA	RATE AND MECHANISM	VAGUS EFFECT	DRUG TREATMENT	ELECTRIC CARDIOVERSION
Sinus tachycardia	SA node rate 100-160; stress	Gradual decrease; returns to previous level	Rest; sedation	Not used
Paroxysmal atrial tachycardia	150-250; irritable ectopic atrial focus	About 50% have sudden cessation; remainder unaffected	Vagus stimulation; sedation; digitalis (in that order)	Treatment of choice (if not due to digitalis)
Atrial flutter	250-350; ectopic focus or circus	Irregular decrease; gradually returns to original rate	Digitalis first; then quinidine	Treatment of choice
Atrial fibrillation	350-500; ectopic focus or circus	Rate slows; irregularity remains	Digitalis to slow rate; quinidine may convert to NSR	Will convert about 80%
Premature contractions	Irritable atrial or ventricular focus	May slow PAC's; no effect on PVC's	If occasional: no treatment; if frequent: quinidine or Pronestyl	Not used
Ventricular tachycardia	150-220; irritable ventricular focus	No effect	Pronestyl intravenously (100 mg/min, up to 2,000-3,000 mg)	Treatment of choice (if not due to digitalis)
Ventricular fibrillation	Probable ectopic or circus	No effect	Electrical defibrillation	Treatment of choice

REFERENCES

Burch, G. E., and DePasquale, N. P. Practical clinical applications of vectocardiography. J.A.M.A., 178:301, 1961.

Ezra, P. S. The normal composite electrocardiogram. Circulation, 24:710, 1961.

Georas, C. S., Dalquist, E., and Cutts, F. B. Subendocardial infarction. Ann. Intern. Med., 111:146, 1963.

Goldberger, E., ed. Progress notes in cardiology. Vector leads. Amer. J. Cardiol., 6:997, 1960.

Grant, R. J. Clinical Electrocardiography: The Spatial Vector Approach. New York, The McGraw-Hill Book Company, 1957.
Heckert, E. W. The clinical value of vectorcardiography. Amer. J. Cardiol., 7:657, 1961.
Johnston, F. D. What is a normal electrocardiogram? Circulation, 24:707, 1961.
Lown, B., Perlroth, M. G., Kaidbey, S., Abe, T., and Harken, D. E. "Cardioversion" of atrial fibrillation, a report on the treatment of 65 episodes in 50 patients. New Eng. J. Med., 269:325, 1963.
Phillips, J. H., and Burch, G. E. Problems in the diagnosis of cor pulmonale. Amer. Heart J., 66:818, 1963.
Roman, G. T., Walsh, T. J., and Massie, E. Right ventricular hypertrophy. Amer. J. Cardiol., 7:481, 1961.

ELECTROLYTE AND FLUID DISTURBANCES

SALT AND WATER

WATER

Water accounts for 45 percent to 70 percent of body weight, or in kilograms, an average of 60 percent of body weight. Approximately two-thirds of total body water (TBW) is intracellular and one-third extracellular.

SODIUM

The osmotic pressure of the extracellular fluid varies proportionately with the sodium concentration in the serum. The normal range of serum osmolality is approximately 290 to 310 mOsm/L. Serum osmolality and serum sodium concentration will be influenced by hyperglycemia, azotemia, and hyperlipemia.

1. Hyperglycemia. Contribution of glucose to serum osmolality = glucose mg per 100 ml × 0.06.
2. Azotemia. Contribution of BUN to serum osmolality = BUN mg per 100 ml × 0.36.
3. Sodium. Contribution of Na^+ to serum osmolality = Na^+ mEq/L × 1.85.

With hyperglycemia and azotemia, the serum osmotic pressure will rise above the intracellular fluid osmotic pressure. As a result, water will migrate out of the cells to dilute the extracellular space. This will lower the concentration of serum sodium. Each increase of 100 mg percent of glucose above the normal value will lower the serum sodium by 2.5 mEq/L.

The osmolality of the urine, a reflection of total molecular content rather than molecular size, is important in evaluating fluid and electrolyte problems. The normal range of urine osmolality is 600 to 1,400 mOsm/L. Specific gravity of the urine will be influenced by glucose, mannitol, and urea.

NORMAL FLUID AND ELECTROLYTE LOSSES

Sodium urinary excretion – 40 to 90 mEq/L per 24 hours.
Potassium urinary excretion – 20 to 60 mEq/L per 24 hours.
Water – Insensible losses – 5 ml/kg per 24 hours.
Sensible losses – 1,500 ml urine output in 24 hours, plus other small amounts in feces, etc.

Sodium and water may be lost or gained in isotonic, hypotonic, or hypertonic proportions.

DEHYDRATION (PURE WATER DEPLETION)

Pure water depletion in excess of sodium loss results in hypernatremia:

CAUSES.

1. Insufficient water intake (coma, impaired sense of thirst).
2. Excessive loss.

   Diarrhea, polyuria due to intrinsic renal disease; diabetes insipidus; water loss due to solute excess (diabetic acidosis, high protein tube feedings).

DIAGNOSIS

1. Skin dry and flushed. Mucous membranes dry. Turgor is normal.
2. BUN, Hct, serum sodium, serum osmolality elevated. Urine volume low, specific gravity high (1.030), urine osmolality high.

TREATMENT. Water, orally or parenterally as 5 percent D/W. Volume of fluid required:

Current volume total body water (L) = 0.6 × body weight (kg)

$$\text{Normal volume TBW (L)} = \frac{\text{Measured serum Na}^+ \times \text{current volume TBW}}{\text{Normal serum Na}^+}$$

(TBW at serum Na^+ 140 mEq/L)

Body water deficit (L) = Normal volume – current volume.

One-third to one-half of calculated fluid requirement may be given in the first 24 hours, depending on patient's cardiac, pulmonary, and renal status. The principle of the above formula is based on the fact that the plasma sodium concentration varies inversely with the volume of extracellular water.

HYPONATREMIA AND FLUID IMBALANCE

Hyponatremia may result from three causes:

1. True sodium depletion (sodium loss greater than water loss).
2. Dilution: overhydration; states with excess total body sodium as congestive heart failure, cirrhosis with ascites, renal disease with edema; artifactual hyponatremia as in hyperglycemia, azotemia, hyperlipemia.
3. Syndrome of inappropriate ADH secretion (SIADH) is characterized by:
   a. Hyponatremia, with serum hypo-osmolality.
   b. Excretion of urine hypertonic to plasma, with continued renal excretion of sodium.
   c. Normal or expanded plasma and extracellular fluid volumes.
   d. Normal cardiac, renal, and adrenal function.

DIAGNOSIS AND TREATMENT

	TRUE SODIUM DEPLETION	DILUTION	INAPPROPRIATE ADH
ETIOLOGY	Loss in GI secretions	CHF	Malignant tumors (lung)
	Salt-losing nephropathies	Cirrhosis	CNS disorders
	Addison's disease	Overload	Pulmonary disease
			Idiopathic
			Myxedema
SYMPTOMS	Weakness, lassitude	Confusion	Confusion
	Confusion, absent thirst	Delirium	Delirium
		Seizure	Seizure
		Coma	Coma
SIGNS			
Skin	Turgor poor	Edema	No edema–good turgor
Weight	Weight loss	Weight gain	Weight gain
Cardiovascular	Hypotension	CHF	–
	Tachycardia		
	Vasoconstriction		

LABORATORY			
Serum Na^+	Decreased	Decreased	Decreased
Hematocrit	Increased	Decreased	Decreased
BUN	Increased	Variable	Low normal
Serum osmolality	Decreased	Decreased	Decreased
Urine Na^+ conc.	Low*	Low	Normal or increased
Urine sp. gr.	High	Low	High
Urine osmolality	High	Low	High
TREATMENT	Sodium** administration	Fluid restriction	Fluid restriction

*Exceptions: Salt-losing nephropathies, Addison's disease.

**Sodium replacement in true sodium depletion.

Sodium deficit = [Normal Na^+ concentration (142 mEq/L) – measured Na^+ concentration (mEq/L)] $\times$ TBW.

Total body water (TBW) = Weight (kg) $\times$ 0.60.

Replace one-third of the deficit in a 24-hour period. Recalculate the sodium deficit the following day and replace one-third of that amount. The concentration of sodium chlorine solution to be administered will depend upon the quantity of fluid to be administered. If acidosis accompanies the sodium deficit, replace a portion of the sodium as sodium bicarbonate, quantity to be determined by the bicarbonate deficit.

POTASSIUM

HYPOKALEMIA

Hypokalemia will result in metabolic alkalosis and may be a result of systemic alkalosis.

The magnitude of potassium depletion cannot be estimated accurately from the serum potassium concentration alone. With a lowering of the serum potassium by 1 mEq/L or more, a deficit of 20 mEq – 400 mEq exists.

CAUSES.

1. Systemic alkalosis, metabolic or respiratory.
2. Potassium loss.
   a. GI tract – diarrhea, fistulas.
   b. through the urine.
      (1) renal tubular dysfunction.
      (2) diuretics.
      (3) 1° aldosteronism.

Hypokalemia may cause a nephropathy characterized by polyuria, alkaline urine, and ultimately diminished glomerular filtration rate and clearances, with degenerative changes and vacuolization in proximal and distal tubules.

TREATMENT. Potassium chloride given orally or parenterally.

The rate of intravenous infusion should not exceed 20 mEq per hour, or more than 200 mEq in 24 hours.

HYPERKALEMIA

The rise in serum potassium concentration is inversely proportional to the urinary output. Hyperkalemia may develop with a urinary output of less than 400 ml/24 hours.

CAUSES.

1. Excess intake.
2. Protein catabolism.
3. Systemic acidosis; metabolic or respiratory.

The electrocardiographic changes of hyperkalemia first become evident at a serum potassium concentration of 6.5 mEq/L.

TREATMENT. See renal failure, acute.

DISTURBANCES IN ACID-BASE BALANCE

Maintenance of acid-base balance and serum pH in physiologic range (pH 7.35-7.45) is determined by several factors:

1. Chemical buffers of the body fluids and cells.
   a. Bicarbonate-carbonic acid buffer system.
   b. Phosphate buffer system.
   c. Protein buffer system.
   d. Hemoglobin buffer system.
   e. Bone buffer system.
2. Respiratory regulatory mechanisms (elimination or retention of CO_2).
3. Renal regulatory mechanisms.
   a. Acidification of phosphate buffer salts.
   b. Reabsorption of bicarbonate.
   c. Secretion of ammonia.

Reference to the Henderson-Hasselbalch equation allows greater understanding of acid-base imbalance and compensatory mechanisms. Expressed schematically:

$$pH = pK + \log \frac{[B^* HCO_3]}{[H_2CO_3 \rightarrow H_2O + CO_2]} \quad \begin{matrix}\text{renal mechanisms} \\ \text{respiratory mechanisms}\end{matrix}$$

*B represents Na^+ or K^+, or other cation.

Renal mechanisms control bicarbonate secretion, respiratory mechanisms control pCO_2 in acid-base regulation.

DISTURBANCES OF ACID-BASE EQUILIBRIUM

RESPIRATORY ALKALOSIS

DEFECT. Respiratory elimination of carbon dioxide, alveolar overventilation.

CAUSES.

1. Hyperventilation syndrome.
2. CNS lesions.
3. Salicylate intoxication.
4. Overventilation with mechanical ventilators.

COMPENSATION. Renal bicarbonate excretion, suppression of ammonia formation, and retention of hydrogen ion.

DIAGNOSIS.

1. Clinical – hyperventilation, tetany.
2. Laboratory – pH ↑, pCO_2 ↓, CO_2 content ↓. The bicarbonate is normal until compensation occurs, then is decreased.

TREATMENT.

1. Sedation.
2. Controlled ventilation with volume cycle respirator.
3. Sedation or curariform drugs.

RESPIRATORY ACIDOSIS

DEFECT. Alveolar hypoventilation, retention of carbon dioxide.

CAUSES.

1. Intrinsic pulmonary disease (emphysema, fibrosis).
2. CNS lesions.
3. Pulmonary restriction.

COMPENSATION. Renal retention of bicarbonate, excretion of hydrogen ions, excretion of ammonia.

DIAGNOSIS.

1. Clinical – hypoventilation.
2. Laboratory. pH ↓, pCO_2 ↑, CO_2 content ↑. The bicarbonate is normal until compensation occurs, then it is increased.

TREATMENT.

1. Adequate airway.
2. Control of secretions.
3. Assisted ventilation.

METABOLIC ALKALOSIS

DEFECT. Loss of H^+, excess bicarbonate.

CAUSES.

1. Excessive intake of base (milk alkali syndrome).
2. Loss of fixed acid (vomiting, nasogastric suction).
3. Potassium depletion (aldosteronism, diuretics).

COMPENSATION. There is some respiratory compensation with carbon dioxide retention. However, the major compensatory mechanisms are renal bicarbonate excretion, suppression of ammonia formation, retention of hydrogen ion.

DIAGNOSIS.

1. Clinical – muscular weakness, ileus, tetany.
2. Laboratory – pH ↑, pCO_2 normal, hypokalemia, CO_2 content ↑. The serum bicarbonate is increased. Urine pH alkaline, except with hypokalemic alkalosis, when paradoxical aciduria may exist.

TREATMENT. Correction of the etiologic factor. Potassium chloride, ammonium chloride. Diamox administration for bicarbonate elimination, particularly in treating the compensatory metabolic alkalosis of the respiratory acidosis syndrome.

LACTIC ACIDOSIS

An excessive accumulation of lactic acid with resultant severe acidosis occurs in a number of clinical circumstances such as diabetes mellitus, hypoxia, shock states, following cardiopulmonary bypass, following phenformin administration or without apparent cause. The definitive diagnosis of lactic acidosis depends upon the measurement of plasma lactate concentration. The normal plasma lactate is 1 mmole/L. In most cases a presumptive diagnosis can be made in a setting of severe metabolic acidosis, on the basis of history, clinical features, and routine serum pH and electrolyte measurements.

The presence of an anion gap is suggestive of lactic acidosis, though such a gap may be seen in diabetic ketoacidosis, uremia, methyl alcohol poisoning and salicylate intoxication. The anion gap or concentration of unmeasured anions is calculated by subtracting the sum of chloride and bicarbonate concentrations from the serum sodium and potassium concentrations. If hydrogen ions have been added to the extracellular fluid with any anion other than chloride (i.e., β-hydroxybutyrate, lactate, sulfate phosphate) a widening of the gap will be observed. Normally, the anion gap will be 15 mEq/L.

Management is directed to the underlying disturbance. Treatment consists of the administration of sodium bicarbonate. Resistance to alkali therapy is characteristic of lactic acidosis. Doses of 200 to 400 mEq sodium bicarbonate over a period of a few hours may be required.

In situations where such large quantities of sodium as sodium bicarbonate may be contraindicated, peritoneal dialysis is preferred. The standard commercially prepared peritoneal solutions contain at least 40 mEq/L lactate and may perpetuate the lactic acidosis. Peritoneal dializing solution containing sodium bicarbonate, D/W, and sodium chloride can be readily prepared.

METABOLIC ACIDOSIS

DEFECT. Retention of fixed acids, loss of bicarbonate.

CAUSES. Acid excess (diabetic acidosis, uremia, lactic acidosis as in shock or phenformin administration, methanol poisoning, salicylate intoxication), loss of base (diarrhea, fistulas, renal tubular acidosis).

COMPENSATION. Pulmonary elimination of carbon dioxide (Kussmaul; respirations). Renal retention of bicarbonate.

DIAGNOSIS.

1. Clinical – depends on etiology. Kussmaul respirations.
2. Laboratory – pH ↓, serum bicarbonate low, carbon dioxide content low, hyperkalemia may exist. The pCO_2 will be normal until compensation occurs, then pCO_2 low.

TREATMENT.

1. Treatment of causative factor.
2. Bicarbonate administration to raise serum bicarbonate to 20 mEq/L. In chronic acidosis (i.e., uremia), do not correct for bicarbonate less than 10 mEq/L unless symptomatic, then do not correct above serum bicarbonate 17 mEq/L.

HCO_3^- deficit =

$$\left[\begin{matrix}\text{Desired } HCO_3^- \text{ conc.} & - \text{ measured } HCO_3^- \text{ conc.} \\ (20 \text{ mEq/L}) & (\text{mEq/L})\end{matrix}\right] \times \text{TBW (partial)}$$

Partial TBW = Weight (kg) × 0.40.

3. Tris buffer. THAM.
4. Dialysis (see section on RENAL DISEASE).

A. Metabolic acid-base abnormalities superimposed on respiratory acid-base disturbances are frequently difficult to evaluate. Recently, considerable interest has arisen in the development of significance bands (physiologic response curves) that define the range of metabolic acid-base values to be expected with a specific respiratory acid-base disorder. These physiologic "steady state" conditions characterizing the range of extracellular hydrogen and bicarbonate ion concentrations are best applied in acute states of hypercapnia and hypocapnia. Chronic, steady state conditions have not been evaluated in humans.

A significance band encompassing carbon dioxide tensions between 15 and 90 mm Hg may be used for assessing complicating metabolic components in acute respiratory acid-base disorders (see Significance Band Figure). A metabolic alkalosis may compensate for primary respiratory acidosis by two major mechanisms: 1) generation of bicarbonate by the titration of body buffers within a few hours, and 2) renal acid excretion and reabsorption of bicarbonate within 1 or 2 days. Primary

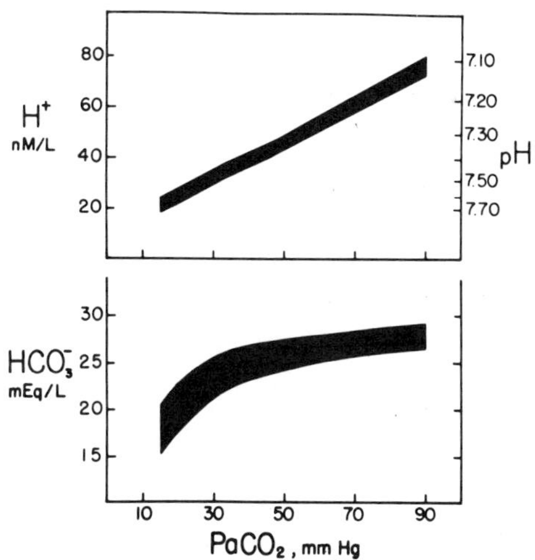

Combined significance band for acute hypocapnia and acute hypercapnia in man. (From *New Eng. J. Med.* 280:122, 1969.)

respiratory alkalosis is compensated by a metabolic acidosis by buffering mechanisms and by renal excretion of bicarbonate.

The response to a given reduction of $PaCO_2$ will lie within a zone that is approximately 6 nM/L wide for hydrogen ion and approximately 5 mEq/L wide for bicarbonate. The response to a given rise of $PaCO_2$ will be within a zone that is 7 nM/L wide for hydrogen ion and approximately 3 mEq/L wide for bicarbonate. Although valucs that lie outside the significance band indicate the presence of a mixed acid-base disturbance, values that fall within the significance band do not necessarily indicate the presence of uncomplicated acute respiratory acid-base disturbance.

IMPORTANT EQUIVALENTS

1. Penicillin G potassium contains 1.7 mEq K^+ per million units.
2. Penicillin G sodium contains 1.5 mEq Na^+ per million units.
3. 1 g Na^+ = 43 mEq Na^+.
4. 1 g NaCl = 17 mEq Na^+.
5. 600 mg $NaHCO_3$ = 7 mEq Na^+ + 7 mEq HCO_3^-.
6. 39 mg K = 1 mEq K.
7. 1 unit whole blood contains 1 mEq K^+/L for each day of age.

REFERENCE

Waters, W. C., Hall, J. D., and Schwartz, W. G. Spontaneous lactic acidosis. Amer. J. Med., 35:781, 1963.

ENDOCARDITIS, BACTERIAL

DIAGNOSIS

PREDISPOSING FACTORS AND CAUSATIVE ORGANISMS

Preexisting rheumatic valvulitis is the site of bacterial endocarditis in 40 to 60 percent of cases in most series. The mitral valve is most often infected (80 percent of cases) with mitral regurgitation the most common lesion. In decreasing frequency of involvement is the aortic valve (60 percent) followed by combinations of the aortic and mitral valves (40 percent) and the tricuspid valve in 18 percent of cases.

Approximately 10 to 20 percent of patients with bacterial

endocarditis have congenital heart disease. The most commonly involved lesions are interventricular septal defects and patent ductus arteriosus, followed by pulmonic stenosis and the tetralogy of Fallot. Interatrial septal defects are rarely infected. Recent reports indicate that apparently normal valves may become involved in 39 percent of cases of endocarditis. This is particularly true in the elderly patient.

The portal of entry of endocarditis is often not apparent. An obvious source of infection is most common in acute endocarditis. In subacute bacterial endocarditis dental manipulation or upper respiratory infection are the most common portals of entry. Genitourinary tract instrumentation or infection and obstetrical procedures are important causes of endocarditis due to enterococci. The prolonged use of continuous intravenous catheters may lead to valvular infection with staphylococci or fungi. Narcotics addiction with intravenous administration of contaminated material is a frequent predisposing factor. In these cases the disease is usually acute and most commonly involves the tricuspid valve with fungi and staphylococcus as predominant organisms.

Endocarditis is a serious complication of prosthetic heart valve replacement occurring in 8 to 12 percent of patients. The most common etiologic agents are staphyloccal organisms (coagulase-negative strains) which have been isolated in 70 percent of cases. Fungi have been isolated in smaller numbers of cases.

The causative organisms in cases reported by Rabinovich, et al. were

Alpha-hemolytic streptococcus	33%
Other streptococci	11%
Staphylococcus aureus	19%
Staphylococcus albus	5%
Fungus	2%
No organisms	26%

Although some cases of infective endocarditis do not conform to the appropriate syndrome on the basis of the responsible organism, classification into subacute and acute endocarditis is clinically important. Rapid diagnosis and treatment of acute bacterial endocarditis is more critical than in the case of subacute endocarditis if survival is to be achieved. Acute endocarditis is a rapidly progressive and lethal disease with a duration of 4 to 6 weeks.

CLINICAL FEATURES

There is a higher incidence of endocarditis in males than in females. Recent studies indicate endocarditis has become more frequent in the older age group in the past 20 years, 60 percent of cases being over the age of 50.

Murmurs are present in 99 percent of cases of SBE. Changing characteristics of a preexisting murmur occurs infrequently. Those who do not have murmurs more frequently have acute bacterial endocarditis due to *Staphylococcus aureus,* with predominantly right-sided (tricuspid) involvement.

Fever is the single most frequent sign of infective endocarditis occurring in 95 percent of cases. The fever may be masked by a terminal phase, renal insufficiency, or by the administration of small quantities of antibiotics, or steroid therapy. Cardiomegaly is present in 75 percent of cases.

Petechiae and subungual hemorrhages occur in 19 to 40 percent of the patients. Osler nodes, minute, painful, tender nodules of the fingers and toes, are thought to represent a hypersensitivity state. They are found in 10 percent of patients. Janeway lesions are painless, red-blue hemorrhagic lesions a few millimeters in diameter which occur in the palms and soles in 5 percent of patients. Fundiscopic abnormalities consisting of flame-shaped hemorrhages, retinal thrombosis, Roth spots, petechiae and other evidence of emboli are found in 17 percent. Larger emboli to the peripheral, visceral, and cerebral vessels occur in 33 percent of patients. Right-sided endocarditis may be complicated by pulmonary embolization with septic infarction.

The appearance of clubbing of the fingers depends on the duration of the illness and appears in 12 to 50 percent of patients. The spleen is palpable in 40 to 60 percent of patients. The size of the spleen is directly proportional to the duration of the illness.

The kidney is the second most common site of embolization. Renal failure is usually present in the late stages of endocarditis and may be due to glomerulonephritis, rather than the more commonly occurring renal infarction or focal embolic glomerulonephritis. The patient may be afebrile and negative blood cultures may be obtained during renal failure.

Cardiac decompensation is a poor prognostic sign and is the most common cause of death. Myocarditis is probably important in determining the prognosis of endocarditis. Myocardial microabscesses may complicate the clinical course and embolic coronary artery occlusion has been reported in a small percentage of patients.

The survival rate of bacterial endocarditis is approximately 75 percent and is directly related to the duration of delay in therapy, the etiologic organism, and the presence or absence of congestive failure.

LABORATORY FINDINGS

Blood cultures may be negative in 10 to 20 percent of patients. Cultures may be negative because of prior antibiotic therapy, right-sided endocarditis, or the presence of renal insufficiency. Six blood cultures should be obtained within a 48-hour period. Correlation with the temperature curve is not important, since the bacteremia is constant.

Normochromic normocytic anemia occurs in 50 to 80 percent of reported cases. Although the white cell count may be elevated, it is frequently normal and may even be low. Elevation of the erythrocyte sedimentation rate is seen in 90 percent and rheumatoid factor may be elevated in 50 percent. Phagocytic histiocytes found in blood obtained from the ear lobe in 30 percent may be of diagnostic value in the presence of negative blood cultures.

TREATMENT

An unexplained fever of more than a week duration in a patient with a cardiac murmur justifies the presumptive diagnosis of bacterial endocarditis. Splenomegaly or evidence of embolization increases the suspicion.

1. Treatment should begin, as soon as the blood cultures have been drawn, with 20 million units of aqueous penicillin I.V. and streptomycin, 1.0 g I.M. per 24 hours.
2. If an organism is isolated appropriate adjustment in therapy is made on the basis of sensitivity. Tube dilution sensitivity titers are essential to achieve bactericidal levels of an antibiotic. When infection is due to *Streptococcus viridans* or sensitive nonhemolytic streptococcus, 5 to 10 million units of penicillin G I.V. daily for 4 weeks may be effective. Moderately resistant nonhemolytic streptococci and enterococci necessitate an increase of penicillin to 20 million units with 2.0 g of streptomycin daily for 6 weeks.
3. Infection with sensitive staphylococcus requires the use of 8 million units of penicillin G per day for 7 weeks. In resistant staphylococcal injections, sodium methicillin, 2 to 4 g q. 6 h. I.V. for 7 weeks is employed. If infection persists, vancomycin, 1 g I.V. q. 12 h. should be used for 3 weeks.
4. Fungal infection (candida) may respond to Amphotericin B, 1 mg/kg per 24 hours I.V., to a total dose of 25 mg/kg.
5. In the presence of negative blood cultures, the dosage of penicillin and streptomycin is increased to 100 million units I.V. and 2 g I.M. per day by doubling the dose of penicillin every 72 hours. If there is no response, change to methicillin, 2 g I.V. q. 6 h.
6. Patients allergic to penicillin may be treated with cephalothin, 8 to 12 g per day for 4 to 6 weeks, or vancomycin, 1 g I.V. q. 12 h. for 3

weeks. An alternative approach is the use of penicillin with steroids (prednisone, 60-80 mg/day) to suppress delayed sensitivity reactions. Depending upon the allergic response, the steroids should be discontinued after 7 days.

7. Endocarditis in the presence of a prosthetic heart valve may rarely respond to early and prolonged antibiotic therapy, including penicillinase-resistant penicillins. Valve replacement is a more definitive approach.
8. The lack of improvement of fever may be due to ineffective antibiotics, inadequate dose, slow response (staphylococcus), metastatic abscess formation and drug allergy. Development of a new fever implies embolization, superinfection, or drug allergy.

If there is any doubt as to the efficacy of the antibiotic therapy, it is important to determine whether the concentration of antibiotic in the serum is bactericidal by tube dilution titers of the patient's serum. This is essential in the penicillin-allergic patient on steroids which will mask the clinical response to the antibiotic.

In the presence of renal failure, appropriate reduction in dosage schedules should be instituted. It is also important to note that penicillin G potassium contains 1.7 mEq K^+ per million units and penicillin G sodium contains 1.5 mEq Na^+ per million units.

PROPHYLAXIS OF ENDOCARDITIS

The patient with rheumatic or congenital heart disease undergoing dental extraction or ENT surgery should receive procaine penicillin G, 600,000 units b.i.d. on the day of the procedure and for the 2 subsequent days. If the patient has recently received antibiotic treatment, streptomycin should be added, 1 g daily.

For urologic manipulation, obstetrical procedures, or extensive GI system surgery prophylaxis with procaine penicillin G 2.4 million units I.M. and streptomycin, 2 g I.M., should be given on the day of the procedure and for 2 subsequent days.

In the patient allergic to penicillin, cephalothin, 0.5 g I.M. for each 600,000 units penicillin, or 1 g methicillin may be substituted.

REFERENCES

Cherubin, C. E. The medical sequelae of narcotic addiction. Ann. Intern. Med. 67:23, 1967

____ Baden, M., Kavaler, F., Lerner, S., and Cline, W. Infective endocarditis in narcotic addicts. Ann. Intern. Med., 69:1091, 1968.

Hall, B., and Dowling, H. F. Negative blood cultures in bacterial endocarditis: A decade's experience. Med. Clin. N. Amer., 50:159, 1966.
Lerner, P. I., and Weinstein, L. Infective endocarditis in the antibiotic era. New Eng. J. Med., 274:199, 259, 323, 388, 1966.
Louria, D. B., Hensle, T., and Rose, J. The major medical complications of heroin addiction. Ann. Intern. Med., 67:1, 1967.
Rabinovich, S., Smith, I. M., and January, L. E. The changing pattern of bacterial endocarditis. Med. Clin. N. Amer., 52:1091, 1968.
Soler-Bechara, J., Soscia, J. L., Kennedy, R. J., and Grace, W. J. Candida endocarditis. Amer. J. Cardiol., 13:820, 1964.
Stein, P. D., Harken, D. E., and Dexter, L. The nature and prevention of prosthetic valve endocarditis. Amer. Heart J., 71:393, 1966.

EOSINOPHILIA

Transient or constant eosinophilia (about 10 or more per 100 white blood cells and total eosinophil count elevated over 400 per mm^3) is usually associated with allergic or parasitic diseases.

1. Allergy. Asthma, allergic rhinitis, urticaria, and angioneurotic edema are frequently associated with a modest eosinophilia (5 to 20 per 100 WBC).
2. Parasites. Eosinophilia is especially seen with echinococcus, trichinosis, schistosomiasis, and taenia and ancylostoma infestations. Eosinophilia is less in filariasis, ascariasis, and malaria, and as a rule is absent in amebiasis, unless the liver is involved.

Other less frequent conditions in which eosinophilia may occur are:

3. Infections. May occur in scarlet fever and gonorrhea; and in convalescence from many infections a mild eosinophilia may occur.
4. Skin diseases. Pemphigus and dermatitis herpetiformis are frequently associated with eosinophilia. May also occur in exfoliative dermatitis, eczema, mycosis fungoides, psoriasis, prurigo, and erythema solare.
5. Hematopoietic. Eosinophilia is seen in about 20 percent of patients with Hodgkin's disease. It occurs also with eosinophilic leukemia, myelogenous leukemia, polycythemia vera, pernicious anemia, and postsplenectomy.
6. Miscellaneous. May occur in periarteritis nodosa, erythema multiforme, rheumatic chorea, neoplasms of serous surfaces, bone and ovary, poisoning with lead, hydrogen sulfide, copper sulfate, camphor, and pilocarpine, x-ray irradiation, Loeffler's syndrome, and rarely as congenital, familial, or idiopathic.

REFERENCE

Roberts, W. C., Liegler, D. G., and Carbone, P. P. Endomyocardial disease and Eosinophilia. Amer. J. Med., 46:28, 1969.

ERYTHEMA NODOSUM

Erythema nodosum is characterized by tender red subcutaneous nodules, usually on the anterior legs, fever, arthralgias, and malaise.

ETIOLOGY

1. Beta hemolytic streptococcal infections and rheumatic fever.
2. Idiopathic: approximately 10 to 15 percent.
3. Allergy to sulfa drugs, penicillin, bromides, iodine, aspirin, and phenolphthalein.
4. Less frequent causes include coccidioidomycosis, tuberculosis, and ulcerative colitis.
5. Rare causes are lymphogranuloma venereum, trichophytosis, meningococcemia, gonococcal septicemia, lues, leprosy, histoplasmosis, sarcoid, and systemic lupus erythematosus. Erythema nodosum has been reported as a reaction to the Kveim, Frei, and tuberculin skin tests.

Differential diagnosis includes nodular panniculitis of Weber-Christian, nodular vasculitis, and erythema induratum of Bazin.

REFERENCE

Beerman, H. Erythema nodosum. A survey of some recent literature. Amer. J. Med. Sci., 223:433, 1952.

ERYTHROCYTE SEDIMENTATION

The elevation of the sedimentation rate is a measure of the rate of fall of red blood cells in plasma and is a nonspecific reaction suggestive of underlying organic disease. The rate is altered by the physiochemical properties of the plasma and membrane of the erythrocytes. These properties bring about the aggregation of red blood cells known as "rouleaux formation."

The charges on the red cell membrane are altered by the concentration of the various plasma proteins in relation to each other and are the principal factor affecting rouleaux formation. An increase of fibrinogen, and normal or abnormal globulins causes an increase in the erythrocyte sedimentation rate (ESR), while an increase in albumin causes the cells to fall more slowly. The larger the RBC, the faster the sedimentation rate. The surface area with rouleaux formation is less than the total surface area of the individual cells combined. Hence, they fall faster because less surface area is exposed to the supporting plasma.

The ESR is determined by the Westergren or Wintrobe method; the former being the more popular. Correction for anemia is highly inaccurate and is not necessary. The rate of fall is determined at 1 hour, and an ESR of 100 mm or more is seen only using the Westergren tube which is graded 0 to 200 mm; gradation on the Wintrobe tube ranges only to 100 mm. The normal ESR for the Westergren method is for the male, 0-15 mm/hr; for the female, 0-20 mm/hr. The ESR for the Wintrobe method is for the male, 0-9 mm/hr; for the female 0-20 mm/hr. Values for the elderly and for children tend to be higher. In the pregnant female the ESR starts to rise at 12 weeks of gestation and returns to normal 4 weeks post partum. A marked elevation of the ESR (100 mm or more) may be indicative of underlying inflammatory disease, infection, malignancies, or connective tissue or renal disease. The relative prominence of these conditions causing an elevated ESR depends, of course, on the sample and the diagnostic methods available.

In recent reports a definite diagnosis was made in 95 percent of patients, but 6 percent of patients with extreme elevations may never have a diagnosis established. The incidence of various diagnoses were as follows:

1. Malignancies were seen in 58 percent. In over 90 percent metastasis was discovered on x-ray or at surgery. The types in descending order of frequency are: lymphoma, carcinoma of large bowel, and breast and multiple myeloma.
2. Inflammatory diseases make up 25 percent, of which infection was 33 percent, connective tissue disease 51 percent, miscellaneous inflammation (i.e., colitis) 16 percent. Pneumonia and tuberculosis were found less frequently than in the past.
3. Renal disease was the cause in 8 percent, and was usually associated with azotemia except in patients with the nephrotic syndrome.

The basic workup provided the diagnosis in most cases, viz., history and physical, hemoglobin analysis, CBC, BUN, chest x-ray, and routine urine analysis. Additional studies which were most beneficial are, viz., protein electrophoresis, bone marrow test, x-ray of axial skeleton, liver battery with BSP, lupus erythematosus (L.E.) preparation and biopsy of appropriate tissue.

REFERENCES

Wintrobe, M. M. Clinical Hematology. Philadelphia, Lea & Febiger, 1967.

Zacharski, L. R., and Kyle, R. A. Significance of extreme elevation of erythrocyte sedimentation rate. J.A.M.A. 202:264, 1967

FEVER OF UNDETERMINED ORIGIN (FUO)

DIAGNOSTIC CRITERIA (Petersdorf and Beeson)

1. Temperature above 101°F on several occasions.
2. The fever must have been present for at least 2 and preferably 3 weeks.
3. The diagnosis must remain obscure after 1 week of investigation in the hospital.

ETIOLOGY OF FEVER OF UNDETERMINED ORIGIN

1. Infection (40%): tuberculosis, SBE, pyogenic infections (pyelonephritis, cholangitis, intra-abdominal abscess), malaria, brucellosis.
2. Neoplasm (20%): leukemia, lymphoma, hypernephroma, carcinoma of stomach, liver, pancreas, carcinoma of lung, carcinomatosis.
3. Connective tissue-vascular disease (15%): periarteritis, systemic lupus erythematosus, rheumatoid arthritis, temporal arteritis, thromboembolic disease, relapsing febrile nodular panniculitis (Weber-Christian disease).
4. Miscellaneous (10%): drug fever, periodic disease, and factitious fever.
5. Undiagnosed (10%).

DIAGNOSTIC APPROACH

1. Careful history and physical examination.
2. Evaluation of the fever curve may be of value.
   Intermittent fever is defined as a temperature curve which returns to

normal during the day and reaches its peak in the evening. This is seen in pyogenic infections, tuberculosis, or lymphoma.
Remittent fever – temperature pattern does not return to the base line (98.6°F). Most fevers caused by infectious agents are remittent.
Sustained fever – little variation in temperature.
Relapsing fever. – Bouts of fever are interspersed with afebrile periods. This is seen in Hodgkin's disease, spirochetal infections, malaria.

3. Cultures, hematologic, metabolic evaluation.
4. Chest film and IVP are usually among the first radiographic procedures to be done.
5. Histologic examination of tissue is the single most productive procedure (biopsy, laparotomy).
6. Therapeutic trials are warranted under certain conditions and may occasionally be of value (i.e., antituberculous therapy, heparin therapy of thromboembolic disease, and withdrawal of drugs in drug fever).

It is important to point out that most patients with FUO do not have unusual diseases, but rather uncommon manifestations of common diseases.

REFERENCES

Hermans, P. E., and Baggenstoss, A. H. Fever of undetermined origin (CPC). Proc. Mayo Clinic, 42:50, 1967.

Petersdorf, R. G., and Beesen, P. B. Fever of unexplained origin: Report of 100 cases. Medicine, 40:1, 1961.

Sheon, R. P., and Van Ommen, R. A. Fever of obscure origin. Diagnosis and treatment based on a series of 60 cases. Amer. J. Med., 34:486, 1963.

Sohar, E., Gafni, J., Pras, M., and Heller, H. Familial mediterranean fever. A survey of 470 cases and review of the literature. Amer. J. Med., 43:227, 1967.

FIBROSCLEROTIC SYNDROMES

(Multifocal Fibrosclerosis)

1. Retroperitoneal fibrosis (venacaval obstruction and vasculitis).
2. Chronic mediastinal fibrosis (venacaval obstruction and vasculitis).
3. Pseudo tumor of orbit.
4. Reidel's struma.
5. Sclerosing cholangitis.

REFERENCES

Carton, R.W., and Wong, R. Multifocal fibrosclerosis manifested by

venacaval obstruction and associated with vasculitis. Ann. Intern. Med., 70:81, 1969.
Comings, D. E., Skubi, K. B., Van Eyes, J., and Motulsky, A. G. Familial multifocal fibrosclerosis. Ann. Intern. Med., 66:884, 1967.
Goodwin, W. E., et al. Diagnostic problems in retroperitoneal disease. Ann. Intern. Med., 65:160, 1966.

GASTRIC HYPOTHERMIA

Local gastric "cooling" significantly reduces the need for emergency surgery in patients with massive upper gastrointestinal hemorrhage. A cessation of bleeding is produced in the majority of patients. Its most effective use is in bleeding esophageal varices, peptic ulcer, and gastritis, with less value in stress ulcer and neoplasm.

TECHNIQUE

The stomach is emptied via a Levin tube, which is left in place, on intermittent suction. An esophageal or gastric balloon tied to a double lumen tube is passed orally and positioned snugly against the gastric cardia. The tube is attached to a special hypothermia machine, which pumps fluid at a constant rate and maintains temperature at a constant degree. About 600 ml of 30 percent ethanol or a Silicone solution is introduced into the balloon and circulated at 0° to 4° C. The patient's body temperature is maintained by electric warming blankets.

The Levin tube is irrigated every half hour. Once the bleeding has stopped, the cooling is continued for 36 to 48 hours, gradual rewarming allowed, and the balloon is decompressed and removed.

REFERENCES

Berenson, M. J., Soscia, J., and Grace, W. J. The influence of gastric hypothermia on experimental bacteremia in dogs. Amer. J. Dig. Dis., 10:631, 1965.
Crampton, R. S., et al. Experience with gastric hypothermia for active upper gastrointestinal tract hemorrhage. Surgery, 55:607, 1964.
McHardy, G., et al. An evaluation of gastric hypothermia. Amer. J. Dig. Dis., 9:717, 1964.
Miller, R. E., Moscarella, A. A., and Fitzpatrick, H. F. Local gastric hypothermia. Arch. Surg., 86:272, 1963.

Wangensteen, S. L., et al. Intragastric cooling for upper gastrointestinal bleeding. Ann. N.Y. Acad. Sci., 115:328, 1964.

GASTROENTERITIS

Gastroenteritis is a syndrome of acute onset, consisting of vomiting and diarrhea, either of which may predominate. There may be guarding, severe tenderness, but no other sign of an acute surgical abdomen.

DIFFERENTIAL DIAGNOSIS

1. Viral and nonspecific infections. Only half have fever. Usually over in a day.
2. Alcoholic overindulgence (gastritis only as a rule).
3. Allergy to foods (gluten, seafood, milk).
4. Infections:
   a. salmonellosis.
   b. shigellosis: 24-48 hour incubation, fever. Sulfa effective.
   c. cholera.
5. Toxic reactions:
   a. staphylococcus toxin.
   b. botulism (neurologic signs predominate, gastrointestinal signs may even be absent).
6. Protozoal:
   a. *Entamoeba histolytica*.
   b. *Giardia lamblia*.
7. Parasitic: trichinosis.
8. Miscellaneous: nausea and vomiting may be conspicuous in appendicitis, pregnancy, Addison's disease, and in uremia. Iatrogenic causes of gastroenteritis include the usually explosive and fatal gastroenterocolitis associated with staphylococcal overgrowth in patients treated with broad spectrum antibiotics; also the spectrum of GI complications from oral antibiotics – from mild disturbances through pseudomembranous enterocolitis.
9. The most common cause is of unknown etiology. Viral infections and psychogenic reactions probably account for many of the unknown.

GENERAL PRINCIPLES OF THERAPY

VOMITING. Hypochloremic, hypokalemic alkalosis may develop. If vomiting is severe and a predominant symptom, the patient is given intravenous fluids only, and nothing by mouth. Antiemetic drugs are of value. Compazine, in doses of 5 to 10 mg, I.M., q. 4 h. is quite effective. Dramamine, Marezine, and Bonine are of less value.

DIARRHEA. Tincture of opium, 0.5 to 1.0 ml, q. 4 h., p.r.n., or camphorated tincture of opium (Paregoric), 5 ml, q. 4 h., p.r.n., is of value. Codeine per se is perhaps a most effective drug. Bismuth or Kaopectate may also be used when the patient is not vomiting.

GENERAL. NPO – often necessary for 8 to 12 hours, then 1 oz clear liquid q. ½ h. (tea, broth), then one glass of clear liquid, then toast, pudding, cooked cereals. Avoid opiates until an acute surgical abdomen has been ruled out. Fluid and electrolyte replacement should be employed where indicated. As a general rule, about 1,500 of 5 percent glucose in water, 500 ml normal saline, and 40 mEq of potassium may be given per day. Sedation in the form of parenteral phenobarbital is of value.

SPECIFIC. When a specific diagnosis is established, appropriate antibacterial, antiparasitic, or antitoxic therapy should be instituted (see below).

STAPHYLOCOCCAL FOOD POISONING

Symptoms begin about 2 to 3 hours after ingestion of food containing staphylococcal enterotoxin and consist of the explosive onset of abdominal cramps, diarrhea, vomiting, and acute prostration. The most important therapeutic problem concerns dehydration and shock. Fluid, sodium, and potassium replacement in adequate doses will shorten the attack and prevent shock.

SALMONELLA INFECTIONS

Gastroenteritis occurring in salmonellosis is as a rule generally mild; only a small percent of cases develop typhoidal symptoms. The treatment is generally symptomatic in uncomplicated salmonella gastroenteritis, and the intestinal tract is freed naturally of the organism by diarrhea. Chloramphenicol is not indicated in the milder cases unless extraintestinal manifestations of infection occur. Then chloramphenicol or amphicillin may be used. The specific agent may be one of about 600 serotypes of salmonella, 40 of which are most common.

BOTULISM

Botulism is a rare cause of gastroenteritis; the main clinical manifestations refer to the toxic effects on the nervous system.

Difficulty in swallowing, diplopia, dysphonia, and respiratory distress are outstanding. In this country, outbreaks occur from the consumption of inadequately processed food. Five types of *Clostridium botulinum* are recognized. In order of decreasing frequency they are A, B, E, C, and D. Specific antitoxins are available for each type. In a critically ill patient with good historical and clinical evidence for botulism, at least 50,000 units each of A and B should be given after testing for hypersensitivity. Following this, at least 10,000 units of each is given daily.

REFERENCES

Bennett, I. L., Jr., and Hook, E. W. Infectious diseases (some aspects of salmonellosis). Ann. Rev. Med., 10:1, 1959.

Bowner, E. J. Challenge of salmonellosis: Major public health problem. Amer. J. Med. Sci., 247:467, 1964.

Dack, G. M. Current status of therapy in microbial food poisoning. J.A.M.A., 172:929, 1960.

Kaufmann, F. The Bacteriology of Entero-bacteriaceae. Baltimore, The Williams & Wilkins Co., 1966.

Koenig, M. G., Drutz, D. J., Mushlin, A. I., Schaffner, W., and Rogers, D. E. Type B botulism in man. Amer. J. Med., 42:208, 1967.

Saphra, I., and Winter, J. W. Clinical manifestations of salmonellosis in man: Evaluation of 7779 human infections identified at the New York Salmonella Center. New Eng. J. Med., 256:1128, 1957.

Weil, A. J., and Saphra, I. *Salmonellae* and *Shigellae.* Springfield, Ill., Charles C Thomas, Publisher, 1953.

GASTROINTESTINAL BLEEDING

(Hematemesis and Melena)

The causes of upper gastrointestinal hemorrhage occur in the following order of frequency.

Peptic ulcer	35%
No diagnosis established	20%
Esophageal varices	15%
Acute erosive gastritis	15%
Hiatus hernia with acute esophagitis	10%
Cancer of stomach	1%

Most adults can tolerate a blood loss of 400 to 500 ml without significant symptoms (for example, blood donors). The patient who presents with syncope or shock from blood loss has probably lost 1,500 to 2,500 ml.

With relatively small volumes of blood loss the stools will be tarry black (the word tarry means just this – a black, gooey, unformed stool). In massive upper gastrointestinal hemorrhage the stool may be maroon-colored or even grossly bloody.

During acute blood loss the blood remaining in the vascular channels is unchanged, i.e. the hematocrit will remain normal or occasionally even increase. Hence the character of the stools and clinical status of the patient give one a far better indication of blood loss than does the hematocrit initially. During the days after the hemorrhage there is a shift of fluid into the vascular tree, a dilution of the red cell mass, and a fall in hematocrit. This fall usually (in the absence of transfusion) may continue for at least 10 days even without further bleeding. This is an important point, as the continued fall in hematocrit is often attributed to oozing from the ulcer, whereas it may simply reflect shift in body fluids. The concept of slow leak and oozing of blood from peptic ulcer or esophageal varices is theoretical. More likely the bleeding point either spurts blood or does not bleed at all.

The stools may remain black for 10 days after one hemorrhage. The guaiac test may remain positive for 2 weeks.

Fever as high as 103°F may occur after GI bleeding. The temperature may remain elevated for a week.

Azotemia frequently follows massive GI hemorrhage. It is probably a reflection of a degree of renal functional impairment due to the rapid blood loss (shock kidney).

Electrocardiographic changes (depression of ST segment and inversion of T waves) are common in GI hemorrhage. Angina may be precipitated. The sudden fall in blood pressure may initiate myocardial infarction. On the other hand, the stress of myocardial infarction may precipitate a peptic ulcer with bleeding.

LOCALIZING THE SITE OF THE UPPER GI HEMORRHAGE

Many methods have been used over the years to determine the site of the blood loss. These include various string tests, aspiration of the esophagus, stomach, and duodenum; emergency BSP tests; emergency upper GI x-ray. None of these procedures has proven completely reliable. At the present time we advocate emergency esophagoscopy and gastroscopy using the fiber-optic instruments as a routine. If there is an indication of impending surgery and the site of bleeding is still unknown, emergency splenoportography should be done. It is likely that an emergency upper GI series should be done if time permits before doing an emergency operation. Selective mesenteric arteriography may also be useful.

EMERGENCY MANAGEMENT OF ACUTE UPPER GASTROINTESTINAL HEMORRHAGE

The patient should be placed at bed rest and given nothing by mouth. Adequate sedation to keep the patient quite drowsy is indicated. Replacement of blood in sufficient quantity to maintain the normal vital signs is also indicated. Hematocrit determinations are done every four hours, and an indwelling nasogastric tube is placed in order to determine whether or not bleeding has stopped or has recurred. During this period of time one should do an emergency esophagoscopy and gastroscopy, which will demonstrate a large proportion of the active bleeding points. If the patient is having a massive hemorrhage (that is, one requiring 6 pints of blood or more in 48 hospital hours), the institution of local gastric hypothermia should be considered even though the site of the blood loss may not be known. The only serious contraindication to this procedure is cancer of the stomach. (See also "Ulcer," p. 421 and "Esophageal varices," p. 69.) Any patient with massive gastrointestinal bleeding should be followed by a surgical consultant as well as by his physician.

SALICYLATES AND GASTROINTESTINAL BLEEDING

It is generally believed that frequent doses of aspirin may cause erosive gastritis with blood loss. Some have felt that this is why more GI bleeding occurs in the fall and spring, the seasons of respiratory infections.

ULCER AND STEROIDS

"Steroid ulcers," i.e., gastric ulcers occurring in patients on long-term steroid therapy, are very common (15 to 30 percent) and may cause massive hemorrhage.

GASTROINTESTINAL HEMORRHAGE AND PERFORATED ULCER

It is frequently said that ulcers do not bleed and perforate at the same time. This, however, does occasionally happen (1 percent).

MALLORY-WEISS SYNDROME

This consists of one or more longitudinal tears in the mucosa and submucosa of the cardia, reaching and frequently crossing the gastroesophageal junction. It follows protracted retching, most often in an alcoholic patient. Bleeding may be slight or massive, and is of arterial origin and cannot be controlled with the Sengstaken-Blakemore balloon. Surgical intervention is usually needed.

Gastrointestinal hemorrhage from the rarer causes include polyps of the stomach, tumors of the upper small bowel, Peutz-Jeghers syndrome, biliary tract disease, pancreatic lesions, uremia.

REFERENCES

Bave, A. E. Bleeding from laceration of the cardia. J.A.M.A., 184:139, 1963.

Dagradi, A. E., Broderick, J. T., Juler, G., Wolinsky, S., and Stempien, S. J. The Mallory-Weiss syndrome and lesion. Amer. J. Dig. Dis. (new series), 11:710, 1966.

Hirschowitz, B. I., Luketic, G. C., Balin, J. A., and Fulton, W. F. Early fiberscope endoscopy for upper gastrointestinal bleeding. Amer. J. Dig. Dis., 8:816, 1963.

Katz, D., Douvres, P., Weisberg, H., Charm, R., and McKinnon, W. Sources of bleeding in upper gastrointestinal hemorrhage: A re-evaluation. Amer. J. Dig. Dis., 9:447, 1964.

_____ Douvres, P., Weisberg, H., McKinnon, W., and Glass, G. B. J. Early endoscopic diagnosis of acute upper gastrointestinal hemorrhage. J.A.M.A., 188:405, 1964.

Mallory, G. K., and Weiss, S. Hemorrhages from lacerations of the cardiac orifice of the stomach due to vomiting. Amer. J. Med. Sci., 178:506, 1929.

Weiss, S., and Mallory, G. K. Lesions of the cardiac orifice of the stomach produced by vomiting. J.A.M.A., 98:1353, 1932.

GENETIC DISORDERS

DISORDER	BIOCHEMICAL DEFECT	CLINICAL FINDINGS	LABORATORY	INHERITANCE	TREATMENT	REFERENCES
Congenital adrenal hyperplasia	Six major types C_{21}: hydroxylase defect most common	Virilism; early growth spurt and skeletal maturation in children; primary amenorrhea; more severe types may have salt-loosing syndrome in infancy	Urinary steroids: ↓ Thydroxy-steroid ↑ 17-keto-steroid ↑ Pregnanetriol	Simple autosomal recessive gene	Hydrocortisone 10 mg P.O. b.i.d. or t.i.d. or cortisone 12.5 mg b.i.d. or t.i.d.; salt-retaining steroid in the salt-loosing type	Bongiovanni, A.M., and Root, The adrenogenital syndrome. New Eng. J. Med., 2,68:1283, 1342, 1391, 1963.
Testicular feminization	Unknown evidence suggests an end organ defect to testosterone	Phenotypic females; well-developed breasts; female external genitalia; testes usually intra-abdominal; sparseness of axillary and pubic hair. Incomplete type, clitoral hypertrophy. Labial or inguinal testes	Negative chromatin pattern. XY sex chromosomal pattern	X-linked inheritance; autosomal dominant inheritance limited to the male sex	(1) Removal of gonads after puberty; (2) Sex steroids-estrogens after removal of gonads	Morris, J.M., and Mahesh, J.B. Further observations on the syndrome of "testicular feminization," Amer. J. Obstet. Gynec., 87:731, 1963. French, F.A., et al. Testicular feminization. Clinical, morphological and biochemical studies. J. Clin. Endocr., 25:661, 1965.

DISORDER	BIOCHEMICAL DEFECT	CLINICAL FINDINGS	LABORATORY	INHERITANCE	TREATMENT	REFERENCES
Wilson's disease (hepatolenticular degeneration)	Not known with certainty; possibly decreased synthesis of ceruloplasmin	Rigidity, dysarthria, spasticity, tremor; more pathologic than clinical evidence of cirrhosis; golden brown granular pigmentation of limbus of cornea	↑ Excretion of copper ↑ Direct serum-reacting copper ↓ Serum ceruloplasmin aminoaciduria	Autosomal recessive	Penicillamine	Walshe, J.H., and Cumings, J.N. Wilson's Disease: Some Current Concepts. Oxford, Blackwell Scientific Publications, 1959.
Nonglycosuric mellituria	Defect in glycuronic acid oxidation pathway	Asymptomatic mellituria principally found in Jews	1.0-4.0 g of pentose L-xylose excreted daily.			
Pentosuria			Suspect patient with positive reducing test in urine but negative specific test for glucose	Autosomal recessive		

Essential fructosuria	Deficient fructokinase	Benign; asymptomatic	High concentration of blood fructose. Blood lactate and respiratory quotient fails to rise	Autosomal recessive	Not necessary	Marble, A. "Nondiabetic Mellituria." In Joslin, E.P., Root, H.F., White, R., and Marble, A., eds. The Treatment of Diabetes Mellitus, 10th ed. Philadelphia. Lea and Febiger, 1959.
Hereditary fructose intolerance	Deficient hepatic fructose L-phosphate aldolase	Severe hypoglycemia and vomiting; distaste for fruits, sweets	Hypoglycemia and decreased serum phosphorus with I.V. administration of fructose	Autosomal recessive	Elimination of fructose-containing foods	
Renal tubular acidosis	Inability to acidify urine; may be due to diffusion of secreted hydrogen from tubular urine back into blood	Weakness, paralysis associated with hypokalemia, osteomalacia, nephrocalcinosis, renal stones, polyuria	Plasma: ↓ bicarbonate ↓ potassium ↑ chloride Urine: pH $>$ 6 ↑ potassium ↑ calcium ↑ phosphorus	Transient disease of infancy. Usually not familial. Persistent disease usually sporadic but of appreciable familial incidence; dominant transmission described	Alkali (Shohl's Sol)	Randal, R.E., and Targgart, W.H. Familial renal tubular acidosis, Ann. Intern. Med., 54: 1108, 1961.

DISORDER	BIOCHEMICAL DEFECT	CLINICAL FINDINGS	LABORATORY	INHERITANCE	TREATMENT	REFERENCES
Periodic paralysis (hypokalemic type)	Not delineated	Patients normal except for episodic muscular weakness or paralysis without loss of consciousness; begins early in life, peaks in the third decade; attacks induced by carbohydrates, rest, exertion, cold, infection, trauma, fluorohydrocortisone, epinephrine	↓ Serum potassium ↑ Muscle potassium ↑ Excretion of sodium-retaining steroids; 17KS and less commonly 17 OH	Autosomal dominant with complete penetration	Potassium salts, aldactone; avoid high carbohydrate intake	Poskauzer, D.C., and Kerr, D.N.S. Periodic paralysis with response to spironolactone. Lancet, 2: 511, 1961. Cicero, F., Cuddy, R., and Streeter, D.H.P. Periodic paralysis. New York J. Med., 63: 2226, 1963.

Muscular dystrophies	Not identified; one theory that of a defect in permeability of muscle membrane	A group of disorders characterized by progressive atrophy of skeletal muscles: Types: (1) Childhood (Duchenne) heart disease common; (2) Limb-girdle; (3) Fascioscapulohumeral	Creatinuria characteristic of childhood type; not always present in adult form. ↑ Serum aldolase, LDH, SGOT, CPK	Childhood type–X-linked recessive trait Limb-girdle; probably autosomal recessive trait Fascioscapulohumeral autosomal dominant trait	No treatment really effective; digitalis, active exercise, and anabolic steroids have been suggested	Walton, N.J. and Nattrass, F.J. On the classification, natural history and treatment of the myopathies. Brain, 77:169, 1954.
Myotonic dystrophy		Myotonia may be early finding followed by progressive muscular weakness; physical characteristics: expressionless face, ptosis of eye lids, cataracts, nasal voice, alopecia, testicular atrophy; heart disease common	Irregular creatinuria; characteristic after potentials of myotonia on electromyogram	Autosomal dominant		

GLOMERULONEPHRITIS

(See also Uremia)

Glomerulonephritis is best classified into four major types:

1. Acute glomerulonephritis.
2. Rapidly progressive glomerulonephritis.
3. Chronic glomerulonephritis.
4. Focal glomerulonephritis.

ACUTE GLOMERULONEPHRITIS

Acute glomerulonephritis is an acute inflammatory disease of the kidney characterized by hypercellularity of the mesangium of the glomerulus. Males are affected twice as often as females; all ages are susceptible with the highest incidence between the ages of 3 and 7 years. Patients usually present with smoky urine and edema, 1 to 4 weeks after a pharyngeal, respiratory, or skin infection with group A hemolytic streptococci, types 12, 4, 1, and Red Lake strain. Transient oliguria, azotemia, and hypertension may occur. Urinalysis reveals proteinuria, usually less than 5 g per 24 hours, red blood cells, white blood cells, red blood cell and granular casts. Glomerular filtration rate and renal plasma flow are normal or low, filtration fraction is reduced, and TmPAH and TmGlucose are impaired. The complications include congestive heart failure, hypertensive encephalopathy, seizures, sepsis, and the uremic syndrome.

DIFFERENTIAL DIAGNOSIS

1. Glomerulitis: lupus erythematosus, polyarteritis, Schonlein-Henoch syndrome and Goodpasture's syndrome.
2. Toxic nephropathy: exogenous poisons, and drugs.
3. Focal glomerulonephritis.
4. Acute tubular necrosis.
5. Acute pyelonephritis.
6. Malignant hypertension.

EVALUATION

Isolation of group A hemolytic streptococci from the throat or skin and a rising antistreptolysin-O titer (ASO) help establish the diagnosis. Serum complement levels are significantly lowered in almost all cases. Complement may also be low in serum sickness, lipoid nephrosis, trichinosis, systemic lupus erythematosus, Hashimoto's disease, and portal cirrhosis. Percutaneous needle biopsy of the kidney is a valuable diagnostic aide.

TREATMENT

1. Penicillin should be administered for 10 to 14 days.
2. Rest and restriction of activity should be enforced in the hope of preventing chronicity. Gradual return to full activity may be begun in a month or two, even if proteinuria or hematuria persists. If, however, these increase in amount, restriction of activity is again indicated.
3. Diet during the acute oliguric phase:
   a. Fluid intake should be restricted to 400-500 ml a day plus output. Parenteral fluid is best administered in the form of 10 to 30 percent solution of dextrose over a 24-hour period. Daily weight is an excellent check on fluid balance. The patient should not gain weight during the acute phase.
   b. Sodium is restricted to 200 mg or less daily.
   c. Diet should be high in carbohydrate and low in potassium and protein. With severe degrees of oliguria, no protein is given.
   d. When urinary output exceeds 1 to 2 liters per day, dietary restrictions should be removed.
4. Frequent measurements of serum electrolytes (especially potassium) and frequent ECG's should be done. Hyperkalemia is the most serious complication of prolonged oliguria (see pp. 199 and 359).
5. Congestive failure. Slow digitalization is undertaken. Diuretics are usually of little value, and may even be harmful.
6. For convulsions and severe hypertension, reserpine, 2.5 mg, I.M., b.i.d., or apresoline, 5 mg, I.M., b.i.d., is of value. Magnesium administration is hazardous.
7. Dialysis with the artificial kidney is reserved for patients poorly responsive to the above regimes. Dialysis, when indicated, may prove lifesaving (see p. 109).

PROGNOSIS

Proteinuria may persist for 6 months and hematuria for 1 year with ultimately complete recovery.

Children:

82% complete recovery
4% develop rapidly progressive glomerulonephritis
10% develop latent chronic glomerulonephritis
4% die during acute illness

Adults:

60% recover completely
5% develop rapid progressive glomerulonephritis
30% develop latent chronic glomerulonephritis
5% die during acute phase

RAPIDLY PROGRESSIVE GLOMERULONEPHRITIS (SUBACUTE)

Some patients have a history of previous poststreptococcal glomerulonephritis which failed to resolve. Others do not have such a history. Characteristically microscopic hematuria, cylinduria, and proteinuria persist, renal function deteriorates with increasing azotemia and often hypertension. Death ensues weeks or months later. Pathologically the lesions resemble the Schönlein-Henoch syndrome and polyarteritis.

CHRONIC GLOMERULONEPHRITIS

Most cases of chronic glomerulonephritis are detected between the second and fifth decade of life. Some cases had a previous poststreptococcal glomerulonephritis with persistent proteinuria and cellular elements in the urine sediment for approximately 15 years. A terminal stage then ensues with chronic renal failure usually with hypertension. The largest group of patients with chronic glomerulonephritis do not have a history of previous renal disease; they merely present with azotemia and hypertension.

The terminal stage is characterized by hypertension, edema, azotemia, and anemia. Loss of the ability to concentrate the urine is usual and patients pass large quantities of dilute urine. The urine sediment shows red blood cells, white blood cells, and terminally broad casts and renal failure casts. Hyperphosphatemia, hypocalcemia and hypermagnesemia may occur. Metabolic acidosis occurs with diminished serum bicarbonate levels and a tendency to hyperkalemia; the serum sodium usually is normal but may fall in patients with salt-losing nephritis.

PATHOLOGIC DIAGNOSIS

There are two major lesions associated with chronic glomerulonephritis. Chronic lobular glomerulonephritis, most frequently related to streptococcal infections, and the nephrotic syndrome. Chronic idiopathic membranous glomerulonephritis usually begins with the insidious onset of ankle edema in patients without a history of previous streptococcal infection; the incidence of males to females is 4:1.

DIFFERENTIAL DIAGNOSIS

1. Chronic pyelonephritis.

2. Essential hypertension.
3. Arteriosclerosis.
4. Systemic lupus erythematosis.
5. Amyloidosis.
6. Diabetes mellitus.

TREATMENT OF RAPIDLY PROGRESSIVE AND CHRONIC GLOMERULONEPHRITIS

1. Treat the underlying cause, if known, e.g., diabetes, SLE.
2. Diet: protein and potassium restrictions are guided by degree of azotemia, acidosis, and potassium excretion. Salt is restricted in the edematous patient, but salt administration is indicated in those with salt-losing nephritis. At least 100 g of carbohydrate must be provided daily.
3. Fluid balance is determined by output plus 500 to 700 ml per 24 hours insensible losses. Severe fluid restriction may be necessary in edematous patients.
4. Anemia in patients with chronic glomerulonephritis is often best left untreated. Generally transfusions are given only when the patient becomes symptomatic of their anemia, weakness, dyspnea, angina, or active bleeding occurs.
5. Hyperphosphatemia may be treated with Amphogel or Basogel 30 ml t.i.d. P.O.
6. Hypocalcemia rarely is severe enough to require therapy. In fact, treatment of hypocalcemia may be dangerous with precipitation of renal calculi and metastatic calcinosis. Correction of hypocalcemia with the administration of calcium and vitamin D and aluminum hydroxide gel is indicated when clinical signs of hypocalcemia become manifest.
7. Acidosis may be improved by the use of sodium bicarbonate.
8. Characteristically uremic patients have five disturbing symptoms: nocturnal insomia, nausea, vomiting, diarrhea, and tremulousness. Treatment is extremely difficult and one must be cautious about using barbiturates, opiates, and tranquilizers in uremic patients since they are not excreted normally. Coma is frequently the sequelae of indiscriminate administration of these drugs. Caution must be exercised in prescribing any medication to a patient with impaired renal function.
9. Exacerbation of nephritis may occur during the latent chronic phase, usually precipitated by infection, and resulting in transient impairment of renal function. Usually permanent damage does not occur. Peritoneal or hemodialysis may be necessary to tide the patient over periods of increased azotemia.
10. Patients with creatinine clearances of less than 5 ml per minute are now being successfully maintained by repetitive hemodialysis, peritoneal dialysis and renal hemotransplantation.

FOCAL GLOMERULONEPHRITIS

Focal glomerulonephritis is a form of nephritis in which only a certain number of glomeruli show abnormalities while others remain normal. Hematuria and proteinuria occur without edema or hypertension, during the course of various infectious illnesses, such as streptococcal infection of the throat, skin, and uterus, pneumonia, staphlococcal and hemophylus influenza infections, typhoid fever, malaria, and relapsing fever. This lesion is frequently seen in the Schönlein-Henoch syndrome, polyarteritis, lupus erythematosus and Goodpasture's syndrome. Focal embolic glomerulonephritis is the renal lesion of subacute bacterial endocarditis and rarely acute bacterial endocarditis. Treatment is directed at the underlying cause. Significant oliguria and azotemia do not usually occur.

REFERENCES

Kassirer, J. P., and Schwartz, W. B. Acute glomerulonephritis. New Eng. J. Med., 265:736, 1961.

Michael, A. F., et al. Immunosuppressive therapy in renal diseases. New Eng. J. Med., 276:817, 1967.

Perkoff, G. T. The herediatry renal disease. New Eng. J. Med., 277:79, 1967.

Pollak, V. E., Rosen, S., Pirani, C. L., Muekrcke, R. C., and Kark, R. M. Natural history of lipoid nephrosis and membranous glomerulonephritis. Ann. Intern. Med., 69:1171, 1968.

Symposium on uremia. Amer. J. Med., 44, 1968.

GOUT

Gout is a disorder of purine metabolism characterized by hyperuricemia, recurrent acute arthritis, and eventually deposition of urates in joint spaces, bursae, tendons, kidneys, heart, and other tissues. The incidence in the general medical population is estimated between 1 and 5 percent. Gout is rare in premenopausal females.

DIAGNOSIS

HISTORY AND PHYSICAL

1. Joint pain – burning, tingling and warmth, progressing to acute pain with edema and erythema. The classical gouty toe is bright violaceous

red, slightly swollen, and exquisitely tender. The metatarsophalangeal joint of the big toe is involved in 60 to 70 percent of initial attacks (podagra). Hands, wrists, ankles, and knees are frequently involved.
2. Gout is frequently precipitated by obvious physical stress, hard physical labor, or the stress of surgery. Any elderly patient who develops acute arthritis immediately postoperatively probably has gout. Attacks are frequently associated with moderate or heavy drinking.
3. Tophi are the most useful clinical finding, occurring in the helix of the ear and around joints in about 25 percent of patients. These, however, are a manifestation of long-standing disease.
4. Obesity is found in about one half of cases.
5. Gouty patients have a significantly high incidence of diabetes (25 percent) and of hypertensive and arteriosclerotic cardiovascular disease.

LABORATORY

1. Serum uric acid is elevated over 6 mg per 100 ml in about 80 percent of cases.
2. X-ray: "punched out" appearance in tophaceous gout. X-rays, however, are frequently normal.
3. Biopsy of tophi.

Secondary gout refers to symptomatic gout related to other hyperuricemic states. There is no special sex distribution. These include the following.

1. Myeloid metaplasia
2. Polycythemia vera
3. Leukemias
4. Multiple myeloma
5. Pernicious anemia
6. Hemolytic anemias

Other causes of hyperuricemia include renal failure, congestive heart failure, acute infections, malignancies, and drugs including chlorothiazide, penicillin, and pyrazinamide. These factors probably will not precipitate clinical gout except in susceptible individuals.

MISCELLANEOUS

Gouty nephropathy occurs in at least 50 percent of chronic gout and may lead to uremia, which may be the outstanding part of the clinical picture.

TREATMENT

Acute attacks.

1. Colchicine is specific for gout and response to colchicine establishes

the diagnosis.* Dose: 0.5 mg, P.O., q.h., until the pain is relieved or nausea or diarrhea occurs. If after the first dose of colchicine the patient is unresponsive, 1.0 mg may be given for the second and third doses. If diarrhea occurs, paregoric may be employed. Intravenous colchicine is occasionally superior because of quicker action and termination of the attack before onset of gastrointestinal symptoms. The dose is 1 mg, I.V., followed by 0.5 to 1.0 mg, q. 6 h., until toxic symptoms or relief occurs.

2. Other drugs.
   a. Phenylbutazone (Butazolidin) should be reserved for patients intolerant or unresponsive to colchicine. The usual dose is 400 mg, followed by 200 mg, q. 4 to 6 h.
   b. Steroids in acute gouty arthritis are rarely necessary, but in the long-standing, untreated gout resistant to colchicine they may be used effectively (80-100 mg/d for 2 to 3 days.)
   c. Indomethacin (Indocin) 25 mg q.i.d.
3. Interval treatment: Colchicine, 1 to 2 mg, q.d., is the most effective agent for the prevention of attacks.
4. Uricosuric agents: Probenecid (Benemid), 0.5 g, b.i.d., will usually lower serum uric acid and promote significant uricosuria (50 to 100 percent increase) after several months of use. A large fluid intake is recommended with this drug. Aspirin probably nullifies the uricosuric effect of probenecid, and the two should not be given together.
5. Allopurinol (Zyloprim). This agent blocks xanthine oxidase and thus the formation of uric acid from xanthine and hypoxanthine. The drug is recommended where there is decreased renal function and to avoid the urolithiasis of uricosuric agents. The dose is 200 to 400 mg daily.

REFERENCES

Gutman, A. B. The significance of the renal clearance of uric acid in normal and gouty man. Amer. J. Med., 37:833, 1964.

Hall, A. P., Barry, P. E., Dawber, T. R., and McNamara, P. M. Epidemiology of gout and hyperuricemia. Amer. J. Med., 42:27, 1967.

MacLachlan, M. J., and Podnan, G. P. Effects of food, fast and alcohol on serum uric acid and acute attacks of gout. Amer. J. Med., 42:38, 1967.

O'Duffy, J. D., and Scherbel, A. L. Treatment of gout and urate calculi with allopurinol. Report of three representative cases. Cleveland Clin. Quart., 35:145, 1968.

*Sarcoid arthritis has been reported to respond to colchicine.

HALLUCINOGEN ABUSE

Any number of drugs can produce hallucinations, but the term "hallucinogen" is generally confined to those substances which produce psychologic changes in a high proportion of subjects exposed to the drug without producing the gross impairment of memory and orientation characteristic of toxic psychoses or drug-induced deliria. The psychologic changes that are produced mimic, to a large extent, the symptoms of the endogenous, "functional" psychoses, especially the schizophrenias. As a result, they are sometimes termed "psychotomimetric," or "schizomimetic"; others favor the term "psychedelic" (mind-manifesting) to avoid the perplexing question of how good a facsimile of spontaneously occurring psychosis is the state induced by hallucinogens. Others term them "M.A.D." (mind-altering drugs) or "consciousness-expanding" drugs. Even as used in the more strict sense, however, many hallucinogens are known: marijuana, mescaline (peyote), lysergic acid diethylamide (LSD), adrenochrome, harmine, tetrahydrocannabinol, di-isopropyl fluorophosphate (DFP), tetraethylpyrophosphate (TEEP), N-allylnormorphine, bufotenin, psilocybin (from mushrooms), ololiuqui (from morning glory seeds), dimethyltryptamine (DMT), STP, and even nutmeg (myristica).

None of the hallucinogens is addictive, at least insofar as physical dependence is concerned, although some tolerance develops to each of them (and usually, cross-tolerance to other members of the group as well, perhaps because the indole ring is a basic structural unit common to all of them). The ones most frequently abused at the present time are marijuana, LSD, and STP. The last two are the most powerful of the entire group.

LSD-*25*; D-LYSERGIC ACID DIETHYLAMIDE. Known popularly as "acid," the Big A, or the Cube; its source is Ergot, *Claviceps purpurea,* a fungus growing on cereal grains. It can be synthesized, however, and is relatively easy to obtain because its manufacture is not a complicated process. In New York, it is sold as a colorless, odorless liquid that is usually dropped onto a cube of sugar in a dose of about 250 μg. Effects are manifest usually within 30 minutes after ingestion, with a peak during the second and third hours, and lasting generally for a total of eight to ten hours. Peak effects include any of the following: hallucinations, feelings of depersonalization, other-worldly sensations, a torrent of thoughts and intensification of feelings with simultaneous lessening of "wanting" or "striving," disconnected images including thrusts of awareness of one's own being, and marked impairment of judgment. Users seek particularly for some kind of mystical union with the unknown, spiritual ecstasy, and rapture. They talk about their trips providing them with a "unitive" religious experience, a oneness with self, with others, with the universe, and with God; a feeling that no matter what one's inner thoughts and visions, they are experienced by everyone else on the drug; a conviction of communication that often they have never experienced in real life.

The major complications of a "trip" are related to the unpredictability of drug effects, which may have different effects on the same subject at different times.

1. Panic reaction, with overwhelming terror, sometimes suicidal ideas (and actions), occasionally outbursts of aggressiveness or homicidal rage – this complication is popularly termed a "bad trip."
2. Persisting, extended, and in some cases perhaps even irreversible psychosis; this probably occurs only in latent schizophrenics or in those otherwise predisposed.
3. Delayed reactions and reappearance of acute psychotic symptoms hours or days after ingestion of the drug, when the subject is no longer under supervision or control.

Treatment: Acute psychotic symptoms generally respond favorably to phenothiazines (e.g., I.M. chlorpromazine); extended psychotic episodes require the same treatment as would be given for any schizophrenic decompensation.

STP. The name for this compound was borrowed by users from that of a commercial additive (although some maintain that it is an acronym for Serenity-Tranquility-Peace). STP was developed as DOM for experimental use in mental patients; chemically, it is 4-methyl 2, 5 dimethoxy-α-methyl-phenethylamine, and is related to mescaline and amphetamine. It is used mainly on the West Coast and is said to have a more powerful mind-distorting effect than LSD even though it is less potent on a weight-for-weight basis. Effects are similar to those described for LSD; its chief difference from the latter is that the psychotic symptoms it produces do not respond to phenothiazines, which may actually aggravate symptoms.

LSD users, and probably STP users as well, demonstrate a significant increase of chromosomal abnormalities (analogous to those produced by excessive irradiation) that persist for at least 6 months after ingestion. What the ultimate significance of this may be to reproduction occurring during that period is unknown.

The chief known hazard of LSD and STP administration is not so much the precipitation of a schizophreniclike state, but in decreasing emotional and effective controls and inducing a persistent state of altered consciousness. The risk appears greater in subjects with emotional lability and psychopathic features than in those with a thought disorder. Indeed, the risk appears greatest in precisely those for whom the compounds have been made most attractive by the press and pseudoscientific enthusiasts.

HEART DISEASE, CONGENITAL

CLASSIFICATION

Congenital heart disease is best classified according to peripheral oxygen saturation into acyanotic, usually acyanotic (or late cyanotic), and cyanotic groups. Each of these can be further subdivided into those associated with normal, increased, or decreased pulmonary blood flow. Pulmonary blood flow may be estimated from routine chest x-rays taken in the PA and lateral position. Note especially the hilar regions on the lateral films. A hypoplastic hilum indicates reduced pulmonary blood flow, as do reduced vascular markings throughout the lung fields (see below, lesions with reduced pulmonary blood flow).

Prominent hilar areas with reduced peripheral pulmonary markings usually indicate rising pulmonary resistance secondary to pulmonary hypertension.

Surgical intervention is curative or palliative in those conditions labeled with an asterisk in the following outline.

ACYANOTIC

A. With normal pulmonary blood flow.
   1. Pulmonary stenosis with intact ventricular septum (mild cases).*
   2. Endocardial fibroelastosis.
   3. Glycogen storage disease.
   4. Congenital myocarditis.
   5. Coarctation of the aorta.*
   6. Vascular ring.*
B. With increased pulmonary flow.
   1. Patent ductus arteriosus (shunt L to R).*

   2. Interatrial and interventricular septal defects (shunt L to R).*
   3. Anomalous drainage of the pulmonary veins.*
   4. Pulmonic stenosis with interatrial septal defect (mild cases).*
   5. Aortic-pulmonic window (shunt L to R).*

C. With decreased pulmonary flow.
   1. Ebstein's malformation.* This consists of downward displacement of the tricuspid valve into the right ventricle, with "atrialization" of the ventricle, enlargement of the atrium, and decreased pulmonary blood flow.
   2. Pulmonic stenosis (with intact ventricular septum).*

USUALLY ACYANOTIC (LATE CYANOSIS). This group includes all septal defects which may, later in the disease, be associated with a right to left shunt. They are patent ductus arteriosus, aortic-pulmonic window, and the intracardiac septal defects.

CYANOTIC.

A. With increased pulmonary flow.
   1. Eisenmenger's complex is in essence a ventricular septal defect with right-to-left shunt. In addition an overriding aorta, right ventricular hypertrophy, and a normal pulmonic infundibulum, valve, and artery are present (the artery may be dilated).
   2. Transposition of the great vessels.
   3. Tricuspid atresia.
   4. Common truncus.

B. With decreased pulmonary flow.
   1. Tetralogy of Fallot * is identical to Eisenmenger's complex, save that in the former the pulmonary artery, valve, or infundibulum is stenotic.
   2. Tricuspic atresia with interatrial septal defect.
   3. Ebstein's malformation plus a patent foramen ovale.*
   4. Transpositions with pulmonic stenosis.*
   5. Pulmonary stenosis with an interatrial septal defect.*

MISCELLANEOUS

1. Ventricular septal defects (20 percent), tetralogy of Fallot (11 percent), patent ductus arteriosus (10.7 percent), and atrial septal defects (9.6 percent) are the most common congenital anomalies. Together these four comprise slightly more than half of all congenital heart disease.
2. If a cyanotic patient with a congenital cardiac malformation has decreased pulmonary vascular markings but no cardiomegaly, the most likely diagnosis is the tetralogy of Fallot. Other possibilities include tricuspic atresia, single ventricle with pulmonary stenosis, and pseudotruncus. This group is most amenable to procedures such as the Blalock-Taussig, Potts-Smith and Brock pulmonary valvulotomy. With increased pulmonary vascular pulsations and cardiomegaly, surgical procedures are of much less value. Banding of the pulmonary artery may be of aid.

3. Lutembacher's disease consists of atrial septal defect plus mitral stenosis.
4. Taussig-Bing syndrome is composed of
   a. aorta arising from right ventricle
   b. pulmonary artery arising from both ventricles
   c. high ventricular septal defect
   d. right ventricular hypertrophy.
5. The causes of congenital idiopathic cardiac hypertrophy are
   a. endocardial fibroelastosis
   b. congenital myocarditis
   c. rhabdomyoma
   d. glycogen storage disease
   e. left coronary artery arising from pulmonary artery
   f. lesions of the coronary arteries (medial hypertrophy and intimal fibrosis, necrosis of the media).

The following table (pages 238-239) outlines the usual or classic findings in the more common – and a few of the rarer – congenital cardiac anomalies.

Ventricular septal defects (20 percent), tetralogy of Fallot, and patent ductus arteriosus (each approximately 11 percent), and atrial septal defects (about 10 percent) are the most common anomalies. Combined, these four conditions comprise more than half of all congenital heart disease.

REFERENCES

Kincaid, O. W. Approach to the roentgenologic diagnosis of congenital heart disease. J.A.M.A., 173:637, 1960

Michaels, L., and Parkin, T. W. Mild congenital heart defects. J.A.M.A., 174:491, 1960.

Rudolph, A. M., and Nadas, A. S. The pulmonary circulation and congenital heart disease. New Eng. J. Med., 267:1022, 1962.

CONDITION:	PULMONARY VASCULARITY	SHUNT	CYA-NOSIS	HEART SOUNDS AND MURMURS	FLUOROSCOPY AND X-RAY	ELECTRO-CARDIOGRAM
Patent ductus arteriosus	Increased pulmonary arterial vascularity			Continuous "machinery"	Hyperpulsatile aorta; engorged lungs	LV enlargement
Atrial septal defect		L → R	0	Systolic Ejection murmur, pul. area	RV+1 –; flooded lungs	Diastolic overload RV (RSR′ V_1)
Ventricular septal defect				holosystolic murmur max LSB 4 I.S.	LV Enlargement, LA may be.	LV enlargement
Complete transposition				systolic murmur LSB P_2 nl. or mod. ↑	Mod. cardiomegaly, narrow waist heart flat or concave P.A. seg.	RV enlargement
Truncus arteriosus	(Pulmonary (Systemic Art. Flow 2/1 or more)	Admixtures	+	Harsh systolic murmur LSB, 2nd sound single	Pul. art. segment may be flat or convex; enlarged heart; LA may be ↑	R, L, or (usually) biventricular enlarged
Total anomalous pul. venous connection to right heart				P_2 usually ↑ & split, noncharacteristic systolic murmur	'Figure of 8' 'Snowman heart'	RA ↑, RAD, RV systolic overload
Tetralogy of Fallot	Diminished pulmonary artery vascularity			Prominent Systolic murmur, LSB. P_2 ↓	'Coeur en Sabot'. P.A. seg. concave. Overriding orrt. sided aorta	RV enlargement, no RA enlargement
Ebstein's malformation		R → L	+	Sounds, gallop or triple rhythm, LSB or apex	'Box shape'. Massive cardiomegaly. RA ↑ ↑	RBBB. Peaked P. Waves
Tricuspid atresia (with pul. hypoplasia)				Variable	Cardiomegaly usually mod. to marked. LA ↑	LV enlargement, LAD Peaked P Waves. No RV ↑

Mitral stenosis	Increased pulmonary venous vascularity (Kerley's lines may be present)			Diastolic murmur and thrill apex. P_2 ↑ and split	LA, RV and pul. art. Seg. all enlarged	Rt. axis deviation, LA and RV Enlargement
Cor triatriatum		0	0	Soft systolic murmur LSB	RV and pul. trunk enlarged	RV enlarged, tall notched P Waves
Severe aortic stenosis, or coarctation				See aortic stenosis and coarctation below		
Endocardial fibroelastosis				Gallop rhythyms and murmur mitral insuff. (from CHF)	Moderate to marked cardiomegaly. LV ↑, LA may be ↑	Arrhythmias and bundle branch blocks
Coronary art. from pulmonary art.				Usually none	Normal. Requires angiocardiogram	Ant. wall infarct (Q. I, avl, v_5, v_6, + ST-T changes) LV enlargement
Isolated pulmonic valve stenosis	Normal pulmonary vascularity	0	0	Systolic ejection murmur and thrill P_2 split, delayed, 2nd component ↓	RV enlarged. P.A. segment dilated	RV enlarged, systolic overload, prominent R V,
Coarctation of the aorta				Systolic murmur entire precardium and between scapulae	In older children and adults, rib notching and 'reversed 3' sign	LV enlargement and 'strain' pattern
Aortic stenosis				Systolic murmur aortic area to neck Early systolic click	LV enlarged with post-stenotic dilated aorta	LV enlargement and 'strain' pattern.

HEART SOUNDS AND MURMURS

HEART SOUNDS

Identification of the first and second heart sounds must be emphasized, for on their proper recognition depends the accurate time of murmurs, gallop rhythms, ejection clicks, and knocks. In addition, accurate timing of these auscultatory phenomena facilitates the recognition of the normal third and fourth sounds.

The *first heart sound* is attributed to closure of the atrioventricular valves and tensing of the ventricular muscle; the *second sound* to the closure of the semilunar valves and to a small vascular component when the blood is ejected into the aorta and pulmonary artery.

The first and second heart sounds each consist of two components. The first sound has a mitral and tricuspic component. Slight asynchrony is normally present in closure and causes the sound to split. The mitral sound normally precedes the tricuspid. The second sound has aortic and pulmonic components. During expiration, these valves close synchronously, but during inspiration aortic closure usually precedes pulmonic. Due to negative intrathoracic pressure during inspiration there is increased filling of the right side of the heart with a consequent delay in ejection of blood from the right side. At times confusion results in determining which is louder (A_2 or P_2). This cannot be determined by comparing the intensity of the second sound in the aortic and pulmonic areas because the aortic component may be equally well heard at both sites.

It is important to evaluate the intensity of each component during inspiration. By such a maneuver they can be separated and correctly evaluated. In atrial septal defect the split is wide and fixed, and respiration has little or no effect. Paradoxical splitting of the second sound – that is, an increase with expiration and decrease with inspiration occurs in a) left bundle branch block and b) aortic stenosis.

VARIATIONS IN THE INTENSITY OF THE HEART SOUNDS

APICAL FIRST SOUND.

Increased:

1. mitral stenosis
2. fever
3. tachycardia
4. short PR interval
5. anemia
6. hyperthyroidism

Decreased:

1. cardiac decompensation
2. myocardial infarction
3. shock
4. long PR interval (0.22 sec or more)
5. pericardial effusion
6. pulmonary emphysema

Varying intensity:

1. complete heart block
2. ventricular tachycardia
3. atrial fibrillation and flutter with varying block
4. paroxysmal atrial tachycardia with variable block

Increased P_2:

1. mitral stenosis
2. left ventricular failure
3. some forms of congenital heart disease associated with pulmonary hypertension

Increased A_2:

1. systemic hypertension
2. coarctation of the aorta

Decreased A_2:

aortic stenosis

The *third sound* is best heard in young individuals and is frequently brought out by exercise when not heard at rest. It is low pitched and short and heard at the end of the first third of diastole, which in time occurs at the end of the period of rapid ventricular filling. It is probably due to rapid early diastolic filling. In a very small percentage of normal individuals the *fourth heart sound* is heard. It is due to ventricular filling following atrial contraction and is heard just before the first heart sound.

GALLOP RHYTHMS

Ventricular gallop (S3, protodiastolic or rapid filling gallop) occurs approximately 0.12 second to 0.16 second after the second heart sound. It is a low-pitched sound usually faint and overlooked. It may be inconstant or transient. At times it can be seen and felt. It is best heard with the bell of the stethoscope at the apex and the lower left sternal border with the patient turned on the left side.

Since it may be heard in the absence of heart disease as the normal physiologic third heart sound of youth, it does not necessarily mean heart failure. It is heard in arteriosclerotic heart disease, hypertensive cardiovascular disease, primary myocardial disease and in conditions of diastolic overload. The application of tourniquets to the extremities or assuming the vertical position can alter the intensity of the ventricular gallop sound and even cause it to disappear. The opening snap of the mitral valve is not affected by these maneuvers. The ventricular gallop is not heard in tight mitral stenosis because this lesion prevents rapid ventricular filling.

Atrial gallop (S4, presystolic gallop or late filling gallop) is the type most often heard in the patient with heart disease. It is a low frequency sound occurring just before the first heart sound and best heard with the bell of the stethoscope near the lower left sternal border in the fifth interspace or at the apex. The atrial gallop is most commonly heard in patients with systemic and pulmonary hypertension, ASHD, primary myocardial disease, and aortic and pulmonic stenosis, in some normal patients, or, in general, in patients in states of systolic overload.

Summation gallop (quadruple rhythm) results when both the ventricular and atrial gallop sounds are heard. When the heart rate increases diastole is shortened, and these two sounds come closer together and eventually fuse, resulting in an easily audible sound heard in middiastole. Fusion usually occurs at rates over 100 per minute. The resultant sound may be mistaken for a middiastolic murmur. Slowing of the heart rate by carotid sinus massage will separate the fused third and fourth components of summation gallop and help to differentiate it from a middiastolic murmur.

Pericardial knock occurs 0.08 to 0.12 second after the second sound, and thus may be easily confused with the opening snap of mitral stenosis. In general it is louder than the opening snap, increases with inspiration, is widely transmitted, and occurs earlier than the gallop. It occurs in any condition in which there is a sudden check to ventricular filling such as constrictive pericarditis, subendocardial fibrosis, or amyloidosis of the heart.

Split second heart sound is due to delayed closure of the pulmonic valve in relation to the aortic valve. Both components of the split second sound are high pitched and heard best with the diaphragm, which is not true of the ventricular gallop. In addition, the split sound is best heard at the base with the patient upright, while gallops are best heard at or near the apex with the patient recumbent.

The opening snap of mitral stenosis occurs 0.04 to 0.12 second after the second heart sound. It differs from other gallop sounds in that it is shorter, higher pitched, and heard best over the left ventricular impulse with the patient recumbent in the left lateral decubitus position. It may be further differentiated from a ventricular gallop sound in that it is usually associated with a snapping loud first heart sound and a diastolic rumble. It cannot be diminished in intensity or made to disappear, as the ventricular gallop can, by pooling of blood through the application of tourniquets or changing position. An opening snap and a gallop in the same ventricle are mutually exclusive, because the slopes of the filling curves in a snap and in a gallop are just the opposite.

Ejection sounds are systolic in timing and may vary in intensity depending on inspiration or expiration. Pulmonary ejection sounds are loudest in expiration and softest with inspiration. They are heard best over the pulmonic area and are caused by the upward doming of a congenitally deformed pulmonic valve, as in pulmonic stenosis, or to dilation of the pulmonary artery as in pulmonary artery hypertension and idiopathic dilation of the pulmonary artery. Aortic ejection sounds vary less with respiration and are heard best over the aortic area, the left sternal border and at the apex. They are heard in congenital aortic stenosis and with dilation of the aorta.

Systolic clicks occur later in systole than ejection sounds. They may be single or multiple and are associated with pleuropericardial disease (when single) or mild mitral insufficiency (when multiple). In the latter case they are produced by snapping of the chordae tendinea.

CARDIAC MURMERS

In evaluating the diagnostic significance of murmurs it is necessary to describe them in relation to their timing in the cardiac cycle, their intensity, duration, location, transmission, and any peculiar musical qualities they may possess. A murmur may fall between the first and the second heart sounds (systolic) or between the second and the first sounds (diastolic).

SYSTOLIC MURMURS

Holosystolic murmurs are true regurgitant murmurs extending completely from the first to the second heart sound, since pressure in the donor chamber is always higher than in the recipient chamber during systole. This murmur is usually accompanied by a thrill. The holosystolic murmur of mitral insufficiency is best heard at the apex; that of tricuspid insufficiency is loudest at the tricuspid area and augments with inspiration. The murmur produced by a ventricular septal defect is best heard at the fourth to fifth left intercostal space along the left lower sternal border.

Ejection murmurs are midsystolic murmurs. They begin an interval after the first heart sound, rise to peak intensity, and wane before the second sound. In the phonocardiogram this murmur has a diamond shape configuration. The aortic systolic ejection murmur is heard over the aortic area, the carotids, along the left sternal border, and at the apex. When associated with a thrill it is characteristic of aortic stenosis. It may also be heard in severe aortic insufficiency secondary to increased blood flow over the aortic valve. The pulmonary systolic ejection murmur of pulmonic stenosis is localized to the pulmonary area and the third left intercostal space. The murmur of an atrial defect, due to augmented blood flow over the pulmonic valve, is also ejection in type. Systolic murmurs of musical quality are associated with congestive heart failure and dilated aorta.

Late systolic murmurs begin in late systole, rise to a crescendo and end with the second heart sound. They are commonly preceded by systolic clicks and are due to mild mitral insufficiency. They may occur after a myocardial infarction due to papillary muscle dysfunction.

Early systolic murmurs begin in early systole and end before the second heart sound. This type of bruit is most commonly heard in patients with small muscular ventricular septal defects and those with pulmonary hypertension and ventricular septal defects.

DIASTOLIC MURMURS

Presystolic murmurs (late diastolic) begin in the last third of diastole, are crescendo in quality, and end with the first heart sound. When due to mitral stenosis the murmur is best heard over the left ventricular impulse with the patient supine in the left lateral decubitus position. The apical diastolic murmur heard in aortic insufficiency (Austin-Flint murmur) is due to the regurgitant stream of blood striking the aortic cusp of the mitral valve. The presystolic murmur of tricuspid stenosis is identical with the mitral stenotic murmur, but is best heard over the tricuspid area and augments in intensity with inspiration.

Early diastolic murmurs begin after the second heart sound. When due to aortic insufficiency they are best heard over the aortic area, along the left sternal border and at the apex. The murmur is loudest at its beginning and then wanes, ending before the first heart sound. The early diastolic murmur attributed to pulmonary insufficiency associated with mitral stenosis (Graham Steell murmur) is similar in time and quality. It may be due to pulmonary artery hypertension or dilation of the pulmonary artery. The murmur of aortic insufficiency is sometimes louder to the right of the sternum than the left. In this case the lesion is probably not due to rheumatic heart disease but more likely to aneurysm of the aorta or an intrinsic aortic lesion such as luetic aortitis or valvular deformity due to bacterial endocarditis.

Middiastolic murmurs begin an interval after the second heart sound. When due to mitral strenosis they are loud and preceded by the opening snap of the mitral valve. When due to active mitral valvulitis the murmur is faint, short, and ends before the first heart sound. This is the Carey Coombs murmur, an early sign of rheumatic mitral valvulitis.

Middiastolic murmurs, functional in origin, due to increased flow over the mitral valve, may be heard in pernicious or sickle cell anemias, thyrotoxicosis, patent ductus arteriosus and ventricular septal defects. The diastolic murmur of atrial septal defect is due to increased flow over the tricuspid valve.

Continuous or machinerylike murmurs wax during systole and early diastole and wane in late diastole, but are characterized by obliteration of the second heart sound by the bruit. The machinery murmur of patent ductus arteriosus is localized in the pulmonary area and is oten accompanied by a thrill. A similar murmur may be heard in aortic-pulmonary window, rupture of the sinus of Valsalva into the right atrium or ventricle, or coronary arteriovenous fistula.

Musical murmurs. The most significant musical murmur is the "dove coo" or "sea gull" murmur which occurs in diastole over the base and along the left sternal border. The usual causes are perforation or eventration of an aortic cusp due to lues or bacterial endocarditis.

Intensity of murmurs may be graded on an arbitrary scale from 1 to 6. Grade 6 can be heard with the stethoscope or ear away from the chest wall. Grade 1 is barely audible with the stethoscope. The intervening grades are subject to personal evaluation of intensity.

The following table (pages 247-248) outlines the more important cardiac murmurs:

SYSTOLIC MURMURS

HEARD BEST	CHARACTER OR POSITION IN CYCLE	TRANS-MITTED	THRILL	CHANGE OF HEART SOUNDS	DIAGNOSIS
Aortic area	Loud, ejection	Neck, occas. Erb's point	Frequent	A_2 soft	Aortic stenosis
Aortic area	Harsh, often musical, ejection	Neck, occas. Erb's point	Infrequent	A_2 may be accentuated	Dilated aorta or valve ring, calcified leaflets, etc.
Pulmonic area	Loud, ejection	Left upper chest	Frequent	P_2 usually soft	Pulmonic stenosis
Upper left sternum	Loud, ejection	All over pre-cordium	Frequent	Wide, fixed splitting of 2nd sound, P_2 increased	Atrial septal defect
Lower left sternum	Holosystolic	All over pre-cordium	Frequent	P_2 may be increased	Ventricular septal defect
Apex	Holosystolic	Axilla	Infrequent	1st sound soft	Mitral insuffi-ciency

DIASTOLIC MURMURS

HEARD BEST	CHARACTER OR POSITION IN CYCLE		TRANS-MITTED	THRILL	CHANGE OF HEART SOUNDS	DIAGNOSIS
Erb's point	Early or holo-diastolic	Blowing	Aortic area	Infrequent	A_2 may be soft	Aortic insufficiency
Apex	Mid and late diastolic (presystolic)	Low-pitched rumbling	Localized	May be present	Accentuated 1st sound, opening snap	Mitral stenosis
CONTINUOUS MURMURS						
Upper left sternum	Usually continuous	Harsh "machinery" systolic accentuation	Left pre-cordium	Usually	None	Patent ductus arteriosus*

*A similar murmur may occur in the rarer conditions of aortic-pulmonic window, coronary artery fistula, rupture of the sinus of Valsalva, and dissecting aneurysm.

HEAT ILLNESS

The following clinical conditions are seen during times of excessive heat:

1. Heat stroke.
2. Heat hyperpyrexia.
3. Heat cramps.
4. Heat exhaustion
   a. Anhidrotic.
   b. Salt deficiency.
   c. Undetermined.
5. Sunburn.
6. Prickly heat.
7. Anhidrosis.
8. Heat neurotic reactions.

HEAT HYPERPYREXIA AND HEAT STROKE. Signs of central nervous system defect characterizes heat stroke. Otherwise, the two phrases above are applied to the same clinical phenomenon. The subject is exposed to excessive temperature, resulting in a body temperature of over 106° F, and dry, hot flushed skin. The clinical picture is frequently that of a sudden collapse, or may be preceded by a few hours of fever, headache, and restlessness. Heat stroke may stimulate a cerebral vascular accident. The neurologic manifestations which distinguish heat stroke from heat hyperpyrexia include coma, delirium, hemiplegia, and convulsions.

The major complicating phenomena, in addition to the obvious cerebral damage, are acute renal failure and serious defects in the blood coagulation systems. (There must be careful monitoring of prothrombin time, bleeding and clotting time, fibrinogen, platelet count.) The treatment is immerision of patient in cold water or the application of cooling blankets until his rectal temperature approaches 101° F.

HEAT CRAMPS. Heat cramps are due to acute salt depletion. The patient is deficient both in water and sodium chloride and generally the best treatment is to give isotonic normal saline.

SALT DEFICIENCY SYNDROME. This is the most often overlooked phenomenon in heat illness; the symptoms are generally attributed to psychoneurosis. The blood and urine show a reduction of sodium chloride.

ANHIDROTIC HEAT EXHAUSTION. This occurs in an individual who is unable to produce any sweat under conditions ordinarily associated with sweating. Generally such a person has spent many months in hot, dry climates. It may be associated with prickly heat. The symptoms are fatigue, throbbing headaches, dizziness, blurred vision, polyuria and polydypsnea. Prolonged overactivity of the sweat glands and their resultant exhaustion seems to be the probably explanation. The treatment is symptomatic; the use of air-conditioned rooms is very useful. The situation, however, will not correct itself for many weeks.

REFERENCES

Editorial: Heat stroke. Lancet, 2:31, 1968.

Ferguson, M., and O'Brien, M. D. Heat stroke in New York City. Experience with twenty-five cases. N. Y. J. Med., 60:2531, 1960.

Sister Michael Marie, and Ferguson, M. Heat illness. G.P., p. 83, 1960.

Schrier, R. W., Henderson, H. S., Tisher, C. C., and Tannen, Richard L. Nephropathy associated with heat stress and exercise. Ann. Intern. Med., 67:356, 1967.

HEMATURIA

Hematuria is distinguished from hemoglobinuria or myoglobinuria by the presence of red blood cells in a urine devoid of blood pigments.

DIFFERENTIAL DIAGNOSIS

1. Bladder, ureters and lower urinary tract: tumor, trauma, tuberculosis, calculi, foreign body, infection (cystitis, prostatitis, urethritis), benign hypertrophy, or carcinoma of the prostrate.
2. Kidney: tumor, trauma, tuberculosis, nephritis, glomerulitis (polyarteritis, SLE, etc.), infection, infarction, papillary necrosis, polycystic disease, calculi, renal vein thrombosis.
3. Other diseases: acute appendicitis, acute salpingitis, carcinoma of the uterus, vagina, or rectum, diverticulitis, blood dyscrasias (leukemia, purpuras, sickle cell anemia, polycythemia), pelvic abscess, serious liver decompensation, drugs (salicylates, sulfonamides, phenacetin, anticoagulants), strenuous exercise.

HEMOCHROMATOSIS

(Bronze Diabetes)

Abnormal iron metabolism with deposition of iron in various body tissues and eventual secondary fibrosis characterizes this disease. It occurs with greatest frequency in males age 45 to 65, and is rare in females. Any tanned diabetic or cirrhotic person is suspect. Etiology is unknown.

DIAGNOSIS

HISTORY AND PHYSICAL FINDINGS

Symptoms and findings relate to the organ or organs involved. The presenting clinical picture may be that of hepatic cirrhosis, congestive heart failure, or both. Pancreatic, hepatic, cardiac, and endocrine manifestions are most common. Symptoms include those of diabetes, weakness, abdominal pain, dyspnea, impotence, and jaundice. About a third of cases have significant alcoholic intake. Physical findings include hepatomegaly, edema, evidence of weight loss, ascites, cardiomegaly, loss of body hair, and skin pigmentation. The last, early in the disease, consists of "tanning" or "bronzing" of the skin, and is due more to increased melanin than iron deposition. However, later in the course a gray or slate color may be seen due to iron. The presence of gonadal hypoplasia lends weight to the diagnosis.

LABORATORY FINDINGS

1. Liver biopsy with stains for iron is the best single test. This is superior to skin biopsy or the Fishback test (intradermal injections of potassium ferrocyanide).
2. Serum iron is usually elevated to 200 mg per 100 ml or more.
3. Additional laboratory findings relate to the various organs involved. Hyperglycemia, glycosuria, deranged liver chemistries, and decreased urinary 17-ketogenic steroids are most common.

DIFFERENTIAL DIAGNOSIS

Includes transfusion hemosiderosis, Laennec's cirrhosis, chronic hepatitis, Addison's disease, Simmonds' disease, Wilson's disease, and argyria.

COURSE

Life expectancy is 4 to 5 years from the time of diagnosis. Pneumonia, hepatic failure, bleeding varices, and congestive heart failure are the usual causes of death. Up to 75 percent of patients develop heart failure.

TREATMENT

Treatment consists of the appropriate diabetic and cirrhotic therapy. In addition, repeated phlebotomies with maintenance of hemoglobin values at slightly anemic levels are of distinct value. Recently chelating compounds for iron have been introduced.

REFERENCES

Moeschlin, S., and Schnider, U. Treatment of primary and secondary hemochromatosis and acute iron poisoning with a new, potent iron-eliminating agent (Desferrioxamine-B). New Eng. J. Med., 269:27, 1963.

Pechet, G. S., and MacDonald, R. A. Idiopathic hemosiderosis, relation to idiopathic hemochromatosis. New Eng. J. Med., 267:6, 1962.

HEMOLYSIS AND HEMOLYTIC ANEMIAS

The normal life span of the erythrocyte is approximately 120 days. Any process which shortens this is termed "hemolytic." However, since the marrow may be capable of increasing its output several fold on demand (seven to eight times for normal marrows), the balance of production against destruction determines the amount of hemolysis which will be characterized by the presence of overt anemia. A state of "compensated hemolysis" is one in which increased destruction is matched by equally increased production, and no anemia is present.

CLASSIFICATION

Hemolytic anemias may be classified in a number of ways, none of them entirely satisfactory. One convenient classification is as follows:

CONGENITAL

1. Hereditary spherocytosis.
2. Hemoglobinopathies.
3. Thalassemic syndromes.

4. Hemolysis associated with a red cell enzyme defect.*
5. Congenital nonspherocytic hemolytic anemia with no demonstrable corpuscular defect.

ACQUIRED

1. Infections (malaria, sepsis).
2. Secondary to other disease (lymphoma, leukemia, neoplasia, systemic lupus erythematosis, liver disease).
   a. with evidence of autoimmune disturbance (positive Coombs' test).
   b. without evidence of autoimmune disturbance.
3. Secondary to drug, with a positive Coombs' test (e.g., penicillin, α-methyldopa, etc.).
4. Idiopathic autoimmune hemolytic anemia.
5. Secondary to isoantibodies (transfusion of incompatible blood, erythroblastosis fetalis).
6. Paroxysmal nocturnal hemoglobinuria.
7. Associated with high titer cold agglutinins (specific and nonspecific).
8. Paroxysmal cold hemoglobinuria.
9. Microangiopathic hemolytic anemia (hemolytic-uremic syndrome, thrombotic thrombocytopenic purpura, following aortic valve replacement, etc.).

LABORATORY EVALUATION

Laboratory tests which suggest or confirm the presence of a hemolytic process include

1. An anemia which is, overall, normocytic and normochromic. This is often better evaluated by examination of the peripheral smear than by measurement of corpuscular constants. At the same time the smear can be inspected for target cells, schistocytes, burr cells, spherocytes, basophilic strippling and polychromatophilia, all of which may be seen in hemolysis.
2. An elevated reticulocyte count in the absence of recent treatment for a specific deficiency. Often more useful than a single observation of the reticulocyte level are serial hemoglobins (or hematocrits) and reticulocyte counts.
   Persistently low or falling hemoglobin level accompanied by elevation or rising reticulocyte percentage is characteristic of hemolysis.
3. Decreased or absent serum haptoglobin.
4. In situations in which significant intravascular hemolysis has occurred plasma hemoglobin levels will be increased.
5. Red cell life span studies, with, for example, Cr^{51}.

*Several of the hemolytic anemias secondary to drug or chemical agent belong in this group–e.g., hemolysis due to sulfonamides or to antimalarials in G-6-PD deficient individuals.

A variety of other studies are often needed to define the etiology of the hemolytic process, and several (if positive) also serve to confirm the presence of hemolysis. Among these are:

1. Sickle cell preparation.
2. Hemoglobin electrophoresis.
3. Measurement of alkali-resistant (fetal) hemoglobin.
4. Coombs' test.
5. Cold agglutinins.
6. Red cell osmotic fragility.
7. Red cell enzyme studies.
8. Test for presence of acid hemolysins (Ham test).

REFERENCE

Osgood, E. E. Antiglobulin-positive hemolytic anemias. Arch. Intern. Med., 107:313, 1961.

HEMOPTYSIS

DIFFERENTIAL DIAGNOSIS

1 Bronchietasis	25%
2. Bronchogenic carcinoma	20%
3. Chronic bronchitis	10%
4. Pulmonary tuberculosis	5%
5. Lung abscess	5%
6. Pneumonia	2%

These six causes represent about two-thirds of patients presenting with hemoptysis. Other less frequent causes include the following:

Congestive heart failure
Pulmonary infarction
Mitral stenosis
Broncholithiasis
Foreign bodies
Bronchial adenoma
Bronchogenic cyst
Metastatic tumors
Trauma to thorax
Blood dyscrasias
Hereditary hemorrhages
Telangiectasis (Weber-Osler-Rendu)
Fungus infections
Parasites (hydatid, ameba, lung fluke)
Aortic aneurysm
Retrosternal goiter
Pulmonary hemosiderosis
Wegener's granulomatosis

HEPATITIS

CAUSES

Infections:
1. Viral (infectious and serum hepatitis), infectious mononucleosis, yellow fever.
2. Bacterial (pneumococci, enterococci, shigellae).
3. Protozoa (amoebae, leptispira).

Toxic and allergic:
1. Drugs (phenothiazones, methyltestosterone, arsphenamine, thiouracil, anticoagulants, sulfonamides, PAS).
2. Chemicals (arsenic, phosphorus, lead, carbon tetrachloride).
3. Alcohol.

Miscellaneous: Collagen disease, ulcerative colitis, congestive heart failure.

INFECTIOUS HEPATITIS

The IH virus causes sporadic and epidemic outbreaks of hepatitis. It is usually transmitted through the intestinal-oral route via contaminated water, milk, or food, but it can also be transmitted by transfusion of whole blood or blood products. Incubation time is 2 to 6 weeks. Children, young adults, and persons in crowded, unsanitary environments are most susceptible. The disease in children is usually much milder than in adults. Liver damage consists of scattered cellular necrosis and lysis with some disruption and inflammation of the bile canaliculi, but with marked sparing of the connective tissue reticulum framework. Clinically, the disease is first manifest by loss of appetite, malaise, nausea, vomiting, diarrhea, and fever of 100° to 103° F. The majority of patients do not progress into the jaundiced phase, and are thought to have a mild upper respiratory or gastrointestinal disease. When jaundice occurs 1 to 3 weeks later, it is first manifest by darkening of the urine. Then a rapidly deepening icterus is noted, with subsidence of the previous constitutional symptoms, so the patient often feels improved. There are light-colored stools. In 70 percent of patients the liver is palpable, smooth, tender, and has a sharp edge. Twenty percent have a palpable spleen. The jaundice increases from its onset to a peak in 3 to 10 days, then gradually clears in 1 to 6 weeks. Strength slowly improves and clinically and biochemically normal levels are usually reached by 4 months.

LABORATORY

Serum transaminase is the best index of hepatic inflammation, and may be the only abnormality in the subclinical anicteric group. In the typical jaundiced patient there is a rapid rise, often to above 500 units. Even though SGPT is slightly more elevated than SGOT, the two can be used interchangeably, and there is no advantage in following both. Serum bilirubin rises to a peak which rarely exceeds 25 mg per 100 ml and then, without reaching a plateau, gradually falls. The direct and indirect fraction rise to about the same extent, although the direct may be higher early in the course. Urinary bilirubin appears quite early, sometimes before serum levels increase; then, strangely enough, the urinary threshold changes, and bilirubinuria disappears while serum bilirubin is high. Cephalin flocculation turns positive in 80 percent of patients, falls quite slowly, and often remains abnormal longer than all other tests. Serum alkaline phosphatase is typically not raised above 30 King-Armstrong or 10 Bodansky units, unless an obstructive phase supervenes. Serum A_2 globulin may become elevated.

TREATMENT

The jaundiced patient is put to bed. He may walk to the bathroom and sit in a chair. Further ambulation is not permitted until bilirubin is 2 mg or less, and transaminase is 40 units or less and has remained so for 1 week. Activity is then slowly increased unless clinical or chemical sign of relapse occurs. Return to work is allowed when the patient's strength returns, provided the liver chemistries remain normal. The usual period of rest is 3 to 4 weeks.

Diet should be high caloric (2,500 to 3,000 Cal), with normal protein (75 to 100 g) and normal fat. If severe symptoms prevent sufficient intake, give I.V. 10 percent glucose in water, 1,000 to 1,500 ml. If the above diet is taken there is no reason to add vitamins or other food supplements.

Isolation: Stool precautions; keep dishes and trays separate; use disposable needles and syringes.

Corticosteroids are used when there is prolonged subacute hepatitis, massive hepatic necrosis, impending coma, or prolonged convalescence with cholangiolitic hepatitis.

SERUM HEPATITIS

Serum hepatitis occurs most often in patients who have been ill with another disease which required surgery or a blood transfusion. Hence, the mortality of serum hepatitis (5 percent as compared to 0.2 percent of infectious hepatitis) is more logically attributed to the severe underlying disease. The clinical picture is identical with that of infectious hepatitis except that the prodromal GI or URI symptoms are usually absent and the onset of jaundice is more gradual. About 1 percent of persons receiving whole blood transfusions develop overt serum hepatitis. It is not transmitted in albumin, gamma globulin, or antihemophiliac globulin.

Incubation period is 2 to 6 months. Laboratory data and treatment are the same as for infectious hepatitis.

PREVENTION OF VIRAL HEPATITIS

Isolation procedures have been listed. Patients are considered infectious for at least one week after jaundice appears. Since both IH and SH patients may be carriers of the virus for an indefinite time, they are not acceptable as blood donors. Unfortunately detection of carriers is difficult because most have had only anicteric hepatitis, and many show completely normal liver chemistries. Gamma globulin 0.01 ml/lb body weight, I.M., given to the family of an IH patient will suppress symptoms but allow subclinical infection to develop with consequent active immunity.

Partial protection against SH may be given to a person by the administration of 10 ml of gamma globulin I.M. repeated in one month.

REFERENCES

Nefzger, M. D., et al. Treatment of acute infectious hepatitis, Amer. J. Med., 35:299, 1963.

Ritt, D. J., et al. Acute hepatic necrosis with stupor or coma: An analysis of thirty-one patients. Medicine, 48:151, 1969.

Tisdale, W. A. Subacute hepatitis, New Eng. J. Med., 268:85, 138, 1963.

PLASMAPHERESIS IN HEPATIC COMA

Since hemodialysis and peritoneal dialysis are ineffectual in hepatic coma and since whole blood exchange transfusions are thought to be helpful, it has been postulated that a protein-bound substance may be responsible for coma. Whole blood exchange in the adult requires large amounts of blood and may place heavy strains upon the blood banks. Plasmapheresis with plasma exchange can be substituted for whole blood exchange. This requires removal of a pint of blood at a time, centrifuging it, and removing the supernatant plasma. Then the patient's own packed red cells are returned to him plus fresh frozen human plasma to replace his own plasma. This technique has a place in patients with coma due to acute hepatic necrosis (acute yellow atrophy) and it may help tide the patient over a crisis until hepatocyte regeneration has occurred.

REFERENCES

Cree, I. C., and Berger, S. A. Plasmapheresis and positive-pressure ventilation in hepatic coma with respiratory arrest. Lancet, 7575:976, 1968.

Lepore, M. J., and Martel, A. J. Plasmapheresis in hepatic coma. Lancet, 7519:771, 1967.

Sabin, S., and Merritt, J. A. Treatment of hepatic coma in cirrhosis by plasmapheresis and plasma infusion (plasma exchange). Ann. Intern. Med. 68:1, 1968.

HEPATOMA

Hepatoma may present six clinical pictures.

1. Typical hepatoma with rapid progression, large tender nodular liver, and frequently jaundice and ascites – 33 percent.
2. Cirrhosis with rapid unexplained deterioration, splenomegaly, ascites, abdominal pain, rapidly increasing and tender hepatomegaly with a venous hum, and massive GI hemorrhage – 25 percent.
3. Occult hepatoma found incidentally at operation, biopsy, or autopsy – 10 percent.
4. Acute abdomen secondary to hemorrhage in a carcinomatous nodule or blood vessel erosion.
5. Acute febrile illness with hepatic pain and tenderness suggesting an abscess, and toxemia.
6. Signs and symptoms referable to distant metastases.

The latter three groups account for 33 percent of cases. About 50 percent of the patients have a major hematemesis as the presenting complaint or at some time during the illness.

Hepatoma occurs more frequently with postnecrotic cirrhosis (up to 10 percent) than with alcoholic cirrhosis (about 1 percent). A cirrhotic patient with a portogram showing thrombosis of the portal vein should be suspected of having hepatoma. Needle biopsy of the liver will diagnose about 50 percent of cases. The accuracy of liver scan is about 70 percent.

REFERENCES

Benner, E. J., and Labby, D. H. Hepatoma: clinical experiences with a frequently bizarre tumor. Ann. Intern. Med., 54:620, 1961.

Elkington, S. G., et al. Hepatoma in cirrhosis, Brit. Med. J., 2:1501, 1963.

Gould, H. Personal communication. Experiences with liver scanning.

Morgan, R. R., et al. Primary liver neoplasms, a review of 20 cases. Amer. J. Digest. Dis., 7:309, 1962.

HYPERTENSION, ARTERIAL

(Hyperpiesis)†

Arterial hypertension is best classified according to diastolic pressure. The *minimal* accepted figure for diagnosis is 90 mm Hg.

Causes of systolic and/or diastolic hypertension are listed below (the asterisks indicate surgically remediable causes).

1. Essential (including malignant).
2. Endocrine *
   a. Adrenal cortex: Cushing's syndrome, primary aldosteronism.
   b. Adrenal medulla: pheochromocytoma.
   c. Ovarian: steroid-secreting ovarian tumors, arrhenoblastoma.
   d. Pituitary: acromegaly.
   e. Uterus: chorionepithelioma.
3. Renal
   a. Arterial: narrowing of renal artery (congenital or secondary to arteriosclerosis *), periarteritis, SLE, scleroderma, embolism,* thrombosis,* aneurysm,* tumor*.
   b. Parenchymal: nephrosclerosis, nephritis, hydronephrosis, amyloidosis, polycysts, infarction, tumors, stones, hypoplasia, eclampsia.

†See also "Renal Hypertension," p. 367.

c. Perinephric: tumors, hematoma, perinephritis.
d. Ureteral: obstruction.

4. Cardiovascular: congestive failure, complete heart block, coarctation of the aorta,* arteriosclerosis.
5. Central nervous system: any state producing increased intracranial pressure, brain stem lesions, and porphyria.

EVALUATION

The suggested minimum evaluation of a hypertensive patient includes the following.

1. History, including familial incidence.
2. Physical, including palpation of the arteries in all extremities, a popliteal blood pressure determination, and ophthalmoscopic exam.
3. Chest x-ray.
4. Electrocardiogram.
5. Complete blood count, urinalysis, blood urea nitrogen, and serum potassium.
6. Where indicated, other studies such as pyelography, urinary catecholamines, differential function tests, and aortography.

The pyelogram is an essential test. If the kidneys are normal in size in the presence of severe hypertension, catecholamine determination should be performed, followed by aortography and the differential function tests.

TREATMENT OF ESSENTIAL HYPERTENSION

In our opinion, most, if not all, patients with sustained diastolic hypertension should be treated.

However, there is no specific treatment for essential hypertension. Furthermore, many patients, particularly older ones, have a good prognosis without treatment and many respond poorly to therapy. For these reasons, some physicians select patients for treatment according to the following categories.

1. Symptomatic: encephalopathy, headache related to diastolic hypertension and cardiac dyspnea.
2. Asymptomatic: retinopathy with choked discs and arterial constriction, sustained diastolic level of 100 mm Hg or more, patients aged 40 or below.

Treatment consists of diet and drugs.

Diet: weight reduction if indicated; low sodium diet (200 to 500 mg).

Drugs (in order of trial):

1. Reserpine: average dose is 0.25 to 0.5 mg, q.d., P.O. Onset of effect with oral reserpine is at least one week. In hypertensive encepha-

lopathy 2.5 mg of reserpine, I.M., is effective within 2 to 3 hours, and lasts for about 12 hours. The drug may be continued even in the face of renal insufficiency, 2.5 mg, I.M., q. 12 h.

2. Hydrochlorothiazide is given. The dose is 50 mg, b.i.d. The patient should be observed for hypokalemia; in the presence of normal renal function potassium chloride may be added, 1 to 3 g q.d.
3. Chlorothalidone (Hygroton) 100 mg q.i.d.
4. Protoveratrine A: dose range is 0.3 to 1.0 mg; the average dose is 0.5 mg, P.O. In hypertensive emergencies 0.12 mg is given intravenously; this is effective for 1 to 2 hours.
5. Hydralazine (Apresoline) may be used in doses of 10 mg, t.i.d., initially and is gradually increased to 200 to 300 mg a day. Above these doses, the syndrome of systemic lupus erythematosus may occur.
6. Ganglionic blocking agents:
   a. Pentolinium (Ansolysen) may be initiated at a dose of 5 mg, four times a day, and increased to 10 to 20 mg, q.i.d., P.O. Used subcutaneously in hypertensive emergencies, 10 to 25 mg will lower the pressure in about 15 minutes and be effective for 3 to 4 hours. Hexamethonium is given in the same doses.
   b. Mecamylamine (Inversine) is given in doses ranging from 2 mg, t.i.d., to 12 mg, q.i.d., P.O.
   c. Chlorisondamine (Ecolid) is active for about 12 hours and is given 50 mg, q.d. or b.i.d., P.O., by gradual increments.
   d. Guanethidine (Ismelin) acts at the nerve-arteriole junction with little central or ganglionic effects. Dose is 10 mg a day, with increments of 10 mg no more frequently than every 7 days, up to a total of 25 to 50 mg, P.O., a day. As with all potent antihypertensives blood pressure should be determined in both the supine and standing positions.
7. Methyldopa (Aldomet) acts by reducing brain serotonin and peripheral norepinephrine. Dose is 0.25 mg t.i.d. increased to 0.5 g or more.

Note. In general, the ganglion-blocking drugs are potent substances with many undesirable side effects. These include orthostatic hypotension, dry mouth, blurry vision, constipation, and impotence. They perhaps are best avoided in the presence of angina pectoris and in renal insufficiency. If chlorothiazide or an analogue is to be used in conjunction, the dose of the ganglionic agent should be reduced by one half.

REFERENCES

Dunstan, H. P., et al. Normal arterial pressure in patients with renal arterial stenosis. J.A.M.A., 187:1028, 1964.

Hagans, J. A., et al. The natural history of hypertension. Amer. J. Med., 28:905, 1960.

Harrison, E. G., Jr., Hunt, J. C., and Bernatz, P. E. Morphology of

fibromuscular dysplasia of the renal artery in renovascular hypertension. Amer. J. Med., 43:97, 1967.
Itskovitz, H. D., et al. The granularity of the juxtaglomerular cells in human hypertension, histologic and clinical correlation. Ann. Intern. Med., 59:8, 1963.
Kaufman, J. J., et al. Upright renal arteriography in the study of renal hypertension. J.A.M.A., 187:977, 1964.
Kirkendall, W. M., et al. Pharmacodynamics and clincial use of guanethidine, bretylium and methyldopa. Amer. J. Cardiol., 9:107, 1962.
Woods, J. S., and Blythe, W. M. Management of malignant hypertension complicated by renal insufficiency. New Eng. J. Med., 277:58, 1967.

HYPOGLYCEMIA

Symptomatic hypoglycemia occurs when the blood sugar falls to about 50 percent or less of the normal fasting level.

Symptoms are referable to:

1. Central nervous system: dizziness, changes in personality or behavior, unconsciousness, coma, signs of cerebrovascular accident, convulsions.
2. Adrenal (hyperepinephrinemia): tachycardia, tremor, sweating, pallor.
3. General: Muscular weakness, ocular paresis, as manifested by diplopia, may be the outstanding symptom.

CLASSIFICATION

Organic – with abnormal secretion of insulin.
1. Insulinoma – islet cell adenoma or carcinoma, rarely islet cell hyperplasia.
2. Spontaneous hypoglycemia of children.

Functional.
1. Hyperinsulinism – physiologic, alimentary.
2. Early diabetes.

Deficient food supply.
1. Starvation.
2. Excess loss from body (lactation, renal glycosuria).
3. Hyperutilization (increased fever, neoplasms).

Hepatic disorders.
1. Cirrhosis, hepatitis.
2. Glycogen storage disease.
3. Ethanolism.
4. Other rare heriditary disorders.

Hormone deficiencies.
1. Hypopituitarism.
2. Hypothyroidism.
3. Adrenal insufficiency.
4. Glucagon and epinephrine deficient response to hypoglycemia.

Pharmacogenic.
1. Excess insulin (iatrogenic or factitious).
2. Oral hypoglycemic agents.
3. Ganglionic-blocking agents.
4. Leucine sensitivity (in childhood particularly).
5. Phenylbutazone, aspirin.

TESTING PROCEDURES

1. *Glucose tolerance test* – main usefulness in patients with functional types with development of reactive hypoglycemia. It does *not,* however, differentiate functional from organic types.
2. *Blood sugars* after overnight fast or more prolonged fast (72 hours). Sugars drawn every 12 hours or whenever symptoms of hypoglycemia appear.
3. *Insulin assays* – fasting hyperinsulinism found 90 percent of patients with insulinism.
4. *Tolbutamide test* (I.V. Orinase test) – 1 g of sodium tolbutamide in 20 ml of 0.9 percent saline given I.V. over 2 minutes.

   Blood sugars are done at 15-minute intervals for first hour and half-hour intervals for next 2 hours. Plasma levels of insulin are measured in fasting state, and at 10-minute intervals for first half hour. Patients with insulinoma experience greater than 50 percent drop in blood sugar from fasting level and remain at low level for duration of tests. An increase in insulin levels greater than 150μU per ml after 20 minutes is almost pathognomonic of insulinoma. *NOTE:* I.V. tolbutamide test may be dangerous in patients with profound fasting hypoglycemia.

5. *Leucine test* – L-leucine, 150 mg per kg body weight ingested over 5-minute period. Amino acid produces hypoglycemia in 40 percent or more of patients with insulinoma and in some infants with idiopathic infantile hypoglycemia.

REFERENCES

Fajans, S. S., Schneider, J. M., Schteingart, D. E., and Count, W. The diagnostic value of sodium tolbutamide in hypoglycemic states. J. Clin. Endocr., 21:371-386, 1961.

Floyd, T. C., Jr., Fajans, S. S., Knopf, R. F., and Donn, J. W. Plasma

insulin in organic hyperinsulinism: Comparative effects of tolbutamide, leucine and glucose. J. Clin. Endocr., 24:747, 1964.
Samols, E. Hypoglycemia in neoplasia. Postgrad. Med. J., 39:634, 1963.
Spurny, O. M., et al. Protracted tolbutamide-induced hypoglycemia. Arch. Intern. Med., 115:53, 1965.
Weisenfeld, S., et al. Hyperinsulinemia in L-leucine-sensitive hypoglycemia in an adult. Amer. J. Med., 31:659, 1961.

DIFFERENTIAL DIAGNOSIS

1. Pancreatic (hyperinsulinism due to islet cell adenoma or carcinoma). The Whipple triad, classic of organic hyperinsulinism, consists of:
   a. Symptoms occurring after fasting or exercise.
   b. Symptoms associated with hypoglycemia.
   c. Symptoms relieved by glucose.
2. Idiopathic (functional hyperinsulinism). This large group accounts for about 70 percent of all cases of hypoglycemia.
3. Insulin administration (overdosage in a diabetic, or surreptitious in a nondiabetic).
4. Alimentary: endogenous hyperinsulinism following rapid intestinal absorption (postgastroenterostomy, postgastrectomy).
5. Hepatic (hepatitis, cirrhosis and diffuse carcinoma).
6. Pituitary (tumors, Simmonds' disease, postoperative).
7. Adrenal (cortical atrophy, granulomas, or neoplasms).
8. Central nervous system (lesions of hypothalamus or brain stem).
9. Fibromas and sarcomas can produce hypoglycemic reactions. Some of these tumors are capable of producing an insulinlike hormone.
10. Renal (severe degrees of renal glycosuria).
11. Severe muscular work.
12. Severe inanition.
13. Idiopathic hypoglycemia of infancy. Some of these cases are due to sensitivity to amino acids such as leucine. The sensitivity is manifested by hypoglycemia.

Idiopathic hypoglycemia, insulin administration, and hepatic causes, together account for 80 to 90 percent of all cases. A glucose tolerance test will usually separate the causes. A nearly flat curve is seen most often with hyperinsulinism (exogenous or endogenous). Functional hypoglycemia results in a sharp decrease in blood sugar at 2 hours, and hepatic lesions show a sharp elevation to diabetic levels. Patients with islet cell tumors (insulinoma) usually manifest their symptoms after periods of fasting. The idiopathic (functional) hyperinsulinism manifests symptoms 1 to 2 hours after meals. About 50 percent of islet cell tumors respond to leucine administration with marked hypoglycemia.

The intravenous tolbutamide (Orinase) tolerance test is used to differentiate hypoglycemic states. After the intravenous administration of 1.0 g of sodium tolbutamide, the following values may be expected:

	30 MINUTES	90 MINUTES TO 3 HOURS
Normal	38-79	78-100
Insulinoma	17-50	40-66
Hepatic	40-66	64-100
Adrenal insufficiency	37-63	78-100
Functional	38-79	78-100

(Numbers refer to blood sugar, expressed as % of the fasting value.)

INFECTIOUS MONONUCLEOSIS

(Glandular Fever)

Infectious mononucleosis is a disease of unknown cause manifested by fever, malaise, lymphadenopathy, splenomegaly, sore throat, palatine petechiae, the appearance of absolute lymphocytosis with atypical lymphocytes, and a positive heterophil titer. This is a disease of young people, with 95 percent of cases occurring before 35 years of age.

The illness has been classified into three overlapping clinical categories.

1. *Glandular*. This is the most common; with diffuse lymphadenopathy. Most suggestive is the presence of posterior cervical and epitrochlear nodes.
2. *Febrile (Typhoidal)*. This category may present a problem in diagnosis when protracted fever without splenomegaly or lymphadenopathy presents.
3. *Anginose*. This is the least common of the three. Abdominal pain due to enlarged mesenteric nodes may be sufficiently outstanding as to present as an acute surgical abdomen.

LABORATORY TESTS

1. Lymphocytes. Save in rare instances, at least 20 of 100 white cells on smear are atypical lymphocytes; and this level is sustained for a week or longer.
2. Heterophil test. The minimum serologic evidence required to make the diagnosis is
   a. with unabsorbed serum, a sheep cell agglutination titer of 1:56;

b. with absorption with guinea pig kidney, a titer of 1:14;
c. after absorption with beef cell antigen, no agglutination of sheep cells should occur.

Using unabsorbed serum only, heterophil titers of 1:56 or over may occur in Hodgkin's disease, sarcoma, polycythemia, agranulocytosis, leukemia, and tuberculosis. Therefore absorption with guinea pig kidney should be done on all titers of 1:56 or over. It is to be noted that the heterophil test may be negative during the first 7 to 10 days of illness.

COMPLICATIONS IN INFECTIOUS MONONUCLEOSIS

Hepatic. The liver is probably involved in every case. Clinical jaundice is rare.

Hematologic complications.
1. Thrombocytopenic purpura.
2. Leukemoid reactions simulating leukemia (1 percent of cases).
3. Acquired hemolytic anemia (22 cases reported).
4. Agranulocytosis (very rare).

Central nervous system (1 percent of cases).
1. Facial diplegia (3 cases).
2. Aseptic meningitis (14 cases).
3. Encephalitis (20 cases).
4. Landry-Guillain-Barré syndrome (18 cases).
5. Peripheral neuropathy (not uncommon).

Miscellaneous
1. Orchitis.
2. Pericarditis.
3. Splenic rupture is an unusual but serious complication. It may occur spontaneously, following exertion, or following palpation by the examining physician. Almost all of the deaths in infectious mononucleosis have occurred from this or the Landry-Guillain-Barré syndrome.
4. Pleuritis, pneumonitis (3 percent).
5. Hematuria (10 percent).
6. Skin rashes of all types have been described (7 percent). The most common is a fine erythematous macular rash.

TREATMENT

Therapy is supportive and nonspecific. However, steroids are specifically indicated in the following situations. The efficacy of cortisone and analogues is primarily due to a lymphocytolytic effect.

1. Massive cervical adenopathy interfering with respiration or swallowing.
2. Seriously ill patients with hyperpyrexia.
3. The more serious complications (massive splenomegaly, Landry-Guillain-Barré syndrome, severe thrombocytopenic purpura, bilateral orchitis, severe pericarditis, meningitis, encephalitis, and marked degree of hemolysis).

REFERENCES

Gerber, P., Hamre, D., Moy, R. A., and Rosenblum, E. N. Infectious mononucleosis: Complement-fixing antibodies to herpes-like virus associated with Burkitt lymphoma. Science, 161:173, 1968.

Nieduman, J. C., McCollum, R. W., Hinle, G., and Hinle, W. Infectious mononucleosis: clinical manifestation in relation to EB virus antibodies. J.A.M.A., 203:203, 1968.

Schumacher, et al. Treatment of infectious mononucleosis. Ann. Intern. Med., 58:217, 1963.

JAUNDICE

Over 90 percent of patients presenting with jaundice will have one of the following:

1. Common duct stone associated with cholecystitis and cholelithiasis (20 to 50 percent).
2. Cirrhosis (10 to 20 percent).
3. Hepatitis (toxic and viral) (10 to 20 percent).
4. Carcinoma (15 to 25 percent).

About 90 percent of patients with jaundice under 20 years of age have hepatitis; over the age of 40 acute infectious hepatitis is unusual.

Miscellaneous (in this group jaundice may occur without hepatic inflammation).

1. Dubin-Johnson syndrome (intermittent jaundice with centrilobular distribution of pigment in the liver).
2. Gilbert's disease (constitutional hepatic dysfunction).
3. Crigler-Najjar syndrome (congenital deficiency in glucuronyltransferase).
4. Physiologic hyperbilirubinemia of the newborn.
5. Lupus erythematosus ("lupoid hepatitis").

REFERENCES

Foulk, W., and Schoenfield, L. Advances in the metabolism of bilirubin. J.A.M.A., 178:398, 1961.

Haemmerli, U. P., and Wyss, H. I. Recurrent intraphepatic cholestasis of pregnancy. Medicine, 46:299, 1967.
Lester, R., and Schmid, R. Bilirubin metabolism. New Eng. J. Med., 270:779, 1964.
Levine, R. A., and Klatskin, G. Unconjugated hyperbilirubinemia in the absence of overt hemolysis. Amer. J. Med., 36:541, 1964.
Schoenfield, L. J., McGill, D. B., Hunton, D. B., Fould, W. T., and Butt, H. R. Studies of chronic idiopathic jaundice (Dubin-Johnson syndrome). 1. Demonstration of hepatic excretory defect. Gastroenterology, 44:101, 1963.

JAUNDICE: BIOCHEMICAL CHANGES

	(HEMOLYTIC ANEMIA)	HEPATO-CELLULAR (HEPATITIS, CIRRHOSIS)	HEPATOCANALICU-LAR (CHOLANGIO-LITIC HEPATITIS) (BILARY CIRRHOSIS)	OBSTRUCTIVE (STONE, STRIC-TURE, TUMOR)
Direct bilirubin	0.2	1-20	1-10	5-40
Indirect bilirubin	1.0-10.0	1-6	1-10	5-40
Albumin	4.5-5	2.5-3	4	4
Globulin	2	2-4	2-4	2
Cephalin flocculation	0	2-4	0-4	0-1
SGOT	40 or less	over 40	40 or less	40 or less
Alkaline phos. (Bodansky)	3-4	4-10	10 or more	10-40 or more
Cholesterol esters	70%	65% or less	65% or less	65% or less
Cholesterol total	100-300	100-300	600-2,000	100-300 or more
Urine bilirubin	absent	present	present	present

LEUKEMIA

The leukemias are characterized by extensive and abnormal proliferations of the white blood cells and their precursors, accompanied by cellular infiltrations into the bone marrow, spleen, lymph nodes, and other body organs.

ACUTE LEUKEMIA

Acute leukemia is most common in children under five, but can occur at all ages. When untreated, it may pursue a very rapid course (average six months). Chemotherapeutic agents can produce remissions and significant prolongation of life can be achieved, especially in children. The outcome, however, remains fatal.

CHRONIC LEUKEMIA

Chronic leukemia is an adult disease. The natural history of this disease is longer, and although treatment may not markedly affect survival, it may have a very marked effect on symptomatology.

REFERENCES

Boggs, D. R., Wintrobe, M., and Cartwright, G. E. The acute leukemias. Medicine, 41:163, 1962.

Bryan, W. R. (Moderator). Viral etiology of leukemia: Combined clinical staff conference at the National Institutes of Health. Ann. Intern. Med., 62:376, 1965.

Burchenal, J. H. Treatment of leukemias. Seminars Hemat. 3:122, 1966.

Dameshek, W., and Gung, F. Leukemia. 2nd ed. New York, Grune & Stratton, Inc., 1964.

Diamond, H. D., and Miller, D. G. Chronic lymphocytic leukemia. Med. Clin. N. Amer., 45:601, 1961.

Galton, D. A. G., Wiltshaw, E., Szur, L., and Daric, T. V. The use of chlorambucil and steroids in the treatment of chronic lymphocytic leukemia. Brit. J. Haematol., 7:73, 1961.

Goh, Kong-oo, and Swisher, Scott. Specificity of the Philadelphia chromosome. Cytogenic studies in cases of chronic myelocytic leukemia and myeloid metaplasia. Ann. Intern. Med., 61:609, 1964.

TREATMENT

TYPE OF LEUKEMIA	STEROIDS	IRRADIATION	CHLORAM-BUCIL	BUSULFAN	6-MP	DRUG* COMBINATIONS
Chronic myelogenous	0	++++	+	++++	++	0
Chronic lymphocytic	++++†	++++	++++	+	0	0
Acute myelogenous	+++ or 0	0	0	0	++	+++
Acute lymphoblastic	++++	0	0	0	++	++++
Acute monocytic	++ or 0	0	0	0	++	++

++++ very effective; +++ fairly effective; ++ effective; 0 ineffective.

*Steroids and 6-mercaptopurine and/or vincristine, and/or methotrexate, with drug alternation or cycling for maintenance of induced remissions.

†Especially for complicating autoimmune hemolytic anemia.

Haut, A., Wintrobe, M. M., and Cartwright, G. E. The clinical management of leukemia. Amer. J. Med., 28:777, 1963.
Osserman, E. F. The plasmocytic dyscrasias. Plasma cell myeloma and primary macroglobulinemia. Amer. J. Med., 31:671, 1961.
Zuelzer, W. W., and Flatz, G. Acute childhood leukemia: A ten-year study. Amer. J. Dis. Child., 100:886, 1960.

LIPID STORAGE DISORDERS WITH NORMAL PLASMA LIPIDS

These are granulomatous diseases characterized by an accumulation of lipid within phagocytic reticuloendothelial cells. In contrast to the hyperlipidemic syndromes associated with xanthoma formation, the plasma lipid levels are normal. The granulomatous lesions may be confined to skin, mucosa and/or tendon. Some types may involve internal organs.

LESIONS WITHOUT SYSTEMIC INVOLVEMENT

DISORDER	PREDOMINANT LIPID	FAMILIAL
Xanthelasma (eyelids)	Cholesterol	Rarely
Giant cell tumor of tendon	Not known	No
Lipogranuloma (scars, sites of inflammation)	Not known	No
Normolipidemic xanthomas (skin)	Probably cholesterol	No

LESIONS WITH SYSTEMIC INVOLVEMENT

DISORDER	PREDOMINANT LIPID	FAMILIAL
Xanthoma disseminatum	Cholesterol	No
Juvenile giant cell granuloma	Probably cholesterol	No
Hereditory tuberous and tendinous xanthomatosis	Cholesterol	Yes
Lipoid dermatoarthritis	Triglyceride	No
Lipoid proteinosis	Lipoglycoprotein	Yes
Gaucher's disease	Glucocerebroside	Yes
Niemann-Pick disease	Sphingomyelin	Yes
Familial xanthomatosis with adrenal calcification (Wolman's disease)	Triglyceride and cholesterol	Probably
Histiocytosis X: eosinophilic granuloma	Cholesterol	No

(bone lesions), Hand-Schüller-Christian (bone, viscera, skin), Letterer-Siwe disease (liver, spleen, lungs)

REFERENCES

Frederickson, D. S. Lipidosis and xanthomatosis. *In* Harrison, T. R. et al., ed. Principles of Internal Medicine. New York, McGraw-Hill Book Company, 1966.

Harlan, W. R., Jr., and Still, W. J. S. Hereditary tendinous and tuberous xanthomatosis without hyperlipidemia. New Eng. J. Med., 278:416, 1968.

HYPERLIPOPROTEINEMIA

A rational classification and understanding of abnormal lipid metabolism can best be attained by considering the lipoprotein transport of plasma lipids. The structural relations of plasma lipids to the protein vehicle is not clear. The two most widely used methods of isolation of lipoproteins are ultracentrifugation and electrophoresis.

There are four groups of lipoproteins of clinical importance.

1. High density or α-lipoprotein.
2. Low density or β-lipoprotein.
3. Very low density or pre-β-lipoprotein.
4. Chylomicrons.

The major lipid components of alpha lipoprotein are phospholipid and cholesterol; the major content of the β-fraction is cholesterol; the prebeta fraction major component is triglyceride with an appreciable amount of cholesterol. The chylomicron fraction consists mainly of triglyceride.

Based on detailed evaluation of hyperlipidemic families, five abnormal phenotypes have been identified primarily by electrophoresis. These primary, or familial types, also have secondary or acquired counterparts having similar clinical and metabolic features. These are summarized in the table below.

The normal range of total cholesterol is 120 to 330 mg per 100 ml. The accepted range for plasma triglyceride is 10 to 190 mg per 100 ml; total lipid normally ranges between 400 to 800 mg per 100 ml.

DIAGNOSTIC APPROACH TO HYPERLIPOPROTEINEMIA

1. Exclude acquired or secondary causes of hyperlipoproteinemia by history and physical examination.
2. Examination of postabsorptive fasting plasma.

TYPE	PLASMA*	PLASMA LIPIDS		ELECTROPHORESIS	GENETICS AND FAMILIAL FEATURES
I Hyperchylomicronemia	Milky	Cholesterol ↑	Triglyceride ↑↑↑	Chylomicrons a, Pre-β, B ↓	Deficiency of postheparin lipolytic activity (PHLA) Expression in childhood
II Hyperbetalipoproteinemia	Clear	↑↑↑	N, ↑	β ↑↑↑	Expression in childhood
III Broad beta disease	Turbid	↑↑	↑↑	Broad β	Expression in adulthood
IV Endogenous hyperlipemia	Turbid	↑, →	↑↑	Pre-β ↑↑↑	Expression in adulthood
V Mixed hyperlipemia	Milky	↑	↑↑	Chylomicron Pre-β ↑↑↑	Expression in adulthood

*Postabsorptive plasma after 12-hour fast. Stored at 4°C.

3. Plasma cholesterol, plasma triglyceride.
4. Lipoprotein electrophoresis.

CLINICAL FEATURES	FAT TOLERANCE AND GLUCOSE TOLERANCE	ATHEROMATOSIS	SECONDARY CONDITION SIMULATING PRIMARY	THERAPY
Lipemia retinalis, eruptive xanthomata hepatosplenomegaly, pancreatitis	F.T.-Abn. G.T.-N.	None	Alcoholism (acute), pancreatitis, diabetes mellitus, hypothyroidism	Fat restriction
Tendon and tuberous xanthoma, xanthelasma, arcus	F.T.-N. G.T.-N.	++++	Hypothyroidism dietary cholesterol, obstructive liver disease, nephrotic syndrome, paraproteinemia	Low cholesterol diet, hypolipemic agents
Planar, tuberoeruptive xanthoma, arcus	F.T.-Abn. G.T.-Abn.	++++		Weight control, low cholesterol diet, hypolipemic agents
Eruptive xanthoma hepatosplenomegaly	F.T.-N. G.T.-Abn.	++++	Diabetes mellitus, pancreatitis, hypothyroidism, paraproteinemia	Weight control, carbohydrate restriction
Lipemia retinalis, eruptive xanthoma hepatosplenomegaly abdominal pain	F.T.-Abn. G.T.-Abn.	None	Alcoholism (acute), pancreatitis, diabetes mellitus	Weight control, balance of low fat and carbohydrate

REFERENCE

Strisower, E. H., Adamson, G., and Strisower, B. Treatment of hyperlipidemias. Amer. J. Med., 45:488, 1968.

LUPUS ERYTHEMATOSUS

Systemic lupus erythematosis (SLE) is a disease of multisystem involvement affecting the blood, blood vessels, and connective tissue. It may be an autoimmune disease.

Blood. Almost any fraction of blood or its constituents may be involved.

1. Anemia (70 percent of cases), sometimes hemolytic (10 percent).
2. Leukopenia (42 percent).
3. Thrombocytopenia (5 to 10 percent).
4. Hypergammaglobulinemia (related to positive flocculation tests), the lupus erythematosus cell phenomenon, and biologic false positive tests for syphilis (20 percent). The LE cell factor is thought to be an immunoglobulin G.
5. Hyperfibrinogenemia.
6. Prothrombin and thromboplastin inhibitors may be increased, producing a bleeding tendency.

Blood vessels. The small blood vessels are spottily involved.

1. Lungs and pleura, producing recurrent pneumonitis and pleuritis (45 percent).
2. Joints, producing arthritis (40 percent).
3. Kidneys (50 percent) (including classic wire-loop glomerular lesions).
4. Skin (butterfly rash, Raynaud's phenomenon) (71 percent).
5. CNS (psychotic episodes, convulsions) (30 percent).
6. Heart (pericardium, myocardium, and endocardium) (30 percent).
7. Lymph nodes (producing adenopathy in 58 percent).
8. Peritoneum and GI tract, usually manifesting as abdominal pain (5 percent).

Systemic lupus erythematosus is a chronic relapsing disease of females from 15 to 40 years of age in 80 percent of cases. It is closely related to the more benign discoid lupus erythematosus. About 10 percent of the latter eventually progress to SLE. Any young woman with arthritis and albuminuria is suspect.

THERAPY

In severely ill patients steroids are the drug of choice. Prednisone, 60 to 80 mg a day, in divided doses, is begun; and this may be increased by 15 to 20 mg every day or two, if necessary, until improvement is noted. In the majority of patients remission will occur, with one notable exception. Moderate or advanced renal involvement may not respond. Azotemia, hematuria, proteinuria, cylindruria, and hypertension are not as a rule benefitted by steroid therapy. Renal involvement carries the most serious prognosis, usually death occurs in 1 to 3 years.

When remission occurs, the steroid dose is gradually withdrawn, or decreased to the smallest dose on which remission is maintained.

Salicylates and antimalarials have a synergistic anti-inflammatory effect and may be employed when tapering steroids.

For mild or moderate degrees of arthritis, modified bed rest and salicylates are indicated. If this fails, the antimalarials hydroxychloroquine sulfate (Plaquenil), 200 mg, t.i.d. or q.i.d., or chloroquine phosphate (Aralen), 250 mg, b.i.d., may be of benefit. Skin manifestations of lupus are also responsive to these drugs.

Occasionally, patients unresponsive to the above drugs, or those with advanced renal manifestations, may be benefited by nitrogen mustard, 6-mercaptopurine or methotrexate. *These are potent anti-inflammatory drugs and must be given with stringent precaution.*

MISCELLANEOUS

It has been noted that tetracycline and its derivatives frequently provoke exacerbations of lupus. Other provocative agents include sunlight, penicillin, sulfonamides, various vaccines, and hydralazine (Apresoline). The hydralazine syndrome is indistinguishable from SLE and occurs with long-term administration of large doses of the drug. This syndrome is usually, but not always, reversible when hydralazine is stopped.

The LE cell phenomenon has been described in the following states:

1. Rheumatoid arthritis.
2. Periarteritis nodosa.
3. Senear-Usher disease (pemphigoid lupus).
4. Scleroderma.
5. Pernicious anemia.
6. Hemolytic anemia.
7. Multiple myeloma.
8. Idiopathic and thrombotic thrombocytopenic purpura.
9. Leukemia.
10. Tuberculosis.
11. Viral hepatitis, "lupoid hepatitis."
12. Amyloidosis.
13. Dermatitis herpetiformis.
14. Penicillin sensitivity.

REFERENCES

Comerford, F. R., and Cohen, A. S. The nephropathy of systemic lupus erythematosus. Medicine 46:425, 1967.

Dubois, E., and Tuffanelli, D. L. Clinical manifestations of systemic lupus erythematosus. J.A.M.A., 190:112, 1964.

Gary, N. E., Maher, J. F., Schreiner, G. E. Lupus nephritis. New Eng. J. Med., 276:73, 1967.

Huang, Chin-Tang, Hennigar, G. R., and Lyons, H. A. Pulmonary dysfunction in systemic lupus erythematosus. New Eng. J. Med., 272:288, 1965.

Johnson, R. T., and Richardson, E. P. The neurological manifestations of systemic lupus erythematosus. Medicine, 47:337, 1968.

Mund, A., Simson, J., and Rothfield, N. Effect of pregnancy on course of systemic lupus erythematosus. J.A.M.A., 183:917, 1963.

Sulkowski, S. R., and Haserick, J. R. Simulated systemic lupus erythematosus from degraded tetracycline. J.A.M.A., 189:152, 1964.

MAGNESIUM

Magnesium is the second most abundant intracellular cation. The human body contains approximately 20 to 30 mg, of which slightly more than one half is in the bones. The normal serum value is 1.5 to 2.5 mEq/L.

The clinical effects of magnesium administration are twofold.

1. Nervous system depression, central and peripheral.
2. Cardiac conduction is prolonged.

Hypermagnesemia is almost always iatrogenic. It may occur in renal failure and Addison's disease. Like potassium, the excretion of magnesium in the urine is obligatory. Hence in situations of *prolonged* low magnesium intake (vomiting, gastric suction, starvation) magnesium deficiency is likely to occur. At least 10 to 14 days of no intake are required to produce magnesium deficiency. The best indicator of magnesium deficiency is a 24-hour urine examination for total magnesium. The normal value is 14 to 20 mEq/24 hours. The serum magnesium may be normal in the presence of total body depletion of magnesium.

The syndrome of magnesium deficiency is manifested by the following.

1. Muscle twitching, hyperactive reflexes.
2. Tremors.
3. Tetany (occasionally).

4. Delirium, hallucinations.
5. Confusion, disorientation.
6. Convulsions, coma.
7. Fever, sweating, tachycardia, and anxiety.

TREATMENT

In acute cases intravenous magnesium sulfate may be given to a maximum of 3 g/1,000 ml of 5 percent glucose in water over a 3-hour period or longer, not to exceed approximately 8 g in 24 hours. Intramuscular doses are 1.0 g, b.i.d. A good urinary output is a prerequisite for use of this drug.

REFERENCES

Barnes, B. A., Cope, O., and Gordon, E. B. Magnesium requirements and deficits: An evaluation in two surgical patients. Ann. Surg., 152:518, 1960.

Freeman, R. M., and Pearson, E. Hypomagnesemia of unknown etiology. Amer. J. Med., 41:645, 1966.

Vallee, B. L. The magnesium deficiency tetany syndrome in man. New Eng. J. Med., 262:155, 1960.

Wacker, W. E. C., and Parisi, A. F. Magnesium metabolism. New Eng. J. Med., 278:658, 1968.

____ Magnesium metabolism. New Eng. J. Med., 278:712, 1968.

____ Magnesium metabolism. New Eng. J. Med., 278:772, 1968.

____ Moore, F. D., Ullmer, D. D., and Vallee, B. L. Normocalcemic magnesium deficiency tetany. J.A.M.A., 180:161, 1962.

MALABSORPTION STATES

Malabsorption means failure of the small bowel mucosa to assimilate adequately a nutrient or nutrients. The most obvious clinical manifestation of malabsorption is steatorrhea (10 percent or more of ingested fat excreted in the stool).

ETIOLOGY

Digestive defects.

1. Pancreatic disease (chronic pancreatitis, carcinoma, cystic fibrosis).
2. Hepatobiliary disease (cirrhosis, common duct obstruction).
3. Postsurgical states (gastrectomy, gastroenterostomy, gastroileostomy).

Absorptive defects.

1. Small bowel disease (tropical sprue, celiac disease, Whipple's disease, lymphoma, regional enteritis, tuberculosis, amyloid, scleroderma, multiple diverticula). Celiac disease is also called "nontropical sprue" and "gluten sensitivity."
2. Postsurgical states (resection of over 50 percent of small bowel, blind loops, strictures, internal fistula).
3. Postradiation therapy.
4. Disaccharide deficiency, e.g., lactose deficiency.

CLINICAL MANIFESTATIONS

Depending on the malabsorbed nutrient, the following states may appear.

1. Steatorrhea and diarrhea. Steatorrhea is always present during exacerbations but may be notably absent during remissions. Diarrhea, on the other hand, may be absent even during exacerbations. Fifty percent or more of the daily fat intake may be passed in a single daily semiformed stool.
2. Hemorrhagic states due to vitamin K malabsorption resulting in hypoprothrombinemia.
3. Tetany (calcium malabsorbed).
4. Osteomalacia and osteoporosis (calcium malabsorbed).
5. General malnutrition.
6. Edema (hypoproteinemia).
7. Anemia may be megaloblastic due to vitamin B_{12} or folic acid deficit, or hypochromic due to inadequate iron absorption.
8. Peripheral neuritis, related to decreased vitamin B_1, B_{12}, and folic acid.
9. Glossitis and cheilosis, related to multiple vitamin deficits.
10. Amenorrhea, related to general malnutrition and secondary hypopituitarism.

DIAGNOSIS

DETECTION OF EXCESS FAT IN THE STOOLS. The presence of steatorrhea is best detected by the following tests.

1. Odor and gross appearance of the stool. The characteristic rancid odor and creamy or silver gray color of the stool may be diagnostic. The stool floats.
2. Microscopic staining of the stool for neutral fat and soaps.
3. Intake-excretion studies with quantitative chemical determination of fecal fat (3-day fat balance study).

DEMONSTRATION OF FAULTY ABSORPTION.

1. Radioisotope studies of fat absorption. The most valuable of these is the triolein-oleic I^{131} test.

	TRIOLEIN I^{131} BLOOD	OLEIC I^{131} BLOOD
Digestive defects	↓	Normal
Absorptive defects	↓	↓

2. Vitamin B_{12} labeled with Co^{60} has been used in combination with intrinsic factors to distinguish between pernicious anemia and other malabsorptive states.
3. Carbohydrate absorption defect. The urinary excretion of D-xylose after ingestion of 25 g is 4 g or more in the normal individual. In malabsorptive states due to impairment of absorption (i.e., small bowel disease) less than 4 g is excreted.
4. Lactose absorption defect. This may be demonstrated by giving the patient 50 to 100 g of lactose P.O. and following his blood lactose curve. In lactose deficiency, the curve will be flat. Biopsy specimens of the small bowel may be obtained via the endoral route and tested for lactase content.

X-RAY STUDIES. In malabsorption states, small bowel x-rays may show dilation, segmentation, and thickening of bowel loops; hypersecretion and hypermotility (increase in transit time) may also be present. These changes are most marked in sprue, lymphosarcoma, and Whipple's disease.

SMALL BOWEL BIOPSY. Several peroral techniques have been developed facilitating biopsy of small bowel mucosa. In the primary malabsorptive states (celiac disease) the mucosa shows flattening with short, blunted, "clubbed" villi. In the others the biopsy findings are normal.

Other tests, including the glucose tolerance test and the vitamin A tolerance test, have been employed but are of less value.

THERAPY

(See also "Chronic Pancreatitis," p. 295.)

SPECIFIC MEASURES (SPRUE). The gluten-free diet produces clinical and chemical remission in 90 percent of patients with celiac disease. Broad spectrum antibiotics are of value in the blind-loop syndrome. Steroids have been employed with marked benefit in patients with malabsorptive states unresponsive to other measures.

General nutrition and dietary supplementation is of value. The suggested diet is low-fat and high-protein with moderate amounts of carbohydrate, preferably as monosaccharides. Calcium gluconate, 5 to 15 g, q.d.; vitamin D, 25,000 to 600,000 units, q.d.; and intensive therapy with other vitamins may be employed.

REFERENCES

Bolt, R. J., Parrish, J. A., French, A. B., and Pollard, H. M. Adult coeliac disease. Ann. Intern. Med., 60:581, 1964.

Dahlqvist, A. Disaccharide intolerance. J.A.M.A. 195:225, 1966.

____ Hammond, J. B., Crane, R. K., Dunphy, J. V., and Littman, A. Intestinal lactase deficiency and lactose intolerance in adults. Gastroenterology, 45:488, 1963.

Dunphy, J. V., et al. Intestinal lactase deficit in adults. Gastroenterology, 49:12, 1965.

Kalser, M. H. Laboratory aids in diagnosis of steatorrhea. J.A.M.A., 188:37, 1964.

Laster, L., and Ingelfinger, F. Intestinal absorption. New Eng. J. Med., 264:1246, 1961.

MacDonald, W. C., Dobbins, W. O., III, and Rubin, C. E. Studies of the familial nature of celiac sprue using biopsy of the small intestine. New Eng. J. Med., 272:448, 1965.

Newcomer, A. D., and McGill, D. B. Lactose tolerance tests in adults with normal lactase activity. Gastroenterology, 50:340, 1966.

Sleisinger, M. Clinical and metabolic studies in nontropical sprue. New Eng. J. Med., 265:49, 1961.

MEDIASTINAL MASSES

Mediastinal masses may be classified according to location.

SUPERIOR MEDIASTINUM

1. Thyroid. May cause pressure symptoms and brassy cough. The trachea or esophagus may be displaced, or superior vena caval obstruction may result.
2. Thymus. May be associated with myasthenia gravis.
3. Bronchogenic cysts. These are as a rule asymptomatic, and occur along the trachea or bronchi. On x-ray, they appear round or oval with smooth borders.

INFERIOR MEDIASTINUM

Anterior.

1. Dermoid cysts. Symptoms occur from pressure or infection.
2. Thymus.

Middle.

1. Lymphomas are the most common mediastinal tumors. They present as bilateral masses with scalloped borders.
2. Bronchogenic cysts.
3. Sarcoid.

Posterior.

1. Neurogenic tumors on x-ray show as round or ovoid masses with smooth borders. They may cause erosion of ribs or vertebrae, or cause symptoms due to nerve compression (including Horner's syndrome).
2. Mesodermal tumors (fibromas, lipomas, etc.) are usually large and bulky, of various morphology, and productive of few if any symptoms.

In an analysis of 782 cases 90 percent of the mediastinal masses were classified as follows:

Lymphomas	25%
Sarcoid	20%
Metastatic neoplasms and bronchogenic carcinoma	10.0%
Histoplasmosis	7%
Tuberculoma	6%
Hernias, diverticula, and achalasias	5%
Aneurysms	4%
Teratomas and dermoids	4%
Thymus (cysts and thymoma)	4%
Goiter	2.5%
Neurogenic tumors	2%

MISCELLANEOUS

1. Other mediastinal masses include pericardial cysts, vascular abnormalities (AV ring, etc.), coccidioidomycosis, infectious mononucleosis, and traumatic hematoma. Each accounts for 1 percent or less of masses.
2. Lymphomas usually are located in the middle mediastinum but may be anywhere.
3. An accurate clinical diagnosis is made in only half of mediastinal tumors.
4. Of all mediastinal tumors, about two thirds are benign and one-third malignant.

REFERENCE

Lyons, H. A., et al. The diagnosis and classification of mediastinal masses, 1. A study of 782 cases. Ann. Intern. Med., 51:897, 1959.

MENINGITIS

Meningitis is inflammation (usually due to infection) of the meninges. Infection may occur via the blood stream (meningococcus, pneumococcus), by direct extension (paranasal sinuses, ear), by retrograde thrombophlebitis, or by spinal fluid pathways.

There are four important clinical features of meningitis.

1. Headache.
2. Stiffness of the neck (with or without a positive Brudzinski or Kernig sign).
3. Mental confusion exists in varying degrees from slight cloudiness of mentation to overt delirium.
4. Fever.

In addition neurologic manifestations may occur. These include convulsions, hemiplegia, papilledema, and oculomotor paralysis.

BACTERIAL MENINGITIS

With the single important exception of tuberculous meningitis, the bacterial meningitides are characterized by the following:

1. Polymorphonuclear leukocytosis in the cerebrospinal fluid.
2. Frequently, grossly cloudy fluid. (At least 200 cells must be present before any change in the spinal fluid can be seen by the naked eye.)
3. Decrease in CSF sugar.
4. Protein is always elevated.

If all age groups are considered (including pediatric cases) the usual organisms are:

Meningococcus	10%
Pneumococcus	10%
H. influenzae	15%
Streptococcus	10%
Gram-negative bacilli	7.5%
Staphylococcus	7.5%

Multiple organisms	15%
Unknown organisms	20%
Total	95%

Other rarer forms include brucella, salmonella, Friedlander's bacillus, pasteurella, diphtheroids, and *Listeria monocytogenes.*

In the absence of head trauma and severe debilitating disease, meningococcus and pneumococus account for practically all bacterial meningitis of adults.

The mortality, variously reported from 30 to 68 percent, is unfavorably influenced by the presence of coma, pneumonia, or age over 60.

VIRAL MENINGITIS

This group is characterized by the following:

1. Lymphocytosis in cerebrospinal fluid.
2. Only rarely is the fluid cloudy.
3. Protein and sugar are as a rule normal.

The usual causes of viral meningitis are as follows:

1. Lymphocytic choriomeningitis.
2. Poliomyelitis.
3. Mumps.
4. Infectious mononucleosis.
5. ECHO groups.
6. Herpes simplex.
7. Coxsackie group.

TREATMENT

BACTERIAL. Penicillin is given in massive doses (24 million units in 5 percent glucose in water per 24 hours) for *pneumococcic* meningitis. The same dose is effective against *meningococcic* meningitis. The penicillin may be given in 5 percent glucose in water, 6 million units, q.i.d.

For *meningococcic meningitis* Gantrisin or sulfadiazine may be used. Gantrisin is less likely to crystallize in the kidneys or ureters. The adult dose of Gantrisin is 3 to 4 g initially, then 1 to 2 g, q. 4 h. The drug may be given P.O., I.M. or I.V. A significant proportion of meningococcic meningitis recently reported from army installations is due to type B and C organisms which are sulfonamide-resistant. However, large doses of penicillin G are effective.

When the organism cannot be identified, massive penicillin therapy should be started. When the organism is identified, one or other of the above drugs may be discontinued.

H. influenzae meningitis responds well to chloramphenicol in intravenous doses of 0.5 g, q. 6 h. This organism is a very rare cause of meningitis in adults (26 reported cases).

In children chloramphenicol is almost invariably started initially, as *H influenzae* is the most common causative agent of meningitis. When the causative organism is not immediately identified, chloramphenicol and massive penicillin therapy are generally begun together.

REFERENCES

Swartz, M. N., and Dodge, P. R. Bacterial meningitis – A review. New Eng. J. Med., 272:725, 1965.

Whitecar, J. P., Reddin, J. L., and Spink, W. W. Recurrent pneumococcal meningitis. New Eng. J. Med., 274:1285, 1966.

Wilson, F. M., Lerner, A. M. Etiology and mortality of purulent meningitis. New Eng. J. Med., 271:1235, 1964.

MONOCYTOSIS

DIFFERENTIAL DIAGNOSIS

Monocytosis exists when 15 or more monocytes are found per 100 white blood cells.

1. Infections
   a. tuberculosis.
   b. subacute bacterial endocarditis.
   c. brucellosis.
   d. typhoid.
   e. syphillis.
   f. measles.
   g. rickettsial infections.
   h. infectious mononucleosis (atypical lymphocytes).
2. Thyrotoxicosis.
3. Carbon tetrachloride poisoning.
4. Lymphomas.
5. Monocytic leukemia.
6. Recovery phase of agranulocytosis (can go as high as 90 percent).

MULTIPLE MYELOMA

Multiple myeloma is a disease associated with plasma cell tumors of the bone marrow. The characteristic findings are:

1. Anemia.
2. Lytic bone lesions (skull, clavicles, ribs, spine, pelvis). Occasionally diffuse demineralization of the skeleton will be seen instead of, or in addition to, discrete lytic lesions.
3. Abnormalities of the serum proteins.
4. Increased plasma cells in the marrow.

The disease occurs, typically in middle-aged and elderly individuals, with a 2:1 ratio of males to females.

The abnormalities of the serum proteins may be:

1. An "M spike" in the globulin area on serum protein electrophoresis. This is usually γA or γG.
2. Hypogammaglobulinemia for all γ globulins except the "M spike."
3. Bence Jones protein may be found in the urine.
4. Twenty percent of patients will have hypogammaglobulinemia *without* an "M spike." Bence-Jones proteinuria will be found in these patients.

Other important abnormalities which are frequently found are:

1. Recurrent bacterial infections.
2. Hypercalcemia.
3. Hyperuricemia.
4. Renal insufficiency.
5. Amyloidosis.

PROGNOSIS

Prognosis for life is generally 2 to 3 years. Occasionally, in cases surviving long enough, amyloidosis may occur.

TREATMENT

Transfusions and analgesics may be employed when indicated. Irradiation of painful bony areas is generally successful.

Melphalan and Cytoxan have been valuable agents, and significant improvement (symptomatic and objective) has been observed in from one-fourth to one-half of patients adequately treated with these drugs. Steroids are generally reserved for management of hypercalcemia if it occurs. Careful attention to hydration to prevent and treat hypercalcemia and hyperuricemia and their complications is mandatory.

REFERENCES

Berlin, N. I. (Moderator). Neoplastic plasma cell (Clinical staff conference). Ann. Intern. Med., 58:1017, 1963.

Brody, J. I., Beizer, L. H., and Schwartz, S. Multiple myeloma and myeloproliferative syndromes. Amer. J. Med., 36:315, 1964.

Carbone, P. P., Kellerhouse, L. E., and Eehan, E. Plasmacytic myeloma. A study of the relationship of survival to various clinical manifestations and anomalous protein type in 112 patients. Amer. J. Med., 42:937, 1967.

Edwards, G. A., and Zawadzki, Z. A. Extraosseous lesions in plasma cells myeloma: Report of six cases. Amer. J. Med., 43:194, 1967.

Speed, D. E., Galton, D. A. G., and Swan, A. Melphalan in the treatment of myelomatosis. Brit. Med. J., 1:1664, 1964.

PRIMARY MYOCARDIAL DISEASE

The term "primary myocardial disease" is confusing because of diverse terminology and unwieldy classification. The condition appears under many names; myocardiopathy, cardiomyopathy, diffuse myocardial disease, idiopathic cardiac hypertrophy, primary cardiomegaly, and the big heart syndrome. Primary or idiopathic myocardial disease is at present the preferred designation. The term "primary myocardial disease" should probably be limited to heart diseases of unknown etiology and to heart diseases not associated with systemic disorders or metabolic derangements.

Primary myocardial disease, as seen clinically, is the approaching end stage of myocardial reaction to infectious, toxic, hormonal, or autoimmune mechanisms still unidentified. Such disease factors produce a similar clinical course and pathologic findings. For these reasons, Friedberg's simple classification of dividing the condition into the primary or idiopathic group and the secondary myocardiopathies is preferred.

In the primary group the etiology is unknown or if suspected, as in alcoholic myocardiopathy, myocardial involvement dominates the pathologic findings and the clinical course. It is classified as follows:

1. Idiopathic myocardiopathy.
2. Familial cardiomegaly.
3. Alcoholic myocardiopathy.
4. African endomyocardial fibrosis.
5. Postpartum heart disease.
6. Endocardial fibro elastosis.

Despite the diverse causes of primary myocardial disease, the clinical course, signs and symptoms are strikingly similar whether the myocardial reaction is due to inflammation, toxic, vascular, or metabolic factors and the result, namely, dilation, hypertrophy, degeneration, and fibrosis, produces the same clinical course though the etiology differs. In adults symptoms usually appear between the ages of 20 and 50 – the years when both rheumatic and arteriosclerotic symptoms also appear.

The first clue to primary myocardial disease in most patients is unexplained cardiomegaly noted by routine x-ray examination. Biventricular enlargement is common and the left atrium is often enlarged; hence, it is confused with rheumatic heart disease. The signs and symptoms of biventricular failure are common and often accompanied by hypertension which is confused with hypertensive cardiovascular disease. In primary myocardial disease, however, the blood pressure usually falls to normal when congestive failure is relieved. In general, an enlarged heart, congestive failure and gallop rhythms, and multiple arrhythmias are most common in primary myocardial disease.

In most patients, atrial or ventricular gallops or both are frequent. With tachycardia the rumbling quality of a summation gallop may simulate the murmur of mitral stenosis. Apical holosystolic murmurs are caused not by valvulitis as in mitral insufficiency, but by ventricular dilation. Unlike the true valvular murmur of rheumatic mitral insufficiency, the intensity of the apical systolic murmur of primary myocardial disease decreases with improved compensation. Aortic ejection murmurs due to left ventricular outflow tract obstruction may result from hypertrophied muscle. Aortic diastolic murmurs are extremely rare and valvular calcification is not present. A wide variety of arrhythmias are common features of primary myocardial disease. Changing arrhythmias early in a clinical course associated with cardiomegaly and failure should alert one to this disorder.

Thromboembolic phenomena in both the pulmonary and peripheral circulation are more common in this disease than in rheumatic or arteriosclerotic heart disease. Fourteen of 26 autopsied cases had mural thrombi; five had systemic and six pulmonary embolism. With advanced failure the pulmonary emboli may arise from the pelvic or leg veins. The pattern of inferior or anterolateral myocardial infarction is often present in primary myocardial disease because of the electrical characteristics of fibrotic myocardium.

Treatment consists of rest, salt restriction, and diuretics. Digitalis should be used with care since these patients are possibly more sensitive to the drug than patients with other forms of heart disease. Because of the high incidence of thromboembolism and the necessity for prolonged bed rest, anticoagulants should be used. Arrhythmias are treated as usual but they usually recur.

The value of steroids is debatable. Those patients who respond probably represent active carditis rather than the fibrotic end stage of primary myocardial disease.

REFERENCE

Mattingly, T. W. Clinical features and diagnosis of primary myocardial disease. Mod. Conc. Cardiovasc. Dis., 30:677-682, 1961.

NEPHROTIC SYNDROME

The nephrotic syndrome is a clinical entity characterized by massive proteinuria and the excretion of fat bodies. There is a variable tendency toward edema, hypoproteinemia, and hyperlipemia. Protein excretion rates are usually in excess of 3.5 g per 24 hours per 1.73 m^2 body surface area in the absence of depressed glomelular filtration rate. Hypoalbuminemia is present with a serum albumin less than 3.5 g per 100 ml.

ETIOLOGY

The following tabulation lists all the known causes. Those marked with an asterisk are the major causes of the nephrotic syndrome.

1. Glomerulonephritis*: proliferative, membranoproliferative, idiopathic membranous, focal, lobular, lipoid nephrosis.
2. Diffuse and nodular diabetic glomerulosclerosis.*
3. Amyloidosis.

4. Multiple myeloma.
5. Collagen-vascular diseases*: Takayasu disease, polyarteritis, SLE, dermatomyositis.
6. Sickle cell anemia.
7. Renal vein thrombosis.
8. Constrictive pericarditis.
9. Congestive heart failure.
10. Tricuspid valvular insufficiency.
11. Nephrotoxins: mercury, bismuth, gold.
12. Allergens: pollens, bee stings, poison oak, poison ivy, snake bite, wool.
13. Drugs: Tridione and Paradione, insect repellents, "cold pills," serum therapy, globulin and polio vaccine, hydroquinone.
14. Cytomegalic inclusion disease.
15. Syphilis.
16. Malaria.
17. Typhus.
18. Chronic jejunoileitis.
19. Tuberculosis.
20. Subacute bacterial endocarditis.
21. Herpes zoster.
22. Hereditofamilial causes.
23. Pregnancy.
24. Transplant.

DIAGNOSIS

CLINICAL SIGNS

The most common finding is edema which may be subtle and localized or cyclic. A wet retinal sheen may be noted. Muehrckes' lines may be noted on the fingernails. Generalized skin pallor may occur, with localized brown darkening of the skin around the eyes. Hypertension may or may not be present. Some patients present with congestive heart failure, coma, or seizures.

LABORATORY FINDINGS

1. Elevated ESR.
2. Elevated serum cholesterol, cholesterol esters, triglycerides, phospholipids and low density lipoproteins.
3. Decreased serum albumin.
4. Proteinuria, red blood cells, hyaline, granular and cellular casts, doubly refractile fat bodies, oval bodies and droplets of neutral fat. Selected patients may have a "telescoped urinary sediment."
5. Renal biopsy is of importance for diagnostic, therapeutic, and prognostic determinations.

THERAPY

Therapy is directed at the edema, the underlying renal cause, and secondary complicating illnesses. Whenever possible specific therapy is employed.

1. Edema
   a. Low sodium diet (0.5 mg Na^+).
   b. High protein diet (unless patient is azotemic).
   c. High caloric diet.
2. Steroid: Immunosuppressive therapy. Treatment with steroids and/or immunosuppressive drugs has been beneficial in lipoid nephrosis and lupus nephritis with the nephrotic syndrome.
3. Specific therapy is available for constrictive pericarditis, congestive heart failure, malaria, syphilis, subacute bacterial endocarditis, and tricuspid stenosis.

PROGNOSIS

The prognosis generally depends on the underlying cause (SLE, diabetes, amyloid, etc.) of the nephrotic syndrome. The outlook for patients with lipoid nephrotis tends to be good but poor for those with membraneous glomerulonephritis.

REFERENCES

Churg, J., Grishman, E., Goldstein, M. H., Yunis, S. L., and Porush, J. G. Idiopathic nephrotic syndrome in adults. A study and classification based on renal biopsies. New Eng. J. Med., 272:165, 1965.

Gary, N. E., Maher, J. F., and Schreiner, G. E. Lupus nephritis: Renal function after prolonged survival. New Eng. J. Med., 276:73, 1967.

Maher, J. F., and Schreiner, G. E. Clinical aspects and pathology of toxic nephropathy. Proceedings of the III International Congress of Nephrology, 2:276, 1967.

Rosenman, E., Pollak, V. E., Pirani, C. L. Renal vein thrombosis in the adult: A clinical and pathologic study based on renal biopsies. Medicine, 47:269, 1968.

NONDISEASE

Nondisease is present when a specific condition is suspected in a patient but is not established by further appropriate investigation. The most striking examples of nondisease are the mimicking syndromes, such as non-Cushing's disease in a patient with obesity, moon face, facial hair, and buffalo hump, the nonvirilizing syndrome with excessive facial hair, and non-Addison's disease in a normally pigmented hypotensive patient. On further investigation the patients prove not to have the disease originally suspected. In short, they have nondisease – normal variations, laboratory errors, and overinterpretation of x-rays; physical signs contribute to the groups of nondisease when the errors are recognized and corrected.

The importance of the concept of nondisease is in management and treatment, or rather nontreatment if the latter has been started. Treatment is never that indicated for the corresponding disease. It consists in explaining to the patient the nature of his nondisease.

REFERENCE

Meador, C. K. The art and science of nondisease. New Eng. J. Med., 272:92, 1965.

OSMOMETRY

Osmometry is a measure of concentration of solute per kilogram of water, not per total volume of solution. Normal serum osmolality is 285 to 290 mOs/kg. Serum osmolality in combination with serum sodium can be useful in distinguishing different types of hyponatremia.

SODIUM	OSMO-LALITY	INDICATES	BECAUSE
Low	Normal	High lipids or other fatty artifacts	These are not soluble, do not affect osmolality, but do affect total volume; sodium is only apparently low.
Low	High	Particles causing increased concentration, e.g., uremia, hyperglycemia	Particles are both soluble and cause increased volume; sodium is apparently low.
Low	Low	Too little sodium or too much water	Sodium concentration per total water is low.

The ratio of sodium (mEq/L) to osmolality (mOsm/kg) falls in the range:

$$\frac{\text{Na}}{\text{Osm}} = 0.43 \text{ to } 0.50$$

If the ratio is lower than 0.43, increased amount of total solute is indicated; e.g., uremia. In dilutional hyponatremia (too much water) the ratio tends to be normal since all constituents are affected equally. In true hyponatremia with reduced sodium, the osmolality will be near normal and the ratio below 0.43.

Another useful formula is:

$$\text{Calculated osmolality} = 1.86\ \text{Na} + \frac{\text{glucose}}{18} + \frac{\text{BUN}}{2.8}$$

In normal cases, the calculated osmolality will be about 5 to 8 mOsm less than the measured value. Excessively high differences in calculated and measured values have been reported in acutely ill and terminal cases, and have been reported to indicate a poor prognosis.

PANCREAS, DISEASES OF

PANCREATITIS WITH ACUTE CHOLECYSTITIS

In many of the patients with acute cholecystitis, acute inflammation of the pancreas occurs. Calculi in the ampulla of Vater cause diversion of bile into the pancreatic ducts, which activates pancreatic enzymes. Only rarely, however, does acute necrosis of the pancreas occur. The symptomatology of acute cholecystitis usually dominates the clinical picture. The serum amylase may be quite high (800 to 1,200 units). The treatment is that of acute cholecystitis.

ACUTE HEMORRHAGIC PANCREATITIS

(Acute Pancreatic Necrosis)

The mechanism of this illness is not clear. Some cases are associated with the impaction of gallstones in the ampulla of

Vater, subsequent release of pancreatic enzymes, and necrosis of the gland. In some patients no gallstones or obstructions to the pancreatic ducts can be found.

The clinical picture is striking and violent. The onset is sudden with severe abdominal pain and vomiting. Circulatory collapse is frequent with falling blood pressure and rapid weak pulse. The temperature may be quite high. The physical findings vary from mild upper abdominal tenderness to the physical signs of boardlike abdomen. Frequently the findings are indistinguishable from perforated peptic ulcer. In the differential diagnosis flat films of the abdomen to rule out perforated ulcer must be done. The serum amylase is always high (800 units or more) if the test is done within 48 hours of the onset of symptoms. The serum calcium is low on the fifth and sixth days reflecting sequestration of calcium in areas of fat necrosis.

A purple discoloration of the abdomen (periumbilical or in the flanks) is occasionally seen. This is the Grey-Turner sign, suggesting, but not specific for, acute pancreatitis.

Therapy is symptomatic. In addition, steps are taken to reduce stimuli to pancreatic secretion, i.e., anticholinergic compounds. Continuous gastric suction is of value. The clinical course is protracted. Mortality is high. Marked electrolyte derangements occur. Hyperglycemia may occur, but only rarely is this of sufficient magnitude to require therapy in itself.

CHRONIC PANCREATITIS

This is a chronic disorder of the pancreas with fibrosis of the gland and destruction of endocrine and exocrine glandular tissue. The presenting manifestation will vary according to the degree of destruction of the gland and according to which of its functions is most deranged. Hence the diagnosis is occasionally made in an asymptomatic person by the accidental discovery of calcification of the pancreas. In some patients the major clinical problem is steatorrhea. In others a pancreatic cyst may become large enough to be the presenting problem.

The most troublesome aspects of this illness are intermittent attacks of acute pancreatitis, which may vary from very mild to very severe. In some patients the attacks progress inexorably to the point where almost continuous pain is present in the epigastrium, presumably due to fibrosis extending beyond the pancreas to involve the solar plexus. Associated with this are the sequelae of chronic pain, i.e., loss of appetite, reduced food intake, loss of weight and strength. As most of these patients are chronic alcoholics, disturbance of behavior is frequent. An abnormal glucose tolerance curve is frequently seen. These patients are easily addicted to opiates and every effort must be made to avoid their use for chronic, recurrent pain.

TREATMENT

Therapy includes abstinence from alcohol and good general hygienic measures for living. Removal of gallstones, if present, is mandatory. When pain becomes intractable many surgical procedures are available, no one of which is predictably successful.

The steatorrhea of chronic pancreatitis is managed by a low-fat diet, antispasmodic drugs, and pancreatic enzyme replacement. These enzymes must be given in large doses and are only moderately successful. These drugs are pancreatin, 4 g daily; Viokase, 3 g daily; Cotazym, 900 mg, 4 to 6 times daily.

ISLET CELL TUMORS OF THE PANCREAS

These neoplasms are made up of cells originating in the island of Langerhans. They may be "nonfunctioning," i.e., do not secrete hormones, or they may secrete hormones quite actively. The tumors may be carcinomatous or benign and may present with symptoms and signs of pancreatic exocrine dysfunction and biliary tract obstruction or may be entirely asymptomatic. Functioning islet cell tumors may be divided into three main categories: 1) insulin-producing (insulinomas), 2) gastrin-producing (Zollinger-Ellison), and 3) nonbeta islet cell tumor, nongastrin producing.

INSULINOMA. These are beta cell tumors of the islands of Langerhans and are characterized by Whipple's triad:

1. Attacks of nervous or gastrointestinal disturbances coming on in the fasting state associated with –
2. Hypoglycemia with readings below 50 mgm%.
3. Relief of symptoms by the ingestion of glucose.

The symptoms of hyperinsulinism appear with fasting; early morning attacks are common. The simplest provocative test is complete fasting which should induce an attack within 24 hours in most patients. The intravenous injection of tolbutamide may be used for diagnosis, but it is hazardous, requiring close observation of the patient and instant availability of glucose for intravenous administration. So-called functional hypoglycemia almost never causes loss of consciousness or convulsions. The treatment for insulinoma is surgical excision. These tumors are extremely vascular, and can be seen by selective visceral angiography thereby obviating the necessity for blind resections of the pancreas.

GASTRIN-PRODUCING ISLET CELL TUMORS. These are responsible for gastric hypersecretion and the Zollinger-Ellison syndrome. The latter is a rare disorder manifested by severe recurrent peptic ulceration of the upper GI tract. The tumor, of nonbeta islet cell origin, is not associated with abnormalities of glucose metabolism. These tumors can be responsible for profound gastric hypersecretion and a fulminating ulcer diathesis. Any patient with previous gastric surgery and an atypical pattern of peptic ulcer in the distal duodenum or the upper jejunum is suspect. Following surgery the early reappearance of an ulcer which is resistant to therapy is characteristic. These patients have a remarkable gastric hypersecretion and may secrete as much as 300 to 400 ml of gastric juice per hour, as opposed to the normal gastric secretion of 20 to 60 ml. Any patient presenting with fulminating and recurrent peptic ulceration and gastric hypersecretion should have surgical exploration of the pancreas. The tumor secretes gastrin.

Removal of the tumor may cure the condition. If excision is not possible, if the tumor is malignant, or if there are metastases, the treatment of choice is total gastrectomy which removes the target organ.

NONBET, NONGASTRIN AND NONINSULIN SECRETING TUMORS. These are rare and produce the syndrome of severe diarrhea, electrolyte depletion, and malabsorption. Excision of the tumor appears to be the treatment of choice.

REFERENCES

Doubilet, H., and Mulholland, J. Surgical treatment of chronic pancreatitis, J.A.M.A., 175:177, 1961.

Ellison, E. H., and Wilson, S. D. Zollinger-Ellison syndrome: Reappraisal and evaluation of 260 registered cases. Ann. Surg., 160:512, 1964.

Gregory, R. A., Grossman, M. I., and Tracy, H. J. Nature of gastric secretogogue in Zollinger-Ellison tumors. Lancet, 2:543, 1967.

____ Tracy, H. J., and French, J. M. Extraction of gastrin-like substance from pancreatic tumors in case of Zollinger-Ellison syndrome. Lancet, 1:1045, 1960.

Johnson, T. A., and Kalser, M. H. The pancreas, contribution of clinical interest, Gastroenterology, 39:469, 1960.

Lepore, M. J. The management of pancreatic insufficiency. Med. Clin. N. Amer., 44:3, 827,833, 1960.

Longmire, W. P., Jr., moderator. Islet cell tumors of the pancreas. The UCLA Interdepartmental Conference. Ann. Intern. Med., 68:203, 1968.

McGuigan, J. E., and Trudeau, W. L. Elevated serum levels of gastrin in Zollinger-Ellison syndrome. New Eng. J. Med., 278:1308, 1968.

Murray, J. S., Paton, R. R., and Pope, C. E., II. Pancreatic tumor associated with flushing and diarrhea: Report of a case. New Eng. J. Med., 264:436, 1961.

Whipple, A. O. The surgical therapy of hyperinsulinism. J. Int. de Chir., 3:237, 1938.

Zollinger, R. M., and Ellison, E. H. Primary peptic ulcerations of jejunum associated with islet cell tumors of pancreas. Ann. Surg., 142:709, 1955.

____ and Moore, F. T. Zollinger-Ellison syndrome comes of age. Recognition of complete clinical spectrum and its management. J.A.M.A., 204:361, 1968.

PARATHYROID DISEASE

(See also "Calcium," p. 46)

HYPERPARATHYROIDISM

Hyperparathyroidism is due usually to adenoma, less commonly hyperplasia, and rarely carcinoma of the parathyroid gland. It has been aptly described as "a disease of stones, bones, abdominal groans, and psychic moans."

STONES. In this country, where milk drinking is prevalent, renal stones occur more frequently than skeletal manifestations. Almost half of the patients with hyperparathyroidism have single or recurrent calculi. As many as 5 to 10 percent of patients presenting with renal stones may be found to have hyperparathyroidism.

BONES. Vague local or generalized bone pains, bone cysts, pathologic fractures, and skeletal deformities may occur. X-ray changes include bone resorption in the phalanges and outer third of the clavicles, giant cell tumors in the skull or mandible, osteoporosis, typical osteitis fibrosa cystica, and absence of the lamina dura.

ABDOMINAL GROANS. Peptic ulceration occurs in about 10 to 25 percent of patients. (Incidence in general population: 5 to 10 percent.) Slightly over 1 percent of all patients with peptic ulcers may have hyperparathyroidism. Pancreatitis and pancreatic calcifications on x-ray are not infrequent. Nausea, vomiting, and abdominal pain not due to ulcer or pancreatis are frequent. This seems to relate to hypercalcemia per se. Epigastric pain intensified by large amounts of milk should suggest the diagnosis.

PSYCHIC MOANS. Neuropsychiatric symptoms occur frequently and seem to be due to the hypercalcemia itself. Symptoms run the gamut from apathy or irritability to frank psychosis.

DIAGNOSIS

1. Hypercalcemia (may be intermittent).
2. Hypercalcinuria (not reliable – found in 30 to 80 percent of patients).
3. Hypophosphatemia (40 to 60 percent may have normal valves).
4. Hyperphosphaturia – decrease tubules reabsorption of phosphate (TRP).
5. Cortisone suppression. Prednisone, 10 mg P.O. q.i.d. for two weeks. A return to normal serum calcium against the diagnosis of primary hyperparathyroidism but continued elevation is not pathognomonic.*
6. Parathyroid hormone assays may be helpful in future.
7. Roentgenologic findings as listed above (generally not demonstrable unless alkaline phosphatase is elevated).

SECONDARY HYPERPARATHYROIDISM

With azotemia, a relative vitamin D deficiency occurs with subsequent lowering of serum calcium. The fall in calcium leads to increased parathyroid hormone secretion and bone changes similar to those occurring in primary hyperparathyroidism may develop. Serum calcium may be normal or low; serum phosphorous may be normal or increased.

HYPOPARATHYROIDISM

The usual cause of hypoparathyroidism is ablation of the parathyroid glands occuring during thyroid surgery. Other causes include neck irradiation, hemorrhage, infection, and idiopathic (about 150 cases of the latter reported). Malabsorption of calcium, such as may occur in steatorrheic states, renal failure, and pseudohypoparathyroidism, should also be considered.

Hypoparathyroidism is manifested by muscle spasm and tetany. There are also alopecia, convulsions, cataract, papille-

*Best tests.

dema, increased intracranial pressure, trophic changes of nails and skin, and various neuropsychiatric symptoms.

The most important difference between the metabolism of calcium and phosphorus in these patients and normal individuals is the inability of the hypoparathyroid patient to excrete phosphate.

Laboratory findings include the following:

1. Hyperphosphatemia with hypophosphaturia.
2. Hypocalcemia and hypocalciuria.
3. ECG indicative of low calcium (prolonged ST interval).
4. EEG shows generally slow activity.
5. X-rays may show growth arrest lines and increased density in the bones and intracranial calcifications.
6. On administration of parathyroid hormone a greater than normal phosphate diuresis occurs (positive Ellsworth-Howard test).

	HYPERPARATHYROIDISM		HYPOPARATHYROIDISM			
	PRIMARY	SECONDARY	PRIMARY	SECONDARY	PSEUDO	PSEUDO-PSEUDO
CAUSE	Adenoma usual; hyperplasia uncommon; carcinoma rare	Renal disease	Idiopathic	Thyroid surgery, neck irradiation	Renal unresponsiveness to parathyroid hormone	Not endocrine but multiple congenital defects
HISTORY	"Stones, bones, abdominal groans & psychic moans"	Renal disease	Tetany and convulsions		May have familial history	
PHYSICAL FINDINGS	May show muscular weakness, flaccidity, and reduced or absent reflexes, lethargy, semicoma with "parathyroid crisis"		Alopecia, trophic nail and skin changes		Round facies, short stature, short metacarpals and metatarsals; ectopic calcifications (exostoses, lens, aorta, etc.)	

LABORATORY FINDINGS						
Serum Ca	↑	Normal		↓	↓	Normal
Serum PO_4	↓	Usually normal, may be ↑		↑	↑	Normal
Urine Ca	↑	↓		↓	↓	Normal
Urine PO_4	↑	↑		↓	↓	Normal
Urea nitrogen	Normal (occas. ↑)	↑		Normal	Normal	Normal
Alkaline phosphatase	Usually normal, may be ↑	↑ may be ↑	Normal	Occas. ↓	Normal, occas. ↓	Normal
Response to parathyroid hormone (Ellsworth-Howard test)	–	–	Positive (phosphate diuresis)		Negative (no phosphate diuresis)	Normal

PSEUDOHYPOPARATHYROIDISM

This is a genetic disorder inherited as an X-linked recessive with variable penetrance. It has been suggested that the primary defect is renal unresponsiveness to parathyroid hormone.

The diagnostic criteria of pseudohypoparathyroidism are as follows:

1. Round facies, short stature, short metacarpals and metatarsals, and ectopic calcifications.
2. Hyperphosphatemia and hypocalcemia.
3. Failure to respond to parathyroid extract, i.e., no phosphate diuresis (negative Ellsworth-Howard test).

PSEUDO-PSEUDOHYPOPARATHYROIDISM

It is present in patients who have the clinical features of pseudohypoparathyroidism but usually have normal serum calcium and phosphorus. However, some patients have developed hypocalcemia later in the course of the disease so that this disorder may not be distinct from pseudohypoparathyroidism.

REFERENCES

Berson, S. A., and Yalow, R. S. Parathyroid hormone in plasma in adenomatous hyperparathyroidism, anemic and bronchogenic carcinoma. Science, 154:907, 1966.

Dent and Watson. Hyperparathyroidism and cancer. Brit. Med. J., p. 218, July 1964.

Keating, F. R., Jr. Diagnosis of primary hyperparathyroidism. Clinical and laboratory aspects. J.A.M.A., 178:547, 1961.

Rasmussen, H. Parathyroid hormone (review). Amer. J. Med., 30:112, 1961.

Symposium: Thyrocalcitonin. Amer. J. Med., 43:000, 1967.

Todd, J. N., Hill, R. S., Nickerson, J. F., and Tingher, J. O. Hereditary multiple exostoses, pseudo-pseudohypoparathyroidism, and other genetic defects of bone, calcium, and phosphorus metabolism. Amer. J. Med., 30:289, 1961.

Uhr, N., and Bezahler, H. B. Pseudo-pseudohypoparathyroidism: Report of three cases in one family. Ann. Intern. Med., 54:443, 1961.

PERICARDITIS

ETIOLOGY

1. Idiopathic or nonspecific (about 25 percent of cases).
2. Infections:
   a. bacterial (pyogenic 16 percent, TBC 7 percent).
   b. fungal (including histoplasmosis).
   c. viral (including Coxsackie group B, types 2, 3, 4, 5).
   d. infectious mononucleosis (rare, 16 cases reported).
3. Collagen diseases, including systemic lupus erythematosus, rheumatoid arthritis, and rheumatic fever (11 percent).
4. Sensitivity states, including serum sickness, autoimmune responses, and various allergies. The postmyocardial infarction syndrome and the postcardiotomy syndrome belong to this group.
5. Inflammations of contiguous structures including myocardial infarction (11 percent), dissecting aneurysm, esophageal disease, and pulmonary disease, especially pneumonia and embolism.
6. Neoplastic.
7. Metabolic disorders, including renal failure (17 percent) and myxedema.
8. Traumatic (1 percent).
9. Pericarditis secondary to x-ray therapy.
10. Cholesterol pericarditis (rare, 12 cases reported).

DIAGNOSIS

DIFFERENTIAL DIAGNOSIS

Admission diagnosis is made correctly in only about 20 percent of cases. Most frequently confused with pericarditis are the following:

1. Myocardial infarction (40 percent).
2. Pneumonia (25 percent).
3. Acute rheumatic fever (5 percent).
4. Pulmonary embolism (5 percent).
5. Acute cholecystitis (2.5 percent).

SYMPTOMS AND PHYSICAL FINDINGS

1. Chest pain depends primarily on involvement of the pleural or

diaphragmatic pericardium. It is often increased by motion, respiration, coughing, or swallowing. Up to 50 percent of patients have *no* pain.
2. Pericardial friction rub is pathognomonic. It is best heard with the patient sitting and leaning forward.
3. Electrocardiographic changes are referable to the epimyocardial involvement. One half to three quarters of patients have either suggestive or typical findings; such as
   a. displacement of the RS–T junction upward;
   b. T wave abnormalities – the ascending limb may be concave early, later may invert;
   c. in chronic pericarditis, low voltage due to calcification with epimyocardial atrophy or to the presence of fluid.
4. Chest x-rays. Serial roentgenograms may show an accumulation of fluid. The minimal amount of fluid recognizable on x-ray is about 250 ml. With further increases the "water bottle" configuration may occur. The pericardiophrenic angle is preserved.
5. Pericardial biopsy is often of great value. It may establish the diagnosis in bacterial, viral, neoplastic, and other causes.

PERICARDIAL EFFUSION

The differentiation between pericardial effusion and cardiomegaly is usually difficult. Only rarely does one see the classic "water bottle" heart which shifts on positioning of the patient. The pericardiophrenic angle is not always obliterated in cardiomegaly without effusion. In the presence of suspected cardiac tamponade, one is justified in doing a pericardiocentesis immediately. Under less pressing circumstances other tests are generally done first for fear of complications of the needling (laceration of the atrium or coronary artery). Intravenous angiography using contrast material is safe and usually clarifies the diagnosis. Intravenous injection of CO_2 is safe and can also be of use. New techniques of "scan" of the heart and the use of sonic devices have not yet been fully evaluated. In cases where the diagnosis of pericardial effusion seems correct, it may be necessary to obtain pericardial fluid for examination and culture. A pericardial tap can then be performed.

PERICARDIAL TAP

This procedure is best done in a fluoroscopy room after sedation with Demerol and pentobarbital. The exploring needle, connected to the chest lead of the ECG by a sterile alligator clamp and wire, is inserted into the pericardial sac by the subxiphoid approach or through the fifth ICS in the MCL. If the needle comes in contact with the epicardium, ST elevation will be recorded by the ECG, and the needle is withdrawn a short distance. The fluid removed is replaced by at least 150 cc of air, and repeat chest x-rays are taken.

REFERENCES

Brawley, R. K., Vasko, J. S., and Morrow, A.N.G. Cholesterol pericarditis. Am. J. Med., 41:235, 1966.

Neill, J. R. Pericardiocentesis electrode. New Eng. J. Med., 264:711, 1961.

Wolff, L., and Grunfeld, O. Pericarditis, New Eng. J. Med., 268:419, 1963.

PERNICIOUS ANEMIA

Pernicious anemia is characterized by involvement of three systems.

1. Blood: megaloblastic anemia, frequently with a slight to moderate hemolysis; leukopenia with neutropenia and sometimes thrombocytopenia.
2. Nervous system: paresthesias, loss of position and vibration sense, and ataxia.
3. Gastrointestinal tract: achlorhydria and diarrhea. Gastric carcinoma occurs with three times the usual incidence.

DIAGNOSIS

Diagnosis is highly likely in the presence of a megaloblastic bone marrow, histamine-fast achlorhydria, response to vitamin B_{12} given parenterally, and the absence of any other cause for B_{12} deficiency. The Schilling test may be helpful in establishing the diagnosis, particularly in cases in which vitamin B_{12} has already been given. In PA there is practically no urinary excretion of orally administered radioactive B_{12} (Co^{57} B_{12}). The excretion becomes normal when the intrinsic factor is given along with radioactive B_{12}.

TREATMENT

Treatment is parenteral B_{12}. There are many successfully used regimens. In one the dose is 1,000 μg B_{12}, I.M., q. for 4 days, then 100 μg, I.M., q. mo. for life. The large initial dose saturates body stores of B_{12}. The liver normally stores about 1,000 to 2,000 g of B_{12}. For this reason it takes approximately 3 to 5 years post total gastrectomy for pernicious anemia to develop.

Addisonian pernicious anemia, by definition, consists of achlorhydria with absent intrinsic factor and megaloblastic anemia. Non-Addisonian pernicious anemia – B_{12} deficiency anemia in the presence of intrinsic factor – may occur in malabsorptive states, *Diphyllobothrium latum* infestation, the blind loop syndrome, and multiple small bowel diverticula.

REFERENCES

Davidson, S. Clinical picture of pernicious anemia. Brit. Med. J., 1:241, 1957.

Spurling, C. L., Sacks, M. S., and Jiji, R. Juvenile pernicious anemia. New Eng. J. Med., 271:995, 1964.

PHEOCHROMOCYTOMA

Pheochromocytoma is a tumor of chromaffin tissue usually occurring in the adrenal medulla. Cases have been recorded, however, with chromaffin tissue occurring in the chest, neck, urinary bladder, aortic chain, and retroperitoneal area. About 5 to 10 percent are bilateral, and 10 percent malignant.

DIAGNOSIS

Hypertension due to pheochromocytoma may be either sustained or paroxysmal. With paroxysmal attacks headache, usually extremely severe, sweating, tachycardia, anxiety, and pallor or flushing are common.

LABORATORY FINDINGS

1. BMR is elevated to + 20 or more in about 50 percent of cases.
2. Frequently impaired carbohydrate tolerance.
3. IVP sometimes demonstrates a mass.
4. VMA (vanillyl mandelic acid) – metabolite of epinephrine and norepinephrine. Normal values are 1 to 10 mg every 24 hours.
5. Metanephrines – major metabolites of epinephrine and norepinephrine. Occasionally positive when VMA is normal. Normal value 1.3 mg every 24 hours.
6. Catecholamines: Normal values for 24-hour urine are 50 mg of epinephrine and 150 mg norepinephrine. Exogenous vasopressors,

fluorescent compounds like tetracycline and certain drugs like α-methyldopa may increase the catecholamine determination.

7. Arteriography by the transfemoral route after preparation with an α-blocking agent (phenoxybenzamine, Dibenzylene) has been helpful in the localization and the diagnosis of pheochromocytoma.

DRUGS.

1. Histamine (0.05 mg of histamine base in 0.5 ml isotonic NaCl, I.V.) is employed when the blood pressure is below 160 mm systolic.
2. Phentolamine (Regitine, 5 mg, I.V.) is used in individuals with sustained hypertension. The test is considered positive if a 35-mm systolic drop and a 25-mm diastolic drop occur.
3. Tyramine test – depends on direct release of catecholamines from nerve endings.
4. Glucagon stimulation test – intravenous injection of 0.5 to 1.0 mg of glucagon may result in pressor response in patients with pheochromocytoma. Pharmacologic tests are seldom needed to make the diagnosis of pheochromocytoma.

False negatives may occur if the systolic pressure is not markedly elevated.

NOTES

1. Suspect pheochromocytoma in these situations:
   a. Patients with sustained hypertension who complain of headaches, sweating, palpitations, and vasomotor phenomena.
   b. Thin hypertensive patients.
   c. Young hypertensive patients.
   d. Recent onset of hypertension.
   e. Hypermetabolism without hyperthyroidism.
   f. Paradoxical reactions to ganglionic blocking agents.
   g. Blood pressure increases under general anesthesia.
2. Neurofibromatosis is associated with pheochromocytoma in a much greater than chance fashion. The presence of café au lait spots in a hypertensive patient is suggestive.
3. Banana ingestion may elevate catecholamine values.
4. About 400 cases of pheochromocytoma have been recorded. It is estimated that about 1 percent of hypertension is caused by this tumor. Perhaps as many as 800 deaths per year are due to undiagnosed pheochromocytoma.
5. Patients with familial pheochromocytoma have higher incidence of bilateral tumors and amyloid medullary carcinoma of the thyroid.

REFERENCES

Lawrence, A. M. Glucagon provocative test for pheochromocytoma. Ann. Intern. Med., 66:1091, 1967.

Rossi, P., Kaufman, L., Ruzicka, F. F., Jr., and Panke, W. Angiographic localization of pheochromocytoma. Radiology, 86:266, 1966.
Sjoerdsma, A., Engelman, K., Waldmann, T. A., Cooperman, L. H., and Hammond, W. E. Pheochromocytoma: Current concepts of diagnosis and treatment. Ann. Intern. Med., 65:1302, 1966.

PLEURAL EFFUSION

Pleural effusions are of two types:

1. Transudates: Congestive, renal or hepatic failure. Sp. gr. less than 1,015; protein less than 3 g/100 ml of fluid.
2. Exudates: Fluid due to disease of the pleura. Sp. gr. greater than 1,015; protein greater than 3 g/100 ml of fluid.

Exception: Myxedema produces a transudate with higher protein content than 3 g per 100 ml.

PLEURAL DISEASE

Usually secondary to other serious disease. Rarely, mesothelioma of pleura.

Pain of *parietal* pleuritis is referred to the skin supplied by the corresponding spinal nerve segment.

Diaphragmatic pleuritis: Central portion: Pain is referred to shoulder strap area and the trapezius region. Peripheral diaphragmatic pleura is supplied from adjacent intercostal nerves. Point tenderness on the chest wall may be found in pulmonary infarction.

Epidemic pleurodynia and trichinosis may involve muscle adjacent to the parietal pleura and produce neither friction rub nor fluid.

ETIOLOGY

1. Bacterial: tuberculosis, bacterial pneumonia, lung abscess, and bronchiectasis.
2. Viral and Rickettsial: atypical Pn (Eaton Agent), viral pneumonia, psittacosis, and Q-fever.
3. Mycotic: coccidioidomycosis, actinomycosis, and blastomycosis.
4. Protozoal: ameba.
5. Malignant: primary mesothelioma, metastatic tumor, and lymphoma.
6. Cardiovascular: congestive heart failure, pulmonary thromboembolism, pericarditis, and superior vena caval obstruction.

7. Lymphatic obstruction: lymphoma, metastatic disease, traumatic chylothorax, and malignant chylothorax.
8. Hypoproteinemia: cirrhosis of liver, nephrosis, and collagen disease.
9. Miscellaneous: ovarian tumor (Meigs' syndrome), pneumothorax, and hemothorax.

DIAGNOSIS

Diagnosis is aided by:

1. Aspiration of the fluid.
2. Biopsy of parietal pleura.
   a. needle – study tissue histologically and bacteriologically.
   b. open pleural biopsy (exploratory thoracotomy) if diagnosis is not evident.
3. Biopsy of lymph nodes.
4. Bronchoscopy.

PROGNOSIS AND TREATMENT

Those of the underlying cause.

TUBERCULOUS PLEURISY

Still the most common cause of pleural exudative disease. Open pleural biopsy may be necessary to establish a diagnosis.

TREATMENT

To the regimen outlined under the treatment of tuberculosis add streptomycin daily for 1 to 2 months if severe systemic symptoms are present. Steroids are used in large effusions and in the very young to prevent fibrothorax and prevent scoliosis. Start with 80 mg prednisone daily, diminish over 2 to 3 weeks to 30 mg, and discontinue after 6 weeks.

Treatment with INH (300 mg/d) should continue for 24 months; discontinue PAS (200 mg/k/d) in 1 year if no pulmonary cavitary disease is present. Discontinue streptomycin (1 g/d) in 1 to 2 months. Patient may be up and about when fluid subsides.

REFERENCES

Starkey, G. W. B. Recurrent malignant pleural effusions. New Eng. J. Med., 270:436, 1964.

Stead, W. W., and Sproul, J. M. Pleural effusion. Disease-a-Month, July, 1964.

PNEUMONIA

Pneumonia may be caused by a variety of infectious agents: bacterial, viral, rickettsial, and fungal.

Viral pneumonia is about as frequent as bacterial, and in young adults accounts for about 90 percent of cases.

ETIOLOGY

BACTERIAL

1. *Diplococcus pneumoniae* 90%
2. Hemolytic streptococcus < 1%
3. *Klebsiella* (Friedlander's) *pneumoniae* < 1%
4. *Haemophilus influenzae* < 0.5%
5. *Staphylococcus aureus* approx. 9.5%
6. *Mycobacterium tuberculosus* pneumonia
7. Others, including *Pasteurella tularensis* and *P. pestis,* and enteric bacteria.

VIRAL

1. Eaton viruses (responsive to tetracycline).
2. Adenoviruses (18 antigenic types, of which types 3, 4, 7, and 7A may cause pneumonia in adults).
3. Coxsackie viruses.
4. ECHO viruses.
5. Myxoviruses.
6. HE viruses.
7. Reoviruses.
8. Coe viruses.
9. J-H virus.
10. 2060 virus.
11. Andrewes viruses.
12. Influenza viruses types A, B, C.
13. Parainfluenza viruses types 1, 2, 3 (children).
14. Psittacosis (ornithosis) responsive to broad-spectrum antibiotics.
15. Pneumonia secondary to rubeola, varicella, smallpox, etc.

RICKETTSIAL

1. Epidemic typhus.
2. Rocky mountain spotted fever.

3. Tsutsugamushi disease.
4. Q fever (pneumonitis is the most characteristic sign of Q fever)

MYCOTIC

1. *Histoplasma capsulatum.*
2. *Blastomyces dermatitidis* (North American blastomycosis).
3. *Coccidioides immitis.*
4. *Nocardia asteroides.*
5. *Actinomyces bovis.*
6. *Aspergillus* sp. (especially *fumigatus*).
7. *Rhizopus oryzae* (mucormycosis).
8. *Cryptococcus neoformans.*
9. *Candida albicans* (monilia pneumonia).

DIAGNOSIS

PNEUMOCOCCAL PNEUMONIA. This is usually preceded by an upper respiratory infection (75 percent of cases). After a few days of coryza and of an increasing cough, suddenly shaking chills (70 percent), high fever (100 percent), and blood-streaked sputum (50 percent) supervene. Pleuritic pain occurs in about 50 percent of cases. On physical examination, consolidation is found in 75 percent of patients, with pleural rub and fluid in about 20 percent of patients each. Sputum culture and blood cultures are positive in about 90 percent and 10 to 20 percent, respectively.

VIRAL PNEUMONIAS. These are contrasted as follows:

1. Fever is as a rule less, and shaking chills are less common.
2. Headache is more outstanding.
3. Hemoptysis occurs in only 5 to 10 percent.
4. Pleural pain is present in only 5 percent.
5. On physical examination, rales without consolidation occur in 75 percent of patients. Clear lungs occur in about 15 percent of patients. Pleural fluid is rare and rub is uncommon (1 to 2 percent).
6. Laboratory evaluation reveals a sputum with a normal flora and a negative blood culture, but cold agglutinins are positive in 25 to 50 percent of cases, with a median titer of 1:32. Eaton agent pneumonia is commonly associated with positive cold agglutinins.

FRIEDLANDER'S PNEUMONIA. This is seen in older men and particularly alcoholics. Aspiration is an important etiologic factor. Acute fulminating pneumonia involving the upper lobes and leading to abscess formation is the usual picture. Jaundice occurs in 15 to 20 percent. The classical brick red or "currant jelly" sputum occurs in 33 to 50 percent of cases. Chest x-ray shows massive lobar consolidation (usually RUL) with downward bulging or bowing of the lesser fissure. Gram stain of the sputum shows short, wide, gram-negative, thickly encapsulated bacilli singly or in pairs. The mortality rate in klebsiella pneumonia is 75 to 80 percent. Classically, this disease, the Waterhouse-Friedrichsen syndrome, and the pneumonic form of the bubonic plague are listed as the three bacterial diseases capable of killing within 24 hours.

STAPHYLOCOCCAL PNEUMONIA. This occurs most frequently in the very young, the aged, and the debilitated. The disease begins most often as an indolent bronchopneumonia with cough, yellow purulent sputum, septic fever, chills, and pleurisy. Single or multiple cavities are a common x-ray finding.

TREATMENT

(See also Antibiotics, p. 13)

PNEUMOCOCCAL PNEUMONIA. Penicillin is the drug of choice. Due to the exquisite susceptibility of the organism to this drug, doses as low as 300,000 units daily are quite effective. The usual dose is 600,000 units t.i.d. In the presence of shock or extreme toxicity, penicillin should be given intravenously initially.

FRIEDLANDER'S PNEUMONIA. The recommended initial regimen is chloramphenicol or amphicillin, 0.5 to 1.0 g, q. 6 h., parenterally, plus streptomycin, 0.5 to 1.0 g, I.M., q. 6 h.

STAPHYLOCOCCAL PNEUMONIA. Staphcillin is the drug of choice. Pending sensitivity studies, the preferred antibiotics are Staphcillin, or Staphcillin plus penicillin G, chloramphenicol, and vancomycin.

VIRAL PNEUMONIA. Treatment is symptomatic. Because of the susceptibility of Eaton viruses and the psittacosis group to tetracycline, this drug may be employed in doses of 250 mg q.i.d.

REFERENCES

Forsyth, B. R., Bloom, H. H., Johnson, K. M., and Chanock, R. M. Etiology of primary atypical pneumonia in a military population. J.A.M.A., 191:364, 1965.

Reiman, H. A. Infectious diseases (review). Arch. Intern. Med., 5:679, 1960; 109:60, 1962.

PNEUMONITIS ASPIRATION

(Mendelson's Syndrome)

The inhalation of gastric contents produces a spectrum of chemical responses varying in severity from a localized aspiration pneumonia to life-threatening asphyxia, shock, or pulmonary edema. The overall mortality is 70 percent. Risk is greatest in patients who vomit or regurgitate when the normal protective reflexes of gagging and glottic closure are lost. Conditions with the highest predisposition occur in 1) the anesthetized patient, 2) drug overdoses, 3) alcoholic intoxication, 4) upper gastrointestinal lesions (i.e., gastric outlet and intestinal obstruction, hiatal hernia, achalasia).

CLINICAL PICTURE

The clinical picture is dependent on whether the gastric contents are particulate or liquid. Large solids usually occlude a major or lobar bronchus. This causes a collapse of a lung, or lobar atelectasis, with subsequent cyanosis, tachypnia, tachycardia, and suprasternal and intercostal retractions. Breath sounds are absent over the nonaerated lung, and x-rays reveal massive atelectasis with tracheal and mediastinal deviation to the occluded side. Unilateral emphysema may occur secondary to the "ball valve phenomena." Obstruction of smaller bronchial radicals may be asymptomatic for a few days until atelectasis arises and becomes infected, along with possible abscess formation.

Inhalation of liquid contents in sufficient volume and low pH produces a clinical picture that differs from the above. A brief period of apnea is followed by severe bronchospasm, pulmonary edema, and shock. X-rays usually show patterns of bronchopneumonia or pulmonary edema. Symptoms may occur hours after aspiration.

PATHOPHYSIOLOGY

The three factors governing morbidity and mortality are 1) pH of the aspirate, 2) the volume, and 3) contamination. The pH is the most important. It has been shown in animal experimentation that aspiration of gastric fluid with $pH > 2.5$ evokes the same benign reaction as saline but as the pH decreases a severe hemorrhagic necrotizing pneumonitis and bronchitis occur. The reaction is maximal at a pH of 1.5; pepsin plays no part in the reaction. The aspirate is distributed rapidly, appearing at the pleural surface in 12 to 18 seconds causing air leaks, pleural effusion, and patchy atelectasis in three minutes. This is followed by a profuse transudate which neutralizes the aspirate in 15 to 30 minutes. Fecally-contaminated gastric contents due to intestinal obstruction at a neutral pH will not give the above clinical and pathologic findings, but severe shock can be anticipated in 24 hours because of absorption of endotoxin. These events are analagous to a "chemical burn," and the morbidity is determined by the area of alveolar surface damaged. Bacterial infection is not an early manifestation of the sterile aspirate. Patients who survive the initial insult may develop a secondary infection in a few days. If food or fecal contamination is present, positive cultures may be obtained in 24 hours.

The hemodynamic alterations recorded are immediate systemic hypotension and elevated pulmonary artery pressure which returns to normal within minutes. Progressive systemic hypotension leading to shock and a low right atrial pressure develop. These changes are explained on the basis of marked hypovolemia due to copious transudation into the lung, giving a decrease in plasma volume, compliance, and tidal volume. These factors are important because the pulmonary edema and shock in this setting are not on the basis of cardiac failure but are due to fluid loss from damaged alveoli and bronchi. Treatment with potent diuretics or phlebotomy aggravate the shock state. Arterial blood gas studies show a marked and rapid fall in PO_2 which is refractory to 40 percent oxygen and only responds to positive pressure with 100 percent oxygen. This indicates an abnormal ventilation perfusion ratio with pulmonary shunting of blood. The severity of the hypoxia is directly proportional to the pH and to the volume of the aspirate, as are the arterial pH and pCO_2; in lethal situations there is a decrease in pH and an increase in pCO_2. The reverse is seen in survivors. Respiratory and metabolic acidosis are usually present. Without an episode of aspiration, the clinical picture will simulate acute left ventricular failure or massive pulmonary embolus. A high index of suspicion is needed to make the diagnosis in the unconscious patient.

TREATMENT

1. Monitor central venous pressure and arterial blood gases.
2. Use tracheal suction and lavage with 5 ml saline times three; lavage with large volume of fluid will depress pO_2 and disperse the aspirate. Test pH of secretion for prognostic value.
3. Try bronchoscopy if character of aspirate is unknown. This is of doubtful value if the aspirate is liquid.
4. Employ intubation or tracheostomy with positive pressure assisted ventilation (100 percent oxygen) to treat pulmonary edema and severe hypoxemia. Arterial pO_2 should be maintained at 85 to 100 mm Hg.
5. Give systemic steroids (dexamethasone 8 mg I.V. or I.M. stat; then 4 mg q. 6 h. for 72 hours); they have beneficial effect in decreasing the severity of the reaction in the first 24 hours. By the fourth day the condition of the lungs is the same with or without steroids.
6. Topical steroids are of no benefit and may even cause pulmonary lesions.
7. Treat shock with volume expanders such as dextran or plasma.
8. Give broad spectrum antibiotic coverage, i.e., penicillin and streptomycin.
9. Employ postural drainage, chest physiotherapy.

REFERENCES

Cameron, J. L., Anderson, R. P., and Zuidema, C. D. Aspiration pneumonia (A clinical and experimental review). J. Surg. Res., 7:44, 1967.

Hammelberg, W., and Bosomworth, P. P. Aspiration pneumonitis. Springfield, Ill., Charles C Thomas, Publisher, 1968.

POLYARTERITIS

(Periarteritis Nodosa, Necrotizing Angiitis, and Wegener's Granulomatosis)

Polyarteritis is a disease of fibrinoid degeneration of medium-sized and small vessels. Symptoms depend upon the organ or organs involved; however, renal involvement is most common, followed by myocardial, gastrointestinal, pulmonary, cutaneous, and neurologic manifestations. About 1,000 cases are described in the world literature. The cause is unknown; however, hypersensitivity is suspected. Included on the suspect list are sulfonamide drugs and penicillin as well as many other drugs. Polyarteritis is closely related to other forms of angiitis, especially temporal arteritis and Wegener's granulomatosis.

DIAGNOSIS

The outstanding findings are:

1. hypertension.
2. eosinophilia.
3. asthma.
4. hematuria.
5. peripheral neuropathy.
6. abdominal symptoms.
7. intermittent fever.

Diagnosis is confirmed by a positive muscle biopsy, which unfortunately shows typical findings in only one third of cases or less.

WEGENER'S GRANULOMATOSIS

Wegener's granulomatosis is a disease closely related to polyarteritis nodosa. It is a focal necrotizing granulomatous vasculitis involving mainly the respiratory tract and kidneys. Clinically, the usual sequence is as follows:

1. Rhinitis and sinusitis, initially mild, but progressing to granulomatous destruction of the nasal passages.
2. Nodular pulmonary granulomas.
3. Focal glomerulonephritis as manifested by albuminuria, hematuria, cylindruria, terminating in uremia.

Approximately 40 to 50 cases have been reported, and the ratio of Wegener's granulomatosis to polyarteritis is about 1:20.

TREATMENT

Treatment of these diseases, in addition to removal of possible offending agents causing hypersensitivity, is corticosteroids in high doses. Cytotoxic drugs have also been experimentally used.

REFERENCES

Alarcon-Segovia, D., and Brown, A. L., Jr. Classification and etiologic aspects of necrotizing angiitides: An analytic approach to a confused subject with a critical review of the evidence for hypersensitivity in polyarteritis nodosa. Mayo Clin. Proc., 39:205, 1964.

Varriale, P., Minogue, W. F., and Alfenito, J. C. Allergic granulomatosis: Case report and review of the literature. Arch. Intern. Med., 113:235, 1964.

POLYCYTHEMIA VERA

Polycythemia vera is a myeloproliferative disorder characterized by excessive production of all the bone marrow elements, but predominantly the erythrocyte.

DIAGNOSIS

Diagnosis depends upon a characteristic clinical and laboratory picture, and exclusion of secondary (pulmonary) and other known causes (fibroids, obesity, renal tumors, and hydronephrosis, and cerebellar tumors).

The outstanding features of the disease are as follows:

1. Red cell count over 6.5 million.
2. Hemoglobin of 18 to 24 g.
3. Hematocrit of 60 mm or more.
4. White cell count frequently over 10,000, with metamyelocytes or myelocytes in the periphery.
5. Platelet count often over 300,000.
6. Splenomegaly in at least 60 percent of patients.
7. Normal arterial O_2 saturation.

COMPLICATIONS

Complications include thrombosis in about 25 percent of patients. This is probably secondary to the high blood viscosity. Hemorrhage occurs in about 15 percent of cases, and for this reason anticoagulants are generally contraindicated. Peptic ulcer (10 to 15 percent) and hyperuricemia, usually without clinical gout, may occur in up to 50 percent of patients. The disease may terminate in leukoerythroblastic anemia, myeloid metaplasia, or chronic myelocytic leukemia (20 percent). Life expectancy is about 5 to 10 years.

TREATMENT

Treatment consists of venesection and radioactive phosphorus therapy.

REFERENCES

Miescher, P. A., ed. Polycythemia. Seminars Hemat., 3:000, 1966.
Valentine, W. N., et al. Polycythemia: Erythrocytosis and erythremia. Ann. Intern. Med., 69:587, 1968.

PORPHYRIA

	ERYTHRO-POIETICA PORPHYRIA	HEPATIC PORPHYRIA ACUTE INTER-MITTENT	CUTANEA TARDA	MIXED
Synonyms	Congenital photosensitive	Acute toxic	Chronic	Combined
Frequency	3%	61%	14%	7%
Age at onset	0-5	10-40	40-80	10-80
Clinical findings	Photosensitivity, erythrodontia, hemolytic anemia, splenomegaly	Abdominal, colic, constipation, psychic disturbance, C.N.S. disturbance, hypertension	Photosensitivity, epidermolysis bullosa, skin pigmentation, hepatic dysfunction	Mixed
Color of urine	Red	Normal (darkens on standing)	Red	Normal or red
Porphobilinogen	Negative	Positive	Negative	Positive in 1/3
Uroporphyrinuria	Type I	Types I and III	Types I and III	Types I and III
Coproporphyrinuria	Type I	Types I and III	Types I and III	Types I and III
Marrow porphyria	Increased	Normal	Normal	Normal
Liver porphyria	Increased slightly	Increased markedly	Increased markedly	Increased markedly

Table from Harrison, Principles of Internal Medicine, New York, McGraw-Hill Book Company, 1958, as modified from Schwartz, S., Clinical aspects of porphyrin metabolism, Vet. Admin. Tech. Bull., TB 10-94, Dec. 1, 1953.

REFERENCE

Perlroth, M. G., et al. Acute intermittent porphyria. New morphologic and biochemical findings. Amer. J. Med., 41:149, 1966.

PORTAL HYPERTENSION

Portal hypertension exists when the pressure in the portal vein, as measured by percutaneous splenic pulp manometry, is 280 mm of saline or higher.

ETIOLOGY

Intrahepatic.

1. Cirrhosis (portal, biliary, postnecrotic, schistosomiasis, kwashiorkor, Wilson's disease, Von Gierke's disease, idiopathic).
2. Hepatic vein occlusion (Budd-Chiari syndrome).

Extrahepatic.

1. Congenital narrowing, obstruction, or cavernomatous transformation of the portal vein.
2. Omphalitis, leading to portal vein thrombosis.
3. Idiopathic thrombosis of portal vein (Banti's syndrome).
4. Mechanical obstruction of the portal vein (pancreatitis, pancreatic cysts, neoplasms, etc.).

BUDD-CHIARI SYNDROME. The Budd-Chiari syndrome follows hepatic vein obstruction of any etiology.

Idiopathic thrombosis is perhaps most frequent in the chronic cases, whereas carcinoma (kidney, pancreas, adrenal, ovary, etc.) is commonest in acute cases. Other causes include the following:

1. Congenital (strictures, fibrosis).
2. Mechanical (trauma, torsion, anomalies).
3. Hematologic (sickle cell anemia, polycythemia vera, leukemia lymphoma).
4. Hepatic (cirrhosis, hepatitis, schistosomiasis, abscess, hepatoma).
5. Acquired vascular disease (endophlebitis, phlebothrombosis, generalized vasculitis).
6. Neighboring diseases (pancreatic cyst, regional lymphadenopathy, subphrenic abscess, gallbladder carcinoma).

The course may be acute or chronic. In the former, abdominal pain is outstanding, followed by hepatosplenomegaly, ascites, jaundice, and frequently hepatic coma and death within 1 to 2 months. Quite often, early in the course of either the acute or chronic form, Bromsulphalein retention is markedly elevated, up to 50 percent or more in 45 minutes.

BANTI'S SYNDROME. The syndrome of hepatomegaly and splenomegaly of unknown cause has been called Banti's syndrome. When all cases of cirrhosis of the liver, lymphoma, etc., are removed, only a few cases remain. These are generally congenital defects in the portal venous system. Portal hypertension then follows, with "hypersplenism" and anemia. Leukopenia and thrombocytopenia may also occur.

REFERENCES

Boyer, J. O., et al. Idiopathic portal hypertension. Ann. Intern. Med., 66:41, 1967.

Callow, A. D., et al. Interim experience with a controlled study of prophylactic portacaval shunt. Surgery, 57:123, 1965.

Clain, D., Freston, J. Kreel, L., and Sherlock, S. Clinical diagnosis of the Budd-Chiari syndrome: A report of six cases. Amer. J. Med., 43:544, 1967.

Merigan, T. C., Jr., Plotkin, G. R., and Davidson, C. S. Effect of intravenously administered posterior pituitary extract on hemorrhage from bleeding esophageal varices. New Eng. J. Med., 266:134, 1962.

Rousselot, L. M., Panke, W. F., Bono, R. F., and Moreno, A. H. Experiences with portacaval anastomosis. Amer. J. Med., 34:297, 1963.

PROPRANOLOL

Propranolol is a beta-adrenergic blocking agent which reduces the rate and contractile force of the heart. The result is a fall in cardiac output, arterial pressure, and arterial blood flow. Decreased left ventricular pressure causes a pressure rise in the left atrium and pulmonary arteries. When under the influence of propranolol, cardiac rate and contractile force are not increased by epinephrine nor norepinephrine. Ventricular arrhythmias including those due to digitalis are prevented by propranolol. The drug is particularly contraindicated in patients with asthma or chronic lung disease for it blocks the bronchodilator action of circulating adrenergic substances.

The main conditions in which propranolol is useful are:

1. Treatment of cardiac arrhythmias. Most tachyarrhythmias are favor-

ably influenced either by slowing of the heart rate or by conversion to a more favorable or to a normal sinus rhythm. About 60 percent of atrial tachycardias may be returned to normal sinus rhythm; an additional 20 percent are sufficiently slowed so as to produce symptomatic and functional improvement. Atrial flutter or fibrillation rarely revert to regular sinus rhythm but at least 75 percent are slowed with subsequent benefit. Ventricular tachycardias respond well. In one half the patients with VPC the ectopic beats are eliminated. In ventricular tachycardia or fibrillation electrical cardioversion is preferred but propranolol should be used when the preferred treatment is not available.

2. Angina pectoris (see page 79). Propranolol is strikingly effective in some patients with angina where combined with isosorbide dinitrate or nitroglycerine for it decreases myocardial oxygen demands. However, because of its negative ionotropic effect it must not be used in incipient or actual cardiac failure, a rule which also holds in treating arrhythmias.
3. Hypertrophic subaortic stenosis. In this situation propranolol reduces the resistance to cardiac outflow. The drug given orally produces symptomatic improvement in 80 percent of patients.
4. Pheochromyocytoma. Elevation of the blood pressure in this condition is well controlled by phentolamine, and adrenergic blocking agent but beta-adrenergic effects of the tumor require propranolol for control.

Administration: whenever possible propranolol should be given orally in doses of 10 to 30 mg every 6 to 8 hours. The intravenous route adds the risk of cardiac standstill, hypotension, and congestive failure. If the intravenous route is necessary the dose should not exceed 1 mg per minute to a total dose of 3 mg. The blood pressure and central venous pressure are guides to administration. Elevation of the latter indicates failure of the contractile force of the heart. With slowing of the heart rate, the drug should be stopped until its effect has been evaluated. With no contraindications a second dose may be given in a few minutes to produce the desired effects. Atropine (0.5 to 1.0 mg) is used to control excessive bradycardia.

Contraindications

1. Congestive failure.
2. Sinus bradycardia.
3. Second degree or complete heart block.
4. Cardiogenic shock.
5. Asthma.
6. Allergic disorders.
7. Reserpine.
8. Monamine oxidase inhibitors.
9. Hypoglycemic states.

REFERENCES

Frieden, J. Propranolol as an antiarrhythmic agent. Amer. Heart J., 74:283, 1967.

_____ Rosenblum, R., Enselberg, C. D., and Rosenberg, A. Propranolol treatment of chronic intractable supraventricular arrhythmias. Amer. J. Cardiol., 22:711, 1968.

Harris, A. Long term treatment of paroxysmal cardiac arrhythmias with propranolol. Amer. J. Cardiol., 18:431, 1966.

Lewis, C. M., et al. Beta-adrenergic blockage. Hemodynamics and myocardial energy. Metabolism in patients with ischemic heart disease. Amer. J. Cardiol., 21:846, 1968.

Stephen, S. A. Unwanted side effects of propranolol. Amer. J. Cardiol., 18:463, 1966.

PROTEINS, SERUM

Normal serum proteins	6-8 g per 100 ml (Total)
Albumin 45-55%	3.5-5.5 g per 100 ml
Globulin	1.5-3.5 g per 100 ml
a_1 5-8%	0.13-0.29 g per 100 ml
a_2 8-13%	0.31-0.89 g per 100 ml
B 11-17%	0.48-1.06 g per 100 ml
G 15-25%	0.63-1.77 g per 100 ml

Mobility of important proteins in globulin range

a_1 – Glycoprotein
Ceruloplasmin

a_2 – α-Lipoprotein
Haptoglobin

B_0 – β-Lipoprotein
Transferrin

Alteration of globulins in disease: In any acute inflammatory process, a_2 globulin is the first protein to become elevated.

1. Hepatic disease. Acute inflammation – increased a_2 globulin. Advanced disease – decreased a_1, a_2, B; increased gamma globulin.
2. Diseases of the reticuloendothelial system – decreased gamma globulin.
3. Renal disease. Infectious – early rise of a_2 globulin. Nephrotic syndrome – $a_1\downarrow$, $a_2\uparrow\uparrow$, B$\uparrow$, gamma$\downarrow$. Uremia – $a_2\uparrow$.
4. Connective tissue disease. $a_2\uparrow$, gamma globulin$\uparrow$.

5. Infectious Diseases. Acute – $a_2\uparrow$, $B\downarrow$, gamma $\downarrow$. Chronic – gamma globulin increased.

HYPERGAMMAGLOBULINEMIA

Hypergammaglobulinemia may be separated into two main forms which are distinct chemically, histologically, and in their clinical counterparts. These types are diffuse hypergammaglobulinemia and hypergammaglobulinemia with M Component.

Diffuse hypergammaglobulinemia is characterized by a diffuse, broad band on paper or cellulose acetate electrophoresis. The clinical forms of diffuse hypergammaglobulinemia are:

1. Chronic infection.
2. Hepatic disease.
3. Connective tissue diseases.
4. Sarcoid.
5. Neoplasms.

Hypergammaglobulinemia with an M Component is distinguished by a single prominent spike on paper or cellulose acetate electrophoresis. The clinical forms of M Component hypergammaglobulinemia have also been termed "plasma cell dyscrasia."

PLASMA CELL DYSCRASIA. According to Osserman, "A plasma cell dyscrasia is considered to represent the excessive proliferation of a single clone of plasma cells, resulting in the synthesis of large quantities of a single protein related to one of the major classes of immunoglobulins and/or the synthesis of excessive quantitites of a constituent polypeptide subunit of one of these proteins (i.e., Bence Jones protein, Heavy chain)."

The proteins elaborated in the plasma cell dyscrasias are structurally similar to the normal immunoglobulins and may be termed "paraproteins."

According to Merler and Rosen, the term "M Component" is defined as "a relatively homogeneous increase in the serum or urine concentration of one, or at most a few, closely related immunoglobulins." M Component and paraprotein are terms that may be equated. They are said to lack antibody activity, implying they are abnormal gamma globulins.

Plasma cell dyscrasias are characterized by:

1. The proliferation of plasma cells in the absence of an identifiable antigenic stimulus (? malignant plasma cells).
2. Elaboration of M-type gamma globulins *and/or* polypeptide subunits of these proteins (Bence-Jones protein, H chain).
3. An associated deficiency in the synthesis of *normal immunoglobulins*.

Classification of plasma cell dyscrasias:

1. Multiple myeloma.
2. Waldenström's macroglobulinemia.
3. Gamma G heavy chain disease.
4. Amyloidosis.
5. Plasma cell dyscrasia of unknown significance.
6. Plasma cell dyscrasia: associated with chronic infection; associated with nonreticular neoplasm.

HYPOGAMMAGLOBULINEMIA, AGAMMAGLOBULINEMIA AND DYSGAMMAGLOBULINEMIAS

1. Physiologic (neonatal).
2. Congenital agammaglobulinemia.
3. Acquired agammaglobulinemia.
   a. Primary.
   b. Secondary.
      (1) Protein-losing states: protein-losing enteropathy, exfoliative dermatides, nephrotic syndrome, hypercatabolic states.
      (2) States causing defective synthesis, neoplasm of lymphoid system.
4. Congenital and acquired dysgammaglobulinemia.
   a. Absent G or A, elevated M (Type I).
   b. Absent A and M, normal G (Type II).
   c. Absent A, normal G and M (Type III).
5. Specific immunologic unresponsiveness.
6. Hereditary thymic aplasia.

IMMUNOGLOBULINS

Immunoglobulins are structurally related serum protein molecules having antibody activity. These proteins are considered gamma globulins because of their relative electrophoretic mobility. Five distinct classes of human immunoglobulins are recognized, IgG, IgA, IgM, IgD, IgE.

Certain physical and chemical properties of four of these immunoglobulins are summarized on page 326.

ELECTROPHORETIC MOBILITY OF THE FOUR MAJOR CLASSES OF IMMUNOGLOBULINS DETERMINED BY PAPER ELECTROPHORESIS

Specific identification of immunoglobulins is obtained by immunoelectrophoresis, involving an antigen-antibody reaction.

	GAMMA G	GAMMA A	GAMMA M	GAMMA D
Synonyms	IgG	IgA	IgM	IgD
Serum Conc. mg per 100 ml	800-1,500	50-200	40-120	1-40
Percentage of total	80%	15%	5-10%	1-3%
Mol. wt.	160,000	160,000	1,000,000	160,000
Svedberg sedimentation coefficient	7S	7S	19S	7S

CHARACTERISTICS OF IMMUNOGLOBULINS

IgG.

1. Antibodies of gram-positive pyogenic bacteria.
2. Antiviral antibodies.
3. Antitoxins.
4. Cryoglobulins.
5. LE cell factor.
6. Fixation to skin receptor sites for skin sensitization.
7. Forty percent intravascular.
8. Active transport across the placenta.
9. Initiates complement fixation.
10. Late initial antibody appearance.
11. Major part of antibody secondary response.
12. Catabolism 3 percent per day.
13. Half-life 25 days.
14. Production 2.3 g per day.

IgA.

1. Isohemagglutinins.
2. Antibrucella.
3. Antidiphtheria.
4. Anti-insulin antibodies.
5. Antithyroglobulin antibodies.
6. Forty percent intravascular.
7. Catabolism 12 percent per day.
8. Half-life 6 days.
9. Production 2.7 g per day.

IgM.

1. Saline isohemagglutinins.
2. Saline Rh antibodies.
3. Cold hemagglutinins.
4. Heterophile antibody.
5. Wasserman antibody.
6. Antibodies to 0 antigen (Endotoxin) of gram-negative bacteria.
7. Rheumatoid factor.

8. First detected antibody after antigen stimulation. As IgG appears, IgM antibody production diminishes.
9. Eighty percent intravascular.
10. Catabolism 14 percent per day.
11. Half-life 5 days.
12. Production 0.4 g per day.

IgD.

1. Little is known about IgD immunologic characteristics. Only 10 cases of multiple myeloma have been reported with IgD as the serum paraprotein.

SYNTHESIS OF IMMUNOGLOBULINS:

Site: Plasma cells found in:

1. Lymph nodes.
2. Spleen.
3. Marrow.
4. Lamina propria of intestine.

The four different classes of immunoglobulins and each subclass are produced by different *clones* of plasma cells. Normally, one clone produces a single protein in response to antigenic stimulation.

STRUCTURE OF IMMUNOGLOBULIN MOLECULE

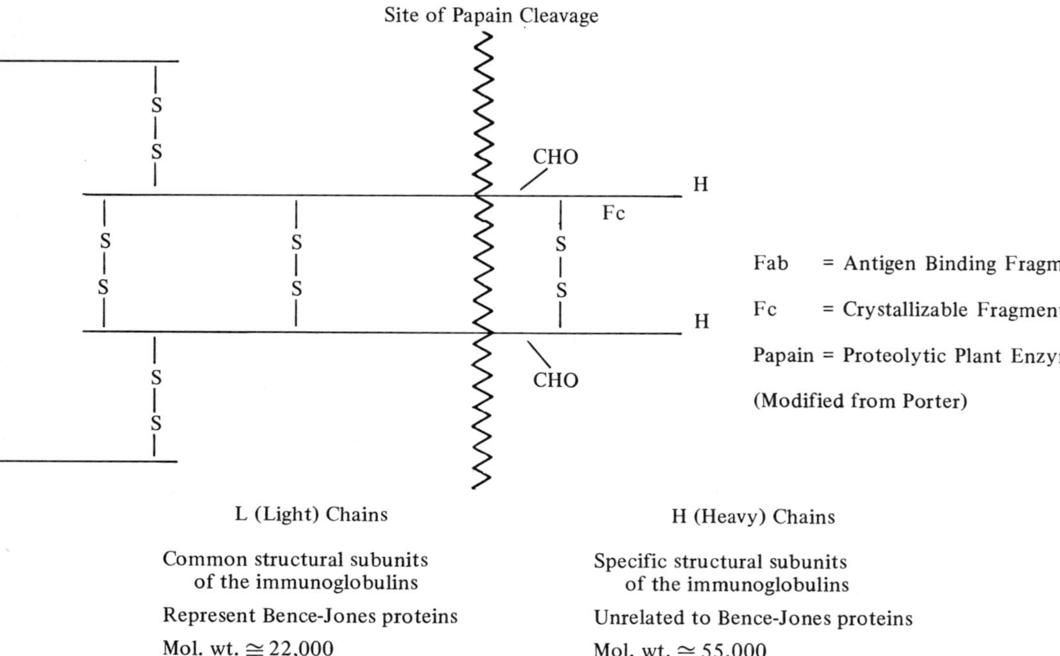

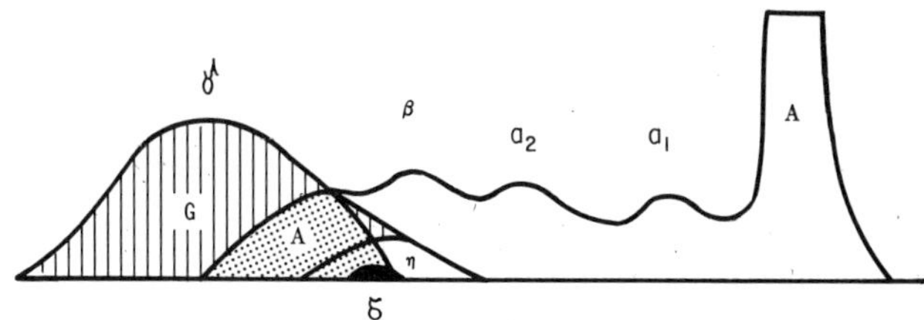

Schematic representation of gammaglobulin molecule as proposed by Porter.

IMMUNOGLOBULIN POLYPEPTIDE CHAINS. There are four forms of heavy polypeptide chains:

1. Gamma.
2. Alpha.
3. Mu.
4. Delta

The form of heavy polypeptide chain determines whether a molecule is IgG, IgA, IgM, or IgD. Two types of light polypeptide chains have been identified. One immunoglobulin molecule contains L chains of the same type: K (Type I), Lambda **λ** (Type II).

Therefore, there are eight categories of serum immunoglobulins:

	TYPE K (I) (MORE COMMON)	TYPE L (II)
IgG	K	λ
	γ	γ
IgA	K	λ
	a	a
IgM	K	λ
	u	u

	TYPE K (1) (MORE COMMON)	TYPE L (II)
IgD	K	λ
	Δ	Δ
IgE		

Gamma H chains of IgG have been determined to be antigenically distinct: Gamma a, gamma b, gamma c, gamma d, and gamma e.

REFERENCES

Fahey, J. L. Antibodies and immunoglobulins. J.A.M.A., 194:71-74, 255-258, 1965.

Janeway, C., Rosen, F. S., Merler, E., and Alper, C. Medical progress; The gamma globulins. New Eng. J. Med., 275:480, 536, 591, 652, 709, 769, 826, 1966.

____ Rosen, F.S., Weber, E. and Alper, C. A.: The Gamma-globulins. Boston, Little, Brown and Company, 1967.

McCallester, B. D., Bayrd, E. D., Hanson, E. G., and McGuckin, W. F. Primary macroglobulinemia. Amer. J. Med., 43:394, 1967.

Metzger, H. The chemistry of the immunoglobulins. J.A.M.A., 202:129-132, 1967.

Osserman, E. Plasma cell dyscrasia. *In* Cecil and Loeb Textbook of Medicine, 12th ed. Philadelphia. W. B. Saunders Company, 1101-1116, 1967.

____ Plasma cell dyscrasia, Amer. J. Med., 44:256, 1968.

Porter, R. R. Hydrolysis of rabbit gammaglobulin and antibodies with crystalline papain. Biochim. J., 73:119, 1959.

Seligmann, M., Fundenberg, H. H., and Good, R. A. A proposed classification of primary immunologic deficiencies. Amer. J. Med., 45:817, 1968.

PSYCHIATRIC DISEASE

(A Guide to Classification)

DISORDERS CAUSED BY OR ASSOCIATED WITH IMPAIRMENT OF BRAIN FUNCTION.

Acute brain syndrome, associated with

1. Intracranial infection.
2. Systemic infection.
3. Drug intoxication.
4. Poisoning.
5. Alcohol.
6. Brain trauma.
7. Circulatory disease.
8. Convulsive disorder.
9. Metabolic disturbance.
10. Intracranial tumor.
11. Idiopathic or uncertain syndrome or disease.

Chronic brain syndrome, associated with

1. Congenital anomalies.
2. Prenatal infection.
3. Birth trauma.
4. CNS lues.
5. Intracranial infection.
6. Brain trauma.
7. Alcohol intoxication (Wernicke's syndrome and Korsakoff's syndrome).
8. CNS atherosclerosis.
9. Convulsive disorder.
10. Senile brain disease.
11. Disturbances of metabolism or growth.
12. Intracranial tumor.
13. Idiopathic or uncertain syndrome or disease.

MENTAL DEFICIENCY.

1. Idiopathic.
2. Heredofamilial.

DISORDERS OF PSYCHOGENIC ORIGIN.

Psychoses.

1. Involutional reaction.
2. Affective reactions: manic depressive, psychotic depressive.
3. Paranoid reactions.
4. Schizophrenic reactions: simple, hebephrenic, catatonic, paranoid, acute or chronic undifferentiated, schizoaffective, childhood, residual.

Psychophysiologic autonomic nervous system and visceral disorders.

1. Skin reaction.
2. Musculoskeletal reaction.
3. Respiratory reaction.
4. Cardiovascular reaction.
5. Gastrointestinal reaction.
6. Genitourinary reaction.
7. Nervous system reaction.

Psychoneurotic disorders.
1. Anxiety reaction.
2. Dissociative reaction.
3. Conversion reaction.
4. Phobic reaction.
5. Obsessive-compulsive reaction.
6. Depressive reaction.

Personality disorders.
1. Disturbances of personality traits or patterns:
   a. Schizoid.
   b. Cyclothymic.
   c. Paranoid.
   d. Compulsive.
   e. Emotionally unstable.
   f. Passive aggressive.
   g. Inadequate.
2. Sociopathic personality disturbances:
   a. Antisocial.
   b. Dysocial.
   c. Sexual deviation.
   d. Addiction to drugs or alcohol.

Transient situational personality disorders.

Brain syndrome, frequently seen in coexistence with medical diseases is evaluated by testing orientation, memory, intellect, judgment, and affect. The *acute brain syndrome* (delirium) is characterized by clouding of the sensorium (disorientation), psychomotor overactivity, perceptual disorders (hallucinations), delusions, mood disorders, and autonomic hyperactivity and fear. These are reversible, based on therapy directed at correction of toxic factors and appropriate sedation.

The *chronic brain syndrome,* usually secondary to organic damage such as chronic alcoholism, neurosyphilis, etc., is generally irreversible. Calculation, learning comprehension, and recent memory are all markedly impaired. These are best evaluated by the serial 7 test, repetition of digits forward and backward, and abstractions such as similarities and differences between a dog and cat, tree and umbrella, etc.

REFERENCE

Wahl, C. W., Golden, J. S., Liston, E. H., Rimer, D. G., and Solomon, D. H. Toxic and functional psychoses: Diagnosis and treatment in a medical setting. Ann. Intern. Med., 66:989, 1967.

PSYCHOTROPIC DRUGS

A psychotropic drug acts on psychic functions, behavior, or experience. For clinical purposes the following definitions are used internationally:

Neuroleptics, also known as "antipsychotics" and formerly "major tranquilizers," have therapeutic effects on psychoses and other types of psychiatric disorders. They also have certain neurologic effects, such as the production of extrapyramidal symptoms.

Anxiolytic sedatives, formerly called "minor tranquilizers," reduce pathologic anxiety, tension, and agitation without therapeutic effects on delusions and hallucinations. They usually increase the convulsive threshold and do not produce extrapyramidal effects; they often have potential for producing dependence.

Antidepressants are effective in the treatment of pathologic depressive states. Drugs in this category have sometimes been called "psychic energizers" and "thymoleptics."

Psychostimulants increase the level of alertness and/or motivation. These effects are usually manifest in normal animals and humans.

Psychodysleptics produce abnormal mental phenomena, particularly in the cognitive and perceptual spheres. They are also called hallucinogens, psychotomimetics, and in some cases psychodelics.

NEUROLEPTICS

PHENOTHIAZINES

Chlorpromazine (Thorazine)
- 25, 50, 100, 200 mg tablets
- 25, 100 mg suppositories
- 10 mg. tsp syrup
- 75 mg to 300 mg spansules
- parenteral form 25 mg/ml

Dosage: 75 mg to 2,000 mg daily in divided doses.

Thioridazine (Mellaril)
25, 50, 100, 200 mg tablets

Dosage: 75 mg to 800 mg daily in divided doses.

Trifluoperazine (Stelazine)
2, 5, 10 mg tablets
2 mg/ml ampules

Dosage: 4 to 20 mg daily in divided doses

Fluphenazine hydrochloride (Prolixin)
1, 2.5, 5 mg.

Dosage: 5 to 20 mg daily in divided doses.

Fluphenazine enanthate (Prolixin Enanthate)

Dosage: Injectable 25 mg per ml twice a month for prolonged action.

BUTYROPHENONES

Haloperidol (Haldol)
1, 2 mg tablets

Dosage: 4 to 15 mg daily in divided doses.

THIOXANTHENES

Thiothixene (Navane)
2, 5, 10 mg

Dosage: 6 mg to 30 mg daily in divided doses.

TREATMENT OF NEUROLEPTIC ADVERSE EFFECTS

Adverse effects result from actions on the central and autonomic nervous systems. They can also be idiosyncratic or allergic. The most frequent side effects of all neuroleptics are extrapyramidal symptoms including parkinsonism, dyskinesia, and akathisia (motor restlessness with inability to sit still or sleep). These reactions are reversible and disappear if dosage is lowered. Rapid control may be achieved by antiparkinsonian drugs:

Benztropine (Cogentin)
2 mg tablets two or three times daily

Procyclidine hydrochloride (Kemadrin)
5 mg tablets once or twice daily

Biperiden (Akineton)
  2 mg tablets; 5 mg ampules. Intravenous injection of 5 mg will promptly relieve dyskinetic reactions.

Most adverse reactions can be controlled by reduction of dosage. Treatment with neuroleptic compounds requires close clinical observation until effective dose levels have been achieved.

ANXIOLYTIC SEDATIVES

Anxiolytic sedatives produce mild sedation when used in small doses and relieve anxiety and tension. Drowsiness, ataxia and dizziness may occur especially during the first few days of administration. Diazepam (Valium) is used intravenously in relief of acute agitation, tremor, and muscle spasm.

The dosages prescribed for patients with histories of alcoholism, drug addiction, or psychoneurosis should be limited to prevent dependency reactions. If patients have been taking large doses for long periods, the drug should not be discontinued abruptly since this may lead to withdrawal reactions similar to those produced by the barbiturates.

Meprobamate (Miltown, Equanil)
  200, 400 mg tablets

  Dosage: 800 to 2,400 mg daily in divided doses.

Hydroxyzine pamoate (Vistaril)
  25, 50, 100 mg

  Dosage: 75 to 300 mg daily in divided doses.

Oxazepam (Serax)
  10, 15, 30 mg

  Dosage: 30 to 120 mg daily in divided doses.

Chlordiazepoxide (Librium)
  5, 10, 25 mg capsules

  Dosage: 15 to 300 mg daily in divided doses.

Diazepam (Valium)
  5, 10 mg tablets
  ampules 2 cc, 10 mg

  Dosage: 10 to 40 mg daily in divided doses.

DEPRESSION

DEFINITION AND DESCRIPTION

Depression consists of a triad of symptoms: 1) dejection of mood, 2) decrease in ideation (decreased thinking and conversation), and 3) decrease in psychomotor activity. In agitated depression (such as seen in involutional melancholia), psychomotor activity increases because of the agitation.

In addition to the triad of symptoms, patients may experience amnesia, weight loss, insomnia, early morning awakening, constipation, fatigue, apathy, hypochondriasis, helplessness and hopelessness, feelings of guilt and worthlessness, and suicidal ideation.

TYPES OF DEPRESSION

Depression is seen in the following clinical entities:

1. Depressed phase of manic-depressive psychoses.
2. Involutional melancholia (change of life depression) – agitated component.
3. Reactive depression (neurotic depression related to a stressful event).
4. Periodic endogenous depressions (many feel this is recurrent manic-depressive psychoses).
5. Senile depression with an agitated component.
6. Depression associated with any brain impairment (as cerebral arteriosclerosis, parkinsonism, brain injury, etc.) with an agitated component.
7. Schizoaffective depression of schizophrenia.
8. Depression associated with alcoholism or alcohol withdrawal may have an agitated component.
9. Depression associated with mental deficiency may have an agitated component.

TREATMENT

ELECTROCONVULSIVE THERAPY. Electroconvulsive therapy (ECT) also known as Electro-Shock Therapy (EST) is still the most effective form of therapy for treatment of depression. The number of treatments necessary depends on 1) the individual patient, 2) the diagnosis, and 3) the development of euphoria, and memory difficulties (the latter being the cut-off point for ECT in most cases).

ECT is a very safe and reliable treatment. There are almost no contraindications except for an acute myocardial infarct, a recent history of serious bleeding, or the presence of a brain tumor. (The last is not an absolute contraindication.)

DRUG TREATMENT. The two major classes of antidepressant drugs are 1) Monamine-oxidase inhibitors (MAO inhibitors) and 2) Dibenzepine derivatives. *Before using these drugs the physician is urged to become thoroughly familiar with their many side effects.*

MAO INHIBITORS

DRUG	DOSE	COMMENT
Isocarboxazid (Marplan)	Daily dose 30-60 mg initially; 10-20 mg after 1-3 weeks	50-80% effective Cumulative side effects mild
Phenelzine sulfate (Nardil)	45 mg reduced to 15-30 mg after 2-6 weeks	More effective in endogenous depression. Complete relief in 80% who respond
Nialamid (Niamid)	75-200 mg reduced to 50-75 after several weeks	Less effective than other MAO inhibitors
Tranylcypromine (Parnate)	20-40 mg reduced to 10-20 mg after 2 weeks	Concomitant use of foods with high tyramine content dangerous; use in hospital setting only*

*See item 10 under Contraindications and Precautions with MAO Inhibitors.

CONTRAINDICATIONS AND PRECAUTIONS WITH MAO INHIBITORS

1. The elderly or debilitated.
2. Cerebrovascular defects.
3. C. V. disease.
4. Hypertension.
5. Pheochromocytoma.
6. Severe headaches.
7. Liver disease or abnormal liver function tests.
8. Simultaneous use of sympathomimetic drugs (cold pills, hay fever remedies, reducing pills).
9. Drugs containing methyldopa, dopamine and tryptophan.
10. *Foods with high tyramine content (cheeses, beer, chianti wines, broad bean pods, chicken livers and yeast extracts). Concomitant use can cause hypertensive crises, or cerebral hemorrhage leading to death.
11. Narcotics, alcohol, hypotensive agents, and CNS depressants.

Note: At least ten days should elapse between discontinuing an MAO inhibitor and instituting the use of a dibenzepine derivative. Hypertensive crises and convulsive seizures and death have resulted from their continued use. All patients on MAO inhibitors should be examined frequently for hyper- or hypotension. Postural hypotension is frequent. Their safety in pregnancy has not been established.

DIBENZEPINE DERIVATIVES (Nonhydrazine, non-MAO inhibitors). Although not as effective as ECT in the treatment of depression the dibenzepine derivatives are the safest antidepressant drugs. They have shown

1. 60 percent good result in all depressions.
2. 74 percent good response in endogenous depressions.
3. 52 percent good effect in reactive depressions.

It takes 5 to 7 days for these drugs to work a therapeutic effect and they should be continued from 3 to 6 months after the depression has subsided. If they are ineffective one must wait at least a week before changing to a MAO inhibitor.

(Each of these drugs should be used in lower dosage in the middle aged or elderly.)

Drug	Daily Dose
Imipramine (Tofranil)	25-300 mg
Desipramine (Norpramin, Pertofrane)	25-300 mg
Amitriptyline (Elavil)	20-300 mg
Nortriptyline (Aventyl)	20-300 mg

No serious complications result from these drugs but numerous side effects can occur.

CONTRAINDICATIONS TO DIBENZEPINE DERIVATIVES. They should not be given with or within at least 10 days of treatment with a MAO inhibitor. Extreme agitation, hyperthermia, hypoglycemia, hypertensive crises, cerebrovascular bleeding, seizures and death have been reported when this caution has not been followed. The drugs are contraindicated in glaucoma, uretheral obstruction or spasm, gastric retention and for the first three weeks of myocardial infarction. The action of thyroid hormones or sympathomimetic drugs is potentiated by the dibenzepine derivatives.

PULMONARY DISEASE

"COIN LESION"

(Solitary Circumscribed Pulmonary Nodule)

By definition this lesion must:

1. Be situated in the substance of the lung.
2. Not be associated with obstructive changes peripheral to the mass.
3. Not display cavitation.
4. Constitute the only significant pathologic change in the lung.

It may occur at any age and is generally an incidental finding on routine x-ray examination in an asymptomatic patient with a negative physical examination.

DIAGNOSIS

1. On physical examination there may be no abnormal findings, or there may be signs of primary disease elsewhere.
2. X-ray characteristics:
   a. Concentric ring or target type.
   b. Popcorn type. These lesions are indicative of a benign granuloma or hamartoma; therefore, they are considered to be benign, safe, and well walled off, if only a fleck of calcium is present in the periphery or eccentrically placed, it may not be benign.
   c. Sharp, well-defined borders. These lesions may not be benign.
   d. More and more primary malignant lesions are seen over a period of several years, without change. One cannot safely exclude primary carcinoma on this basis.
   e. Metastatic lesions are more often multiple but may be solitary.
   f. Tuberculoma, noncalcified, may be due to a blocked inspissated cavity, whose bronchial communication may become patent, and its contents disseminated throughout the lung.
3. Bronchoscopy and cytology are of no value due to the peripheral location of the lesion and the absence of involvement of the major airway.
4. Tomography to demonstrate presence of calcium.
5. Exploratory thoracotomy must be resorted to as a diagnostic tool in order to facilitate histologic diagnosis.

DIFFERENTIAL DIAGNOSIS

The pulmonary nodule may be neoplastic, inflammatory, or vascular in origin.

1. Neoplasms:
   a. Benign – adenomas (usually carcinoid).
   b. Malignant – primary: small bronchogenic Ca.
   secondary: metastatic (colon, kidney, etc.).
2. Inflammatory
   a. Granulomas: histoplasmosis, coccidioidomycosis, tuberculosis.
   b. Chronic: organized pneumonia.
3. Vascular
   Pulmonary AV fistula or dilated pulmonary vessels. These are rare.
4. Organized infarcts

In a study of 156 cases of histologically proved solitary circumscribed pulmonary nodules in patients older than 35 years of age, with a mass greater than 3 cm in diameter, 44 percent of the uncalcified lesions were malignant.

A study of 705 cases was divided into four groups:

	EXPLORED	NOT EXPLORED
1. Calcified on x-ray	16	278
2. Presumed metastatic	23	80
3. Stable or unchanged for 2 years or more	2	35
4. All others	143	128
	184	521

Results were as follows:

1. *Calcified mass* – Forty-two percent of the 705 were calcified. In most cases this was noted on routine x-ray. In five cases calcium was only seen on tomograms. Surgical exploration done only in 16 cases: 13 were granulomas; one was a hamartoma; one was a simple cyst; one was a neurofibroma.
2. *Metastatic masses* – In 103 cases (23 explored) all had primary lesions elsewhere.

Colon and rectum	25
EENT	15
Female genital	14
Kidney and bladder	11
Melanoma skin	7
Female breast	7
Bone	6

Lymphoblastoma	5
Testis	4
Thyroid	3
Neuroblastoma	1
Esophagus	1
Abd. mass – site?	4

3. *Stable mass (unchanged for 2 or more years)* – In 37 cases, two were explored. Although this is not incontrovertible evidence that a lesion is benign, the lesion is more likely to be benign.
   9 cases smaller than 1 cm in size
   17 cases 1-2 cm in size
   7 cases 2-3 cm in size
   2 cases greater than 3-4.5 cm
   Only 2 excised – one was benign: 1 was an adenocarcinoma present for 4 years.
4. *Other masses (271)* – Thorocotomy done in 143: Not calcified, not metastatic presumably, not known to be stable for two or more years. Best advice is to explore!
   Of this group of 271 cases, 91 were malignant.

Bronchogenic Ca	80
Bronchal adenoma	10
Metastatic neoplasm	1

Of the 271 cases, 73 were benign.

Granuloma	47
Hamartoma	11
Cyst	4
Mesothelioma	4
Neurofibroma	2
Lipoma	1
Chronic inflammatory	4

RESULTS OF CALCIFICATION. Laminated or onion skin type or target type is present in a granuloma only; popcorn type practically always signifies a hamartoma. Calcifications in carcinomatous lesions are reported, especially if the calcium is eccentrically or peripherally placed. All solitary lesions should have tomography to demonstrate better the presence of calcium.

PULMONARY CANCER

TYPE	SQUAMOUS	OAT CELL	LARGE CELL	ADENO
% Operable	60%	33%	48%	30%
% Resectable	33%	11%	20%	25%
Five-year survival	12%	1%	5%	11%

REFERENCES

Grood, C. A., and Wilson, T. W. Solitary circumscribed pulmonary nodules: Study of 705 cases. J.A.M.A., 166:210, 1958.
The solitary circumscribed pulmonary lesions due to bronchogenic Ca. Collected Papers of the Mayo Clinic, 50:543, 1958.

PULMONARY EDEMA

Pulmonary edema is due to an exudation of serum into the alveolar spaces because of increased pulmonary capillary pressure (PCP), increased capillary permeability, decreased osmotic pressure of the blood, or a combination of these factors. Though the condition may occur in the presence of normal PCP as in the inhalation of irritant or toxic gases, burns, and the intravenous injection of gold salts, the most important factor is increased PCP, which in turn is due to failure of the left ventricle to eject or to receive the venous runoff from the lungs. When the PCP approaches 30 mm Hg, pulmonary edema is imminent.

TREATMENT

Morphine is, above all, the drug in the treatment of pulmonary edema. The initial dose is 15 mg subcutaneously. In severe cases, 10 mg may be given I.V. It acts by depressing the sensitivity of the respiratory center and by decreasing venous return.

An orthopneic position is assumed instinctively by the conscious patient, and should be provided for one in semicomatose condition to decrease the venous return to the lung.

Though the oxygen saturation may be normal, oxygen by mask, catheter, or a positive pressure apparatus is indicated. The last method is most efficient in counteracting the high PCP and decreasing the venous return to the lungs by increasing the pulmonary alveolar pressure. If not available, oxygen bubbled through an antifoaming agent (50 percent ethyl alcohol) is helpful.

Rapid digitalization with lanatoside C, 0.8-1.2 mg I.V., is effective in patients not previously digitalized. The theoretical objection that its use in pulmonary edema due to mitral stenosis will increase PCP and aggravate the edema is not born out in practice.

Ethacrynic acid 50 mg I.V. is effective in producing prompt diuresis. Mercurial diuretics, I.V., do not have an immediate diuretic effect in pulmonary edema, but within 20 to 30 minutes through an unexplained mechanism they do decrease the pressure on the right side of the heart.

Phlebotomy, either dry by the use of rotating tourniquets, or the actual withdrawal of 300 to 600 ml of blood, is not often necessary, but is at times effective as an adjunct to other measures.

Aminophylline, 0.5 g diluted in 20 ml of water, given by slow intravenous administration, is of itself not effective. We have no experience with hexamethonium advocated by Freidberg in both normal and hypertensive patients in pulmonary edema.

Pulmonary edema in the course of nephritis is due to both LV failure and increased pulmonary capillary permeability. The treatment is as outlined, but mercurial diuretics should not be used.

REFERENCE

Sherry, S. Urokinase. Ann. Intern. Med., 69:415, 1968.

PULMONARY EMBOLISM AND INFARCTION

Pulmonary embolism with infarction is the most prevalent pulmonary disease in general hospitals. Clinical diagnosis is often difficult, though embolism and infarction have been reported to occur in 5 to 15 percent of cases in general autopsy series. They are more frequently found in medical than in surgical patients. In reported series of pulmonary embolization with infarction, 30 percent occurred in the presence of cardiac disease, 40 percent in postoperative cases, and 30 percent in noncardiac medical cases. Infarction follows embolism in only 50 percent of cases.

PREDISPOSING FACTORS

The factors are usually multiple. Prolonged bed rest aggravates all causes.

1. Venous stasis from whatever cause.
2. Immobilization due to surgery and fractures.
3. Congestive heart failure.
4. Pulmonary emphysema (right alveolar thrombus formation).
5. Pregnancy (hypercoagulability state).
6. Acidosis (hypercoagulability state).
7. Arterial hypotension.
8. Endotoxin *(E. coli* and *Salmonella).*

DIAGNOSIS

Dyspnea occurring in 50 percent of cases is sudden in onset, varying from mild discomfort to gasping respiration. Tachypnea is present in 45 percent. There may or may not be pain. The *substernal* pain associated with pulmonary embolism is similar to the pain of myocardial ischemia or pulmonary hypertension. With pulmonary infarction *pleuritic pain* is associated with a friction rub in 10 percent of cases. *Hemoptysis* is usually in the form of blood-streaked sputum. Massive hemoptysis is uncommon. *Fever* usually not above 102° F is common. *Tachycardia* out of proportion to fever and in the absence of other findings may be the only clue. In the clinical setting conducive to pulmonary embolism and infarction any elevation of the pulse or respiration should be weighted with suspicion. *Jaundice* may appear especially with liver dysfunction accompanying congestive failure.

PHYSICAL SIGNS

PULMONARY. Unilateral expansion lag; pleural friction rub; localized chest tenderness.

CARDIAC. Systolic pulsations in the second left ICS; accentuated P_2; systolic and/or diastolic murmurs, second left ICS; gallop rhythm; distended neck veins with or without hepatomegaly; pseudopericardial friction rub in pulmonary embolism.

RADIOLOGIC DIAGNOSIS. Pulmonary embolism without infarction casts no pulmonary shadow, but a prominent pulmonary artery segment and hyperlucent lung may be present on the involved side. With infarction, pulmonary shadows are present and vary from linear streaking or hazy cloudiness to well-defined concave or crescent-shaped densities usually basilar near the costophrenic angles or in the lingula or right middle lobe. The triad of shadow, elevation of the diaphragm, and pleural effusion is not uncommon.

PULMONARY ANGIOGRAPHY

This provides a method of making a positive diagnosis quickly and safely. The following may be noted:

1. Complete obstruction of segmental or lobar branch of the pulmonary artery or total obstruction of the main pulmonary artery.
2. The presence of irregular plaques in the region of the pulmonary artery representing adherent or partially retracted or lysed thrombi.
3. Regional decrease of flow of contrast media at the site of emboli (also seen in chronic lung disease).
4. In some cases, a parenchymal density is also seen (in infarction).
5. If extensive obliteration of the pulmonary vascular bed is suspected, do not use angiography.

RADIOISOTOPE SCANNING IN PULMONARY EMBOLIC DISEASE

Macroaggregated human serum albumin labeled with either I^{131} or Cr^{51} injected intravenously and the accumulation of these macroscopic particles behind an obstruction have permitted their visualization by automatic radioisotope scanning techniques. It offers the advantages of no antigenicity, no aggravation of symptoms, and good visualization of the lungs.

In its clinical application radioisotope scanning is valuable in:

1. Diagnosis of massive pulmonary emboli.
2. Differentiating focal from diffuse pulmonary embolization and diffuse pulmonary disease.
3. Delineating increased radiolucency due to pulmonary embolism without infarction.
4. If scan is positive, one may then do pulmonary angiography.
5. If normal, omit angiography.
6. If massive embolization is suspected, do a scan before attempting pulmonary artery embolectomy.

ELECTROCARDIOGRAPHIC PATTERNS

(See p. 179)

ECG is not very sensitive nor very specific in diagnosing pulmonary embolism.

Observed abnormalities include:

1. Disturbance in rhythm including arterial fibrillation, ectopic beats of various types, heart block, etc.
2. P pulmonale.

3. Positional changes toward right axis, S_1Q_3 pattern, leftward shift of the transitional zone in the horizontal plane, occasional occurrence of tall R-waves in V1-2, right BBB.
4. S-T segment depressions.
5. T-wave inversions in Leads II and III, AVF, V1-4-5.
6. An unusual form in which abnormally inverted T-waves appear in II, III, AVF, V1-4, superimposed on the findings of pulmonary emphysema.
7. S-T segment deviations are probably the most common abnormality encountered, and result from the attendant myocardial ischemia. These in turn are due to associated underlying coronary disease.

BLOOD TESTS

1. Serum LDH is increased in pulmonary thromboembolism.
2. SGOT is normal in the absence of other disease.
3. Hyperbilirubinemia may be present.
4. Arterial pCO_2. If alveolar pCO_2 is decreased and arterial pCO_2 is increased, with the difference equaling 4 mm or more, this may be considered presumptive evidence of pulmonary infarction. This test is positive only in massive infarction.

DEFINITIVE THERAPY

Advocates of pulmonary embolectomy are few. Total successful cases reported in 34 years equal 13.

Requirements are:

1. Surgical "kit" available in OR at all times.
2. Frequent rehearsals.
3. Pulmonary angiograph and radioisotope scanning available preceding surgery.
4. Cardiopulmonary bypass with low-prime bubble oxygenator.
5. Inferior vena cava ligation at same operation.

ANTICOAGULANT THERAPY

Heparin is the drug of choice and may be given I.V., 5,000 - 7,500 units q. 8 h. for 10 to 14 days or subcutaneously. Oral Coumadin may be used after 2 weeks of heparin, for 6 to 12 weeks. Heparin is the drug of choice in cases of pregnancy, since it does not cross the placental barrier. The clinical value of fibrinolysin has not been established. Serum hepatitis is a not infrequent complication of its use.

REFERENCES

Crane, C. Femoral vs. caval interruption for venous thromboembolism. New Eng. J. Med., 270:819, 1964.
Donaldson, G. A., Williams, C., Scannell, J. G., and Shaw, R. S. A reappraisal of the application of the Trendelenburg operation to massive fatal embolism. New Eng. J. Med., 268:171, 1963.
Stansel, H. C., Hume, M., and Glenn, W. W. L. Pulmonary embolectomy: results in ten patients. New Eng. J. Med., 276:717, 1967.
Wacker, W., et al. A triad for the diagnosis of pulmonary embolism and infarction. J.A.M.A., 178:8, 1961.

PULMONARY EMPHYSEMA AND DIFFUSE PULMONARY DISEASE

Emphysema is a disease of unknown cause characterized by obstruction to air flow distal to the terminal nonrespiratory bronchole, with overexpansion of the distal air spaces and destructive changes of the alveolar wall.

ANATOMIC CLASSIFICATION

CHRONIC BRONCHITIS WITH EMPHYSEMA .

1. Centrilobular. Begins in the region of the respiratory bronchiole located in the center of the secondary lobule.
2. Panlobular emphysema. Tends to start in all parts of the secondary lobule.

BULLOUS EMPHYSEMA . Single or multiple large cystic alveolar dilations, often of obscure origin, which may or may not be associated with chronic generalized obstructive emphysema.

1. Air cysts occurring in the upper lobes with a tendency to spontaneous pneumothorax, minimal evidence of bronchitis, only slight disability, which is not progressive. Characterized by normal maximum breathing capacity and increased residual volume.
2. Solitary bulla with healthy lungs, situated in upper lobes and usually free of symptoms, rarely rupture, and normal pulmonary function tests.

3. Bullae associated with diffuse chronic obstructive emphysema. Usually a long history of chronic bronchitis, with disability moderate to severe. All bullae occur in the lower lobes. Clinical and physiologic picture identical with that observed in patients with chronic obstructive emphysema without bullae except that there is less increase in residual volume.

PULMONARY FIBROSIS WITH EMPHYSEMA.

1. Tuberculosis.
2. Sarcoidosis.
3. Pneumoconiosis.
4. Berylliosis.
5. Honeycomb lung.

PHYSIOLOGIC CLASSIFICATION

OBSTRUCTIVE. Pulmonary emphysema is the common example of irreversible obstructive disease; bronchial asthma typifies reversible obstructive disease. Outstanding clinical features are long-standing cough, dyspnea, hyperinflation of chest, decreased breath sounds, and expiratory wheezing (particularly on forced expiration).

RESTRICTIVE.

1. Pulmonary fibrosis may be due to chronic infection and bronchiectasis, pneumoconiosis (asbestosis, berylliosis, silicosis, hemosiderosis, silo fillers' disease, etc.), collagen diseases (particularly scleroderma), sarcoidosis, lymphangitic carcinoma, and Hamman-Rich syndrome.
2. Pleural restriction with entrapped lung.
3. Chest wall restriction due to obesity, kyphoscoliosis, or rheumatoid spondylitis.

ALVEOLAR-CAPILLARY BLOCK. Does not exist as an isolated entity but usually with pulmonary fibrosis.

NEUROGENIC ("PRIMARY") HYPOVENTILATION. Caused by disease of respiratory center, afferent or efferent nerves.

Note: Diffuse pulmonary disease frequently combines several of these physiologic defects. For example, emphysema may begin with pure obstruction, acquire pulmonary fibrosis and consequent restriction, and develop a secondary respiratory center depression as progressive hypercapnia injures the medullary center.

DIFFERENTIAL DIAGNOSIS

	MBC*	VC*	O_2 SAT	CO_2	CHEST FILM
Emphysema	decr.	normal or sl. decr.	sl. decr.	rises as O_2 sat. falls	hyperinflated
Pulmonary fibrosis	normal	decr.	normal	normal or low	fibrosis
Obesity	normal	normal or sl. decr.	low	high	normal
Alv.-cap. block	normal	decr.	normal or sl. decr.	normal or low	fibrosis
"Primary" hypoventilation	normal	normal	decr.	high	normal

*MBC, maximum breathing capacity; VC, vital capacity.

THERAPY IN CHRONIC BRONCHITIS WITH PULMONARY EMPHYSEMA

1. Removal of all bronchial irritants, e.g., any type of dust, air pollution, and tobacco smoking, since they tend to increase mucous formation and airway obstruction.
2. Change of climate is of much less importance than No. 1.
3. Use of antibiotics. There is general agreement on use of penicillin (600,000 u b.i.d) or tetracycline (1.0 g/d) in the treatment of exacerbations of symptoms. Therapy to be continued 2 to 3 weeks. The use of other antibiotics will be determined by the predominating organism and bacteria sensitivity tests.
4. Bronchodilators. This is the cornerstone of therapy. Aerosol therapy – isoproterenol 0.5 ml of 1:200 solution or vaponephrin 0.5 ml diluted with 2 ml of water, and nebulized as a bronchodilator; aqueous Neo-Synephrine, 0.5 percent, 0.5 ml, as a vasoconstrictor or decongestant may be added or used instead of above. The nebulization may be in the form of a hard nebulizer, tank compressor or an IPPB derivative.
5. Iodides are the most common of the various expectorants used. Best results are obtained when given I.V.
6. Aminophylline is best given I.V., 0.5 g/500 ml G/W.
7. Water administered in aerosol form by superheated nebulizer will reduce the viscosity of sputum.
8. Aerosol pancreatic dornase may be effective in the presence of purulent sputum.
9. Acetyl cysteine aerosol therapy is effective for nonpurulent tenacious mucous secretion.
10. IPPB with aerosol therapy is also effective.
11. For severe hypercapnia, hypoventilation, and respiratory acidosis see page 370.
12. In the presence of polycythemia with hematocrits over 57 percent, phlebotomy is of value. Determine level of hemoglobin simultaneously.
13. The use of steroids in the absence of a definite history of allergic asthma is of limited value and is associated with risk, e.g., peptic ulceration with hemorrhage, staphylococcus, influenza, and pneumococcal infection, etc.
14. Oxygen therapy must be administered with great caution for it may lead to stupor and coma.
15. Tracheostomy may be lifesaving in stuporous and comatose patients. The main bedside indication for tracheostomy is the lack of the patient's ability to cough. It facilitates aspiration of secretions. Endotracheal tube with inflatable cuff may be used with automatic cycling positive pressure respirator, such as the Bennett or Bird.

PURPURA

Purpura is a condition in which blood is extravasated into the skin usually because of a qualitative or quantitative platelet defect or because of a defect in the vascular wall. Diagnosis of purpura is outlined in the facing table.

Many other states may produce purpura, the mechanisms for which are poorly understood. Outstanding in this group is uremia. See Diagnosis Table (page 352).

PYELONEPHRITIS

Pyelonephritis is a nonspecific bacterial infection of the renal parenchyma and pelvocaliceal system. It is frequently associated with obstructive lesions of the lower urinary tract. The manner in which bacteria reach the kidney has not been completely resolved. There are three possibilities:

1. Hematogenous spread, which is possible, but uncommon.
2. Ascending spread from the bladder via the ureteral lumen is the most common pathway and is associated with reflux of urine.
3. Lymphatic spread up the ureter; the evidence supporting this is scanty.

PREDISPOSING FACTORS

1. Obstructive lesions of the urinary tract (benign prostatic hypertrophy, calculi, tumor). It appears that the lower in the urinary tract the obstruction occurs, the higher the incidence of infection.
2. Pregnancy. About 6 percent of pregnant women have significant asymptomatic bacteriuria, and, of these, about 40 percent develop acute pyelonephritis if untreated.
3. Instrumentation. Significant bacteriuria occurs in 2 to 5 percent of patients after a single catheterization. After 4 days with indwelling catheters, 98 percent develop significant bacteriuria.
4. Congenital urinary tract anomalies. Polycystic kidney disease, for

DIAGNOSIS OF PURPURA

	BLEEDING TIME	COAGULATION TIME	CLOT RETRACTION	PLATELET COUNT	TOURNIQUET TEST
Thrombasthenia	N – X	N	N – X	N	N – X
Scurvy	N	N	N	N	X
Senile purpura	N – X	N	N	N	X
Sepsis	N – X	N	N – X	N – X	N – X
Allergic purpura (Henoch-Schönlein)	N	N	N	N	N – X
Idiopathic thrombocytopenic purpura	X	N	X	X	X
Symptomatic thrombocytopenic purpura (disease, drug, etc.)	X	N	X	X	X

X = Abnormal
N = Normal

example, is associated with pyelonephritis in about 70 percent of patients.

5. Neurologic diseases. Patients with neurologic diseases who cannot control micturition are susceptible to infection because of the necessity for bladder drainage. Immobilization and demineralization of bones may result in nephrocalcinosis and urinary calculi which by obstructing flow increases the susceptibility of the kidney to infection.
6. Metabolic disease (myxedema, primary hyperparathyroidism, diabetes mellitus, gout, nephrocalcinosis and hypokalemia).
7. Agammaglobulinemia.

DIAGNOSIS

HISTORY AND PHYSICAL EXAMINATION

1. Acute pyelonephritis may present with variegated symptoms. The classic picture is that of abrupt onset of shaking, chills, fever, flank pain, and tenderness with frequency, urgency, and dysuria. Many patients present accompanying upper gastrointestinal symptoms with nausea and vomiting. Particularly in children, the gastrointestinal symptoms may dominate. The disease may mimic acute glomerulonephritis. On examination there is tenderness in the kidney area, anteriorly or posteriorly. Azotemia and hypertension do not occur in uncomplicated acute pyelonephritis.
2. Usually chronic pyelonephritis presents no signs or symptoms referable to the urinary tract but rather with symptoms and physical findings of uremia, anemia, or hypertension.

LABORATORY FINDINGS

1. Urinalysis. Abundance of bacteria, polymorphonuclear leukocytes, red blood cells, clumps of white blood cells, white blood cell casts. The urine may be grossly bloody.
2. Urine Culture. A fresh midstream clean-catch urine containing 100,000 colonies or more per mm^3 of bacteria is significant. A single positive culture in the absence of a significant urinalysis or clinical symptoms is not sufficient for instituting therapy. In 80 percent of cases of uncomplicated acute pyelonephritis the infecting organisms are usually the coliform bacteria, then proteus, pseudomonas, aerobacter, enterococcus and staphylococcus. Mixed infections are quite common.
3. Renal function tests in chronic pyelonephritis reveal hyposthenuria and isosthenuria. The maximal normal urine osmolatity is about 1,300 mOsm/L (sp. gr. 1.032). In chronic pyelonephritis this ability to concentrate the urine is progressively diminished until it reaches a level of about 500 to 700 mOsm/L ("fixed": sp. gr. about 1.010). This defect is related to the loss of normal medullary hypertonicity,

osmotic diuresis, and/or specific lesions involving the distal convoluted tubule and the proximal collecting tubules.

4. Azotemia. When the glomerular filtration rate falls to about one half of normal, a progressive elevation of the blood urea nitrogen occurs.
5. Electrolyte abnormalities.
   a. Both potassium and sodium "losing nephritis" have been described in pyelonephritis as caused by defective tubular reabsorption.
   b. Acidosis, with abnormalities of tubular function, involving hydrogen ion production and exchange and decreased ammonia synthesis and transport, occurs.
   c. With progressive renal failure and oliguria, potassium retention may occur. With the development of edema, usually a dilutional hyponatremia occurs.
6. X-rays of the kidneys (KUB, IUP) and renal biopsy may be of value.

TREATMENT

The success of treatment hinges on early diagnosis, careful examination of the urinary sediment and cultures of the urine. Acute, uncomplicated pyelonephritis is successfully treated in about 90 percent of cases. Chronic pyelonephritis is permanently cured in only about 20 percent of cases.

1. General measures of treatment include adequate hydration and removal of any obstructive element.
2. Specific therapy. Selection of the appropriate antibiotic is made on the basis of bacterial sensitivities. If the patient is septic or toxic when first seen, antibiotic therapy may be instituted prior to report of the cultures. The patient should be started on treatment. After 72 hours urine for culture and sensitivity should be obtained; if this urine is not sterile, then the antibiotic is not effective, and a change in therapy should be made. After two weeks of therapy the patient is taken off the antibiotic and the urine cultured 48 hours later. If this urine is not sterile, the patient should be retreated with another antibiotic to which the organism is sensitive.
3. Chronic pyelonephritis. The patient is treated as above in effort to obtain a sterile urine culture. After cessation of therapy the nonazotemic patient is placed on suppressive therapy consisting of mandelic acid (Mandelamine) 1.0 g q.i.d. If the urine does remain acidic on this regimen, Methionime is added.

REFERENCES

Allen, T. D. Pathogenesis of urinary tract infections in children. New Eng. J. Med., 273:1421, 1472, 1965.

Flanigan, William J. Renal function in chronic pyelonephritis. Southern Med. J., 58:1353, 1965.

Freeman, R. B., Bromer, L., and Smith, W. M. Prevention of recurrent bacteriuria by continuous chemotherapy. Amer. Soc. Nephrology, 1:20, 1967.

Heptinstall, R. H. Experimental pyelonephritis. Proceedings of the III International Congress of Nephrology, 2:128, 1967.

Turck, M., Ronald, A. R., and Petersdorf, R. G. Relapse and re-infection in chronic bacteriuria: II. The correlation between site of infection and pattern of recurrence in chronic bacteriuria. New Eng. J. Med., 278:422, 1968.

QUINIDINE

Quinidine, the dextroisomer of quinine, is a naturally occurring alkaloid of cinchona bark.

CARDIAC ACTIONS

1. Vagolytic.
2. Increases the myocardial refractory period up to 100 percent.
3. Depresses myocardial excitability and contractility. First the atria are depressed, then the AV node, then the ventricles.

USES

1. Conversion of atrial flutter or fibrillation to sinus rhythm after digitalization is complete.
2. In acute myocardial infarction where runs of ventricular premature contractions occur, the VPC's should come two or more in a row and more than once in 60 seconds before the use of quinidine is considered.
3. Quinidine has been employed as a diagnostic and therapeutic agent in the Wolf-Parkinson-White syndrome. By depressing the aberrant pathway normal AV conduction may occur.
4. Ventricular tachycardia.

DOSE

FOR CONVERSION OF ATRIAL FLUTTER AND FIBRILLATION. Quinidine is started in doses of 200 mg, P.O., q. 2 h., for 5 doses on the first day. This is increased to 400 mg, P.O., q. 2 h., for 5 doses on the second day if necessary, and increased daily by 200 mg, q. 2 h., until reversion to sinus rhythm occurs or a maximum of 600 mg, q. 2 h., for 5 doses is reached. Constant careful bedside observation and, where indicated, ECG monitoring must be done before each dose. At doses of 600 mg, q. 2 h., monitoring is mandatory. For this reason the drug is best started at 8:00 A.M. each morning so that the fifth and last dose of each day is given at 4:00 P.M. If the patient fails to respond to 600 mg q. 2 h. × 5, electrical conversion is preferred to giving larger doses. Allow at least 24 hours after the last dose of quinidine.

After conversion of the arrhythmia, maintenance dosage should equal one-half of the conversion dose and is given q. 6 h. For example, if a patient converts to sinus rhythm on a dose of 600 mg q. 2 h., suggested maintenance dose would be 300 mg q. 6 h.

It is to be noted that 80 percent of conversions occur at doses of 600 mg or less q. 2 h.

FOR VENTRICULAR TACHYCARDIA AND VENTRICULAR FIBRILLATION. See page 181.

CAUTION

The elderly, the debilitated, and those with serious heart disease who have rapid ventricular rates with atrial flutter or fibrillation should be digitalized rapidly to control the ventricular rate before quinidine is used. Keep in mind that as long as the ventricular rate is slow, cardiac output will be almost normal and the patient will be in no danger. After digitalization, quinidine treatment is started as above. If digitalis is not first employed, quinidine may slow the atrial rate without effect on the AV node, and more atrial beats will be conducted with resulting very rapid ventricular rate.

Not all persons with atrial flutter or fibrillation need to be converted to sinus rhythm.

1. Many patients tolerate these arrhythmias remarkably well.
2. In long-standing fibrillation, especially when due to advanced arteriosclerotic or rheumatic heart disease, the patient will promptly revert to fibrillation after conversion in spite of continued quinidine.

UNTOWARD EFFECTS

Mild toxic effects occur in up to one third of patients. They include nausea, vomiting, diarrhea, abdominal cramps, and cinchonism as manifested by tinnitus, vertigo, and visual changes.

Severe toxicity or idiosyncrasy is manifested by hypotension, extreme malaise, ventricular ectopic beats, widening of all parts of the P-QRS-T complexes up to 50 percent or more, complete AV block, and ventricular tachycardia or fibrillation. Such serious arrhythmias, called quinidine syncope, occur in 3 to 5 percent of patients. In a sensitive individual, fever, purpura, rashes, or marked hypotension can be induced by as little as 200 mg.

CONTRAINDICATIONS

Contraindications are multiform and are perhaps best listed as major and minor (relative).

MAJOR.

1. Ventricular tachycardia or fibrillation secondary to digitalis.
2. Bundle branch block.
3. Complete heart block.
4. Those conditions listed under severe toxicity and idiosyncrasy.

MINOR OR RELATIVE.

1. During acute infections.
2. In the presence of severe myocardial or valvular disease or advanced failure.
3. In chronic (over 6 months) slow compensated atrial fibrillation, especially in an aged patient.
4. The possibility of embolism secondary to quinidine conversion of atrial fibrillation to sinus rhythm is *not* a contraindication. This risk is minor. Occasionally, anticoagulation is employed prior to attempts at quinidine conversion.

REFERENCES

Sokolow, M. Some quantitative aspects of treatment with quinidine. Ann. Intern. Med., 45:582, 1956.

Wasserman, F. Successful treatment of quinidine and procaine amide intoxication. New Eng. J. Med., 259:797, 1958.

RENAL FAILURE, ACUTE

Acute renal failure refers to acute parenchymal damage associated specifically with reduced renal circulation, or exposure to a nephrotoxin. It is manifested by a sudden marked reduction in urine flow, lasting for days or weeks, following an episode of trauma, poisoning, or severe stressful illness, and is characterized clinically by nitrogen retention, acidosis, and rising serum potassium.

CLASSIFICATION

Over 70 causes of acute renal failure have been described. The six most common are listed here.

1. Postoperative.
2. Obstetrical causes (toxemia, septic abortion, abruptio placentae).
3. Trauma (shock or crush kidney, traumatic nephritis).
4. Severe burns (burn nephritis).
5. Transfusion reactions (hemoglobinuric nephrosis).
6. Nephrotoxins (toxic nephrosis). The list of nephrotoxins includes carbon tetrachloride, ethylene glycol, mercury, bismuth, potassium chlorate, poisonous mushrooms, and sulfonamides.

DIAGNOSIS

The diagnosis of acute renal failure is based on the following two points.

1. Urinary findings. Sp. gr. 1.010, pH 5.0-7.0. The cardinal findings are proteinuria, renal tubular cells, granular hyaline and renal tubular cell casts. Red cell casts may also be present. The urine may contain hemoglobin.
2. Elimination of prerenal and postrenal causes of oliguria and anuria. Correction of preexisting dehydration or elimination of urinary tract obstruction, when present, is therapeutic as well as diagnostic.

If doubt exists as to whether oliguria is prerenal or renal a test with intravenous mannitol may be attempted. When oliguria (< 20 ml per hour output) is detected 20 g of hypertonic mannitol is infused over a 5 to 10-minute interval. If urine flow increases to 40 ml per hour in the next 2 hours, then sustained hydration should be maintained. Additional 20 g infusions of mannitol may be used to maintain the urinary output at 100 ml per minute. Under no circumstances should more than 100 g of mannitol be given in 24 hours. If urinary output does not increase after infusion of 20 g of mannitol, then organic renal failure exists and fluid restriction is imposed. Once parenchymatous damage has occurred, no amount of fluid will promote diuresis until the renal lesion has healed sufficiently to permit urine formation.

CLINICAL SYNDROME OF ACUTE RENAL FAILURE

The clinical course of acute renal failure may be divided into three parts. Shock, if present, is the first phase. It is usually combined with renal vasoconstriction, causing a great decrease in renal blood flow. The second phase (period of little or no urine production) blends in with the first phase and may be evident clinically within a few hours of the inciting cause. This is the oliguric phase, and may last up to 30 days. The third, or diuretic phase, is arbitrarily delineated as the time when the urine volume reaches 400 to 1,000 ml in 24 hours.

The clinical syndrome is shown diagrammatically as follows:

ACUTE RENAL FAILURE

	PHASE		
	SHOCK: ANURIA	OLIGURIA	DIURESIS
Major problem	Shock	Acidosis, hyperkalemia, uremia, cardiac failure	Hypokalemia, uremia
Urine output	0-25 ml	175-250 ml (less than 400 ml)	400 ml or more
Time in days	1-2	2-18	10 or more

THE OLIGURIC PHASE

Attention is usually called to acute renal failure by the sudden development of severe oliguria. During this period there is almost complete renal retention of all waste products, electrolytes, and fluid. The following clinical signs may become evident.

OLIGURIA IS PROMINENT BUT NOT UNIVERSALLY PRESENT. The typical pattern is a profound reduction in urinary flow within a few hours of the precipitating event. Anuria is rare. Generally a volume of 50 ml per day is attained on the second or third day. Thereafter the urinary volume increases slowly until a volume of 350 to 400 ml is attained, after which the volume increases more rapidly. If the period of profound anuria is prolonged (urine output 50 ml or less per day for 3 to 5 days) in a patient who appears to have acute renal failure, then the diagnosis should be questioned and the possibility of urinary tract obstruction investigated. On the other hand, it is to be noted that even a normal kidney may excrete less than 400 ml a day on a fluid-restricted diet. The usual duration of oliguria in severe cases is 10 to 12 days.

CARDIOVASCULAR CHANGES. There are two forms of cardiac dysfunction during the oliguric phase. The first and most frequent is pulmonary edema. The second is the cardiovascular change associated with potassium intoxication.

GASTROINTESTINAL CHANGES. Anorexia, nausea, vomiting, diarrhea, and abdominal distention vary from patient to patient or may be absent, depending upon the seriousness of the uremic state. Gross bleeding is rare.

NEUROPSYCHIATRIC CHANGES. The somnolence of uremia is the most common alteration in the sensorium. Hyperreflexia, twitching, irritability, and asterixis are common. Stupor may progress to profound coma.

FEVER AND LEUKOCYTOSIS. Fever may occur with the initial injury but then the temperature becomes normal. Hypothermia may occur with increasing azotemia. Leukocytosis is almost always present, and may exceed 20,000 cells per cubic millimeter with granulocytes predominating.

ANEMIA. The hematocrit may fall to a value of 20 to 25 percent. The anemia may be due to hemodilution, red cell destruction, or failure of red cell production. Bleeding defects and purpura are common during acute renal failure. Treatment with blood transfusions is not indicated unless the patient has severe symptoms of the anemia or is actively bleeding.

CHEMICAL ABNORMALITIES DURING OLIGURIA. Hyponatremia (serum sodium as low as 115 mEq/L) generally occurs during the oliguric phase. This is probably due to dilution of inorganic ions in body fluids by the administration of water in excess. Untoward effects of the hyponatremia have not generally been recognized. Attempts at correcting the hyponatremia with hypertonic solutions of sodium usually result in the production of cardiac failure. Water restriction rather than sodium replacement is the more physiologic procedure. The low carbon dioxide content represents a metabolic acidosis (uremia and catabolism). Azotemia is variable and progresses rapidly during the first few days of the oliguric phase.

POTASSIUM INTOXICATION. Hyperkalemia is frequently a most serious problem. Potassium intoxication is recognized by an alteration in the sensorium and by signs of cardiovascular and neuromuscular dysfunction. Absence of clinical signs is no assurance that potassium intoxication is not imminent. Serial ECG's and serum potassium determinations should provide adequate warning of progressive hyperkalemia.

TREATMENT OF THE OLIGURIC PHASE

Overhydration must be prevented during the oliguric phase. Daily weight is the best guide. The patient should lose ½ to 1 pound per day. The daily fluid intake should be 5 ml/Kg body weight for insensible losses plus all measurable outputs of the previous day (urine, vomitus and other fluid loss). For each 1° of temperature over 100° F rectally add 10 percent of calculated intake to total fluid intake for the day. Administration of a minimum of 100 g of glucose daily is necessary for protein sparing and for preventing endogenous protein catabolism. Dietary protein, sodium, and potassium should be restricted to minimal amounts. A diet containing 10 g of protein, 200 mg of sodium, 400 mg of potassium and 100 g of carbohydrate is ideal. After two weeks the protein intake must be increased to 30 to 40 g per day in order to provide the essential amino acids. Prior to this the high rate of body catabolism provided the necessary amino acids. With careful management, in the absence of infection, surgery or other stresses the BUN should not rise more than 20 mg/100 ml per day.

MAJOR COMPLICATION

The major threats to life during acute renal failure are 1) hyperkalemia, 2) congestive heart failure, 3) infection, 4) hypertensive encephalopathy, and 5) pericarditis.

TREATMENT OF HYPERKALEMIA

Elevation of the serum potassium results from the liberation of this ion during protein catabolism. Its accumulation in the extracellular space is enhanced by the accompanying acidosis. It is obvious that potassium should be restricted in the diet and not given parenterally unless unusual losses occur. Since there are *no* early signs of hyperkalemia, serial potassium measurements and electrocardiograms should be performed frequently. The ECG findings represent a summation of the effects of relative concentrations of intracellular and extracellular potassium, hydrogen ions, sodium, calcium and magnesium ions on myocardial irritability. The ECG changes which occur with potassium intoxication are covered elsewhere in this book. However, it is worthy to note that the "T" wave elevation of early hyperkalemia may occur only in the precordial and not the standard leads.

Patients with acute renal failure should be treated prophylactically for hyperkalemia, with exchange resins when the serum potassium reaches 5.0 mEq/L. Otherwise the urgency of treatment is dictated by the serum potassium concentration and the ECG changes. A serum level > 7.0 mEq/L must be treated immediately.

If both acidosis and potassium intoxication are present, the most rapid method of reducing the serum potassium level is by the intravenous administration of sodium bicarbonate. Forty-five to 90 mEq of sodium bicarbonate is injected over a period of 5 minutes. If ECG abnormalities persist, the dose may be repeated 15 minutes later. If acidosis is not present, then 200 ml of 3 percent or 5 percent saline may be injected. A 10-percent solution of calcium gluconate, 50 to 100 ml, may be infused with constant ECG monitoring and be equally effective; but administering calcium to patients taking digitalis is hazardous and not advised. The effects of these cations last about 2 hours.

Although the infusion of glucose and water, 250 ml of 25 percent solution, and regular insulin, 20 units, begins acting only 30 minutes later its effectiveness lasts for 4 to 6 hours. This may allow adequate time to begin removing potassium from the patient by gastric suction, potassium exchange resins, or dialysis. The sodium polystyrene sulfonate resin (Kayexalate) exchanges 3 mEq of sodium per gram of resin. The most rapid route of administration is by enema. Thirty to 50 grams of the resin are mixed with 150 ml of 20 percent dextrose and water, instilled rectally and retained 30 to 60 minutes. The procedure is preceded and terminated by cleansing enemas of 20 percent dextrose and water. The serum potassium level may decrease by 0.5 to 2 mEq/h after one enema. Orally the Kayexalate dose is 5 to 20 g q. 6 h. Sorbitol, 20 ml of a 70 percent solution, is administered with each dose to prevent fecal impaction and to produce a mild diarrhea.

Peritoneal or hemodialysis is employed when hyperkalemia is uncontrolled despite good conservative management.

TREATMENT OF CONGESTIVE HEART FAILURE

Congestive heart failure in the patient with acute renal failure is usually secondary to circulatory overload. Unless it is known that the patient has heart disease digitalis should not be used because of its possible toxicity resulting from the body's inability to excrete the drug, and its effect producing rapid changes in potassium and other electrolyte concentrations. Treatment should include salt and water restriction, oxygen, cautious sedation, and, if necessary, dialysis.

PREVENTION OF INFECTION

The major causes of death in patients with acute renal failure are pneumonia and septicemia. Avoidance of indwelling Foley catheters, care in the use of intravenous catheters, and good hygiene are helpful preventative measures. Prophylactic antibiotics are unnecessary. Frequent dialysis may play some role in preventing infection.

TREATMENT OF OTHER COMPLICATIONS

Hypertensive encephalopathy demands urgent treatment with the usual antihypertensive medications. The best treatment of pericarditis is frequent dialysis.

DIFFERENTIAL DIAGNOSIS BETWEEN THE OLIGURIC PHASE OF ACUTE RENAL FAILURE AND SIMPLE DEHYDRATION

Frequently the patient who has had general anesthesia and surgery has a low urine volume during the first 24 postoperative hours. Is this due to renal failure or simply due to failure to supply the patient with adequate fluid intake? In this connection the following comments may be helpful.

1. The usual patient, who has received 2,500 to 3,000 ml of fluid, should have a urine output of 800 to 1,500 ml if he is afebrile.
2. Urine outputs of less than 100 ml/24 hours would be abnormal even in a patient who has no fluid intake.

	ACUTE TUBULAR NECROSIS	DEHYDRATION
Specific gravity	1.010-1.015	1.030
Urine osmolality	300	1.200
$\frac{\text{Urine creatine}}{\text{Plasma creatine}}$ ratio	<8:1	30:1
Urinary sodium mEq/L	40-80	Usually <40
Urinary potassium mEq/L	Less than 15	Greater than 15
Urinalysis	Cylinduria Renal tubular cells Red blood cells	Cylinduria

THE DIURETIC PHASE

The glomerular filtrate is excreted almost unchanged. It is not until a liter or more of this very dilute urine is excreted per day that metabolite removal begins. Hence, it is not uncommon to see a rise in the BUN during the first few days of diuresis. Considerable quantities of sodium, potassium, and chloride are contained in this dilute urine, and the need for their replacement is great. Daily determinations of blood and urine electrolytes, BUN, and water loss are consequently important.

As a rule, if the oliguric phase is of short duration (less than 10 days) the diuretic phase is also short and presents little difficulty. However, if the oliguria is prolonged (15 to 20 days), the diuretic phase requires meticulous attention to fluid and electrolyte replacement. Fluid intake should equal the output plus 400 to 600 ml. Potassium may fall to below normal and require replacement. Protein should be added gradually to the diet.

REFERENCES

Balslov, J. T., and Jorgensen, H. E. A survey of 499 patients with acute anuric renal insufficiency. Causes, treatment, complications, and mortality. Amer. J. Med., 34:753, 1963.

Barry, K. G. Post-traumatic renal shutdown in humans. Its prevention and treatment by the intravenous infusion of mannitol. Mil. Med., 128:224, 1963.

Holmes, J. H. Acute tubular necrosis and its management. Surg. Clin. N. Amer., 43:555, 1963.

Levinsky, N. G. Management of emergencies. VI. Hyperkalemia. New Eng. J. Med., 274:19, 1076, 1966.

Schreiner, G. E., and Maher, J. F. Toxic nephropathy. Amer. J. Med., 38:409, 1965.

FUNCTIONAL DEFECTS OF THE PROXIMAL TUBULE

An abnormal substance present in the urine may result from two mechanisms. In some cases it results from an overflow of a high blood level. For example, in diabetes mellitus, the renal threshold of glucose has been exceeded and the patient has glycosuria. In other instances the excretion of an abnormal substance in the urine results from defective reabsorption of a particular constituent, for example, cystinuria.

The defects of tubular reabsorption, which may be seen in the adult, are:

1. Cystinuria. This is a disturbance in proximal tubular transport of the amino acids, such as cystine, lysine, arginine, and ornithine. There is no other primary renal tubular defect.
2. Hartnup's disease. This is characterized by the presence of a skin rash, episodic cerebellar ataxia, and a proximal tubular defect involving monoamino monocarboxylic acid and acidic amino acids.
3. Glycinuria. A rare condition manifested by excessive excretion of glycine in the urine.
4. De Toni-Debré-Fanconi syndrome. This clinical entity consists of rickets or osteomalacia, glycosuria, diffuse aminoaciduria, hyperphosphaturia, acidosis, and hypokalemia. There are three forms:
   a. The acute form is seen in infancy and childhood, and is usually detected between the ages of 6 months and 1 year. The prognosis is poor with death occurring in the first decade.
   b. The chronic form is usually diagnosed at about the age of two years by the persistence of rickets which are resistant to treatment with vitamin D. These patients also have glycosuria and aminoaciduria, but less commonly than those with the acute form. Death occurs in adolescence.
   c. Patients with the adult form have the same urinary findings as the acute and chronic forms along with symptoms of bone pain and muscle weakness.
5. Aminoaciduria caused by tubular poisoning. Exposure to cadmium and lead have been reported to cause aminoaciduria.
6. Galactosemia. This is believed to be caused by excessive amounts of a galactase-1-phosphate, which is responsible for the inability of the proximal tubule to handle amino acids. The six most common amino acids found in the urine are serine, glycine, alanine, threonine, glutamine and valine.
7. Renal glycosuria. Isolated tubular defect resulting in the inability to reabsorb glucose.
8. Wilson's disease. Presumably, this tubular defect is brought about by the excessive concentration of copper in the kidney. The primary amino acids which are lost in the urine are lysine, threonine, cystine, serine and tyrosine.
9. Other forms of disorder of the proximal tubule are usually seen in children. These include Lowe's syndrome, which is oculocerebrorenal dystrophy, phenylketonuria, and maple syrup urine disease.

FUNCTIONAL DEFECTS OF THE DISTAL TUBULES

SALT-LOSING NEPHRITIS

This may be defined as excessive sodium excretion in the urine, despite normal sodium intake. Most uremic patients lose an excessive amount of sodium in the urine, resulting from a tubular unresponsiveness to aldosterone. In reality the kidney is unable to respond and react normally to salt deficiency, resulting in salt wasting. When salt deficiency occurs from vomiting or diarrhea, the uremic subject is unable to conserve sodium and becomes dehydrated; there is reduction of glomerular filtration and a rise in BUN. Ultimately, death ensues unless infusions of saline or sodium bicarbonate are given. Salt-losing nephritis has been associated with chronic pyelonephritis, cystic disease of the renal medulla, and polycystic kidney disease. It must be differentiated from Addison's disease. The patient may present with signs of severe sodium deficiency, circulatory collapse, loss of skin turgor and muscle weakness. Usually there is a low serum sodium, chlorine, and bicarbonate and high potassium and BUN.

TREATMENT.

Administration of sodium chloride or, if acidosis is present, sodium bicarbonate. Since these patients readily develop water intoxication, all intravenous fluids should be isotonic or in severe cases, hypertonic. After the acute salt loss has been replaced, then the ideal daily salt intake should be determined.

RENAL TUBULAR ACIDOSIS

Renal tubular acidosis is the inability to acidify the urine below a pH of 5.4 under the stimulus of ammonium chloride injection or spontaneous metabolic acidosis. There is an associated fall in blood pH and plasma bicarbonate and an increase in plasma chloride. The defect appears to be in the distal tubules which are deficient in the transfer of hydrogen ion.

1. Infantile form. This form occurs between the ages of 6 and 9 months, symptoms include failure to thrive, loss of appetite, vomiting, and constipation. Often there is radiologic evidence of nephrocalcinosis. The condition is reversible and usually complete recovery occurs.
2. Adult form. In this more serious form of renal tubular acidosis

potassium loss in the urine is responsible for symptoms similar to those seen in periodic paralysis. Bone diseases, either rickets or osteomalacia, and the passage of calculi are not uncommon.

TREATMENT

Infantile form: Modified Shohl's solution (10 g sodium citrate and 6 g citric acid in 100 ml of water). Initially give 15 ml q.i.d. Repeat serum chemistries in 2 weeks and adjust the dose according to the level of plasma bicarbonate which should be maintained at level from 18 to 22 mEq/L. Continue treatment for 1 year then cautiously begin to reduce the dose.

Adult form: A mixture of sodium citrate, sodium bicarbonate, and potassium citrate in amounts from 2 to 8 g daily usually restores the plasma bicarbonate to normal values.

REFERENCES

Elkinton, J. R. Renal acidosis: diagnosis and treatment. Med. Clin. N. Amer., 47:935, 1963.

Relman, A. S. Renal acidosis and renal excretion of acid in health and disease. Advan. Intern. Med., 12:295, 1964.

Wrong, O. Urinary hydrogen ion excretion. J. Clin. Path., 18:520, 1965.

RENAL HYPERTENSION

Some cases of renal hypertension are potentially curable. Within the last decade, diagnosis and surgical treatment of renal hypertension have advanced rapidly. Because of the availability of corrective techniques, early and accurate diagnosis is mandatory.

ETIOLOGY

PARENCHYMAL DISEASE

Pyelonephritis and glomerulonephritis are the usual causes. Because these are essentially bilateral, no surgical approach is feasible as a rule. Rarely unilateral pyelonephritis may cause hypertension, and surgical cure may be possible.

RENAL ARTERY LESIONS

1. Intrinsic
   a. Atherosclerotic plaques.
   b. Segmental mural fibrosis and fibromuscular hyperplasia.
   c. Thrombosis or embolism.
   d. Congenital or acquired stenosis.
   e. Aortic coarctation with renal artery narrowing.
   f. Aneurysm.
   g. Multiple arteries with stenosis or occlusion.
   h. Thrombangiitis.
2. Extrinsic
   a. Kinking and torsion.
   b. External pressure (tumor, fibrous hull, bands, aneurysm, and perirenal hematoma).
   c. Trauma.
   d. Arteriovenous fistula.

Because of the frequently unilateral nature of renal artery lesions the hypertension may be curable by surgical approaches to the artery or by nephrectomy.

DIAGNOSIS

HISTORY AND PHYSICAL

It is to be stressed that in the vast majority of cases there exists no definite historical or physical finding that will separate the renal from other causes of hypertension. The history of hypertension may be long or short, and all ages are represented. Only a few exceptions exist, such as a history of renal trauma antedating the hypertension, or bruit over the renal area in renal arteriovenous fistula. Statistically, however, a majority of the cases fall into the following categories:

1. Onset of hypertension in patients under 30 years and over 45 years, especially in those without a family history of hypertension.
2. Sudden aggravation of previously benign hypertension in any age group.
3. Onset of malignant hypertension without preexistent essential hypertension.
4. History of possible renal vascular accident.

The most helpful clinical sign of renal arterial hypertension is the detection of an upper abdominal bruit; this occurs in approximately 50 percent of patients.

DIAGNOSTIC TESTS

1. Intravenous pyelography is abnormal in 90 percent of patients with proved renal artery stenosis. The 1-, 1.5-, 2-,5, and 15-minute films are used to detect the earliest appearance of dye in the minor calyces. The decreased glomerular filtration rate and urinary volume seen in renal artery stenosis are manifested by delayed visualization of dye on the affected side in 67 percent of patients with proved stenosis. Fifty-eight percent of patients with proved renal arterial lesions showed at least a 1-cm disparity in the length of the long axes of the kidneys. Delayed appearance, decreased density, or prolongation of the nephrogram phase has been noted in 69 percent of patients with renal arterial lesions. The intravenous pyelogram is a highly sensitive and specific test for renovascular disease.
2. I^{131} Radioisotope renogram. This test measures the vascular secretory and excretory phases of the renal handling of the isotope. It is a reasonably sensitive, safe, and simple method of detecting a significant disparity of function between the two kidneys.
3. Renal arteriogram. Percutaneous retrograde transfemoral arteriography serves to locate the anatomic lesion.
4. Split kidney function tests. The patient is placed on a normal sodium diet (3 g sodium) for at least 3 days before the test. Both ureters are catheterized and a glucose, mannitol, or urea infusion is begun. The abnormal side shows a 50 percent decrease in urine volume and a 15 percent drop in sodium concentration. The diagnostic accuracy of individual kidney function tests is equivocal.
5. Measurement of pressor substances. The present data are conflicting and clarification of renin and angiotensin measurements await more specific methodology.
6. Renal biopsy. The histologic findings are varied and of little prognostic value.

TREATMENT

Whether surgical treatment will yield better results than medical treatment in the long-term evaluation is unknown. There are no strict rules for determining who should be treated surgically. Generally, the young and middle-aged patients with severe hypertension are referred for corrective surgery. When feasible, all patients with fibromuscular hyperplasia of the renal artery should be treated surgically. Older patients with generalized atherosclerosis should be treated medically as in essential hypertension. The results of surgical treatment of renal artery stenosis indicate that 50 percent of patients are cured, 26 percent improved, and 18 percent unimproved. The postoperative mortality ranges from 0 to 18 percent with the average about 6 percent.

REFERENCES

Kirkendall, W. M., Fitz, A. E., and Lawrence, M. S. Renal hypertension New Eng. J. Med., 276:479, 1967.

Vertes, V., Gravel, J.A., and Goldblatt, H. Studies of patients with renal hypertension undergoing vascular surgery. New Eng. J. Med., 272:186,1965.

RESPIRATORY ACIDOSIS IN CHRONIC OBSTRUCTIVE LUNG DISEASE, TREATMENT

Respiratory failure is properly diagnosed when carbon dioxide tension rises and oxygen saturation falls. The decrease in oxygen saturation leads to further pulmonary hypertension, polycythemia, and heart failure, but cannot be treated by the usual methods of administering oxygen. Depression of the respiratory center leads to further increase in carbon dioxide tension when oxygen is administered. The physician, therefore, must raise oxygen saturation without further increasing carbon dioxide tension and increasing the respiratory acidosis. The syndrome is frequently precipitated by respiratory infection.

Recent studies have shown that the inhalation of relatively low concentrations of oxygen will raise saturation to normal without raising arterial oxygen tension enough to depress respiration and thus raise carbon dioxide tension. It is suggested that the patient with respiratory failure first be treated with low flow oxygen techniques and careful monitoring of arterial blood gases. Should carbon dioxide tension rise, in spite of low oxygen precautions, respirator therapy is probably indicated.

The following sequence of actions has proven useful:

1. Obtain arterial blood gases and allow the patient to breathe a low concentration of humidified oxygen. This is best accomplished by using a Ventimask which delivers 28 percent to 35 percent oxygen by means of the Venturi principle. If these masks are not available, oxygen may be delivered by nasal catheter at a flow rate of 2 to 4 liters per minute, but no higher. Blood gases should then be repeated

at four hours. If carbon dioxide tension has risen significantly, or if oxygen saturation is not significantly increased, respirator care is probably necessary.

2. The patient should be given antibiotics, expectorants, and a nebulized bronchodilator (Isuprel or Bronkosol) at least every three hours.
3. Should low flow oxygen administration be unsuccessful, or if the patient becomes either obtunded or extremely agitated, respirator care is necessary. An airway should be secured by either oral or nasal intubation – tracheostomy is not generally necessary in this situation. A volume-cycled respirator should provide adequate ventilation. Initially, respirator volume should be adjusted to about 10 ml/kg of body weight. Three types of volume-cycled respirators are currently available. The Emerson and Air Shields both have the advantage of varying the length of inspiration and expiration and of providing for frequent maximal inflations to prevent atelectasis. Occasionally the Air Shields respirator is not able to generate sufficient force to ventilate extremely rigid airways or lungs. This may be recognized by failure to achieve adequate expired volumes as measured by the ventilometer. The Morch respirator is an excellent volume-cycled respirator. When used with a closed airway system delivered volume should be measured with a ventilometer prior to attachment to the patient.
4. Blood gases should be obtained approximately one hour after placing patient on the respirator in order to prevent either inadequate ventilation or hyperventilation. Sedation should be maintained with intravenous meperedine hydrochloride (Demerol) 5 to 25 mg every hour supplemented by promethazine (Phenergan) 25 mg intramuscularly every three to four hours. Diazepam (Valium) 10 mg I.V. 8.h. is also useful.
5. Certain patients with obstructive lung disease and other patients either in shock or with serious pneumonitis are extremely tachypneic. This rapid respiratory rate is very inefficient since much of each tidal breath does little more than ventilate the dead space. In addition, the increased work of breathing may produce a lactic acidosis and further complicate matters. Such a patient is best treated with curare in order to permit complete control of respiration. While curare administration is frequently lifesaving, it should only be undertaken with adequate nursing and physician care since the patient is totally paralyzed and completely dependent upon the respirator.

RHEUMATIC FEVER

The prevention of rheumatic fever depends on the treatment of group A hemolytic streptoccal infections. Commonly the diagnosis of streptococcal infection is made on clinical findings consisting of fever from 101° to 104° F, and sudden onset of sore throat with pain on swallowing. The throat is red and an exudate is usually present. The glands at the angle of the jaw are swollen and tender. A fine scarlatiniform rash occasionally is present. Whenever possible the clinical diagnosis should be verified by throat culture, inasmuch as viral pharynigitis may present with identical findings.

TREATMENT OF STREPTOCOCCAL INFECTION

1. Intramuscularly one injection of benzathine penicillin G (Bicillin), 1,200,000 units; or
2. Intramuscular procaine penicillin, 600,000 units a day for 10 days; or
3. Orally, 200,000 units of penicillin 4 times a day for 10 days.

In patients with penicillin sensitivity sulfadiazine, 1.0 g, should be given 3 times a day for 10 days. Broad spectrum antibiotics are also of value. Whatever the drug, it must be employed for 10 days.

DIAGNOSIS OF RHEUMATIC FEVER

Rheumatic fever is more frequently overdiagnosed than underdiagnosed. Both extremes can be avoided by a rigid application of the Jones criteria (modified) as published by the American Heart Association.

JONES CRITERIA (MODIFIED) FOR GUIDANCE IN THE DIAGNOSIS OF RHEUMATIC FEVER

MAJOR CRITERIA.

1. Carditis, murmur: apical systolic, apical middiastolic, basal diastolic; cardiac enlargement; pericarditis; congestive failure.
2. Polyarthritis.
3. Chorea.
4. Subcutaneous nodules.
5. Erythema marginatum.

MINOR CRITERIA.

1. Fever.
2. Arthralgia.
3. Prolonged PR interval in the ECG.
4. Increased ESR, WBC, or presence of C-reactive protein.

5. Preceding group A hemolytic streptococcal infection including scarlet fever.
6. Previous rheumatic fever or inactive rheumatic heart disease.
7. Elevated or rising antistreptolysin-O titer.

CARDITIS

MURMURS. For a systolic murmur to be significant it must be holosystolic, best heard at the apex, transmitted toward the axilla, and not be altered by respiration or change of position. A basal, decrescendo diastolic murmur is more easily interpreted as a sign of carditis. The low-pitched, short, middiastolic murmur (Carey Coombs), localized at the apex and best heard during expiration in the left lateral position, is valuable in confirming the significance of an apical systolic murmur. The importance of this murmur and the frequency with which it is missed have been emphasized by Feinstein and Spagnuolo.

PERICARDITIS. Pericarditis is present in 12 percent of cases. It does not occur in the absence of valvular involvement.

POLYARTHRITIS

The significance of the word *polyarthritis* is often missed. As the word indicates, two or more joints must be involved to constitute a major criterion. This manifestation is present in 40 percent of childhood rheumatic fever.

CHOREA

Chorea occupies a unique position in the spectrum of rheumatic fever. Whereas carditis and polyarthritis occur 1 to 5 weeks following a group A streptococcal infection, evidence of such a preceding infection is often lacking in chorea. Chorea may not appear for as long as 3 to 6 months following a streptococcal infection without polyarthritis. In conjunction with other signs of rheumatic fever, chorea occurs in 13 percent of cases. The sex predilection is 2.5 to 1 for females. It is rare after the age of 18 except during pregnancy.

SUBCUTANEOUS NODULES

The incidence of subcutaneous nodules varies from 1.2 percent to 14 percent. They last about 3 weeks and may be as many as forty in number.

ERYTHEMA MARGINATUM

Erythema marginatum is the only type of cutaneous change acceptable as a major criterion. It is present in 8 to 12 percent of cases. Purpura, erythema nodosum, and urticaria are neither major nor minor manifestations.

The presence of two major criteria or one major plus two minor criteria indicates a high probability of the presence of rheumatic fever.

In evaluating the *minor criteria* one should keep in mind that arthralgia may not be used as a minor criterion if arthritis is included as a major one. A prolonged PR interval, present in 20 percent of cases, is not acceptable as a minor criterion if carditis is already included as a major one. The erythrocyte sedimentation rate, the C-reactive protein reaction, and leukocytosis are nonspecific reactions. Elevation of one or more of these constitutes only a single minor criterion.

TREATMENT OF RHEUMATIC FEVER

The active treatment of rheumatic fever consists of the following.

1. Rest. In childhood it is easier to order bed rest than to maintain it once the acute phase of fever, polyarthritis, and carditis subside. It may be necessary then to resort to sedation to ensure adequate rest. The average duration of acute inflammatory activity in patients without valvular involvement is 89 days. In patients with valvular involvement the duration is 124 days as measured by the time the C-reactive protein first became and remained negative in the presence of normal vital signs. The sedimentation rate may remain elevated long after all other signs of activity have returned to normal. Strict rest should be continued for at least the period of acute inflammatory activity.
2. Eradication of streptococcic infection.
   a. Procaine penicillin 600,000 units, I.M. q. 12 h. for 10 days.
   b. After the tenth day penicillin, 200,000 units, orally, twice a day. Following the acute stage this should be continued if the patient is not sensitive to penicillin as long as he remains in school, in the armed forces, or is in contact with children.

   Evidence has been accumulating that there is very little difference in the incidence of the streptococcic infection rate per patient year in the oral penicillin and sulfadiazine prophylactically treated groups, being 21.1 percent and 20.7 percent respectively. In the benzathine penicillin treated group the incidence is 7.3 percent. With good prophylaxis the recurrence rate of rheumatic fever per patient year with sulfadazine is 1.9 percent, with oral penicillin 5 percent, and with benzathine penicillin 0.3 percent. Of the oral agents sulfadiazine proved as good as or better than penicillin, though in the study from which these figures are derived the oral dose of penicillin was only 200,000 units daily.

3. Suppression of the acute phase. Salicylates and adrenal steroids are commonly used. Both suppress certain manifestations of the acute phase, notably fever and joint manifestations. The Combined Rheumatic Fever Study Group found no evidence that prednisone was superior to acetylsalicylic acid in preventing residual rheumatic heart disease. However, prednisone suppresses the inflammatory reaction of the acute attack more rapidly than acetylsalicylic acid, and in patients with severe carditis and congestive failure may be lifesaving. The dose of either drug should be sufficient to control the acute phase. Prednisone is given in divided doses of 60 mg daily for about 3 weeks and then gradually withdrawn over a second 3 week period. The dose of acetylsalicylic acid is 50 mg per pound of body weight daily in divided doses for 3 weeks. The drug is withdrawn gradually so as to evaluate the possible recurrence of the acute inflammatory phase. As valuable as these drugs are in controlling symptoms, the duration of activity is the same in those treated as in those not treated.
4. Treatment of *chorea* consists of bed rest for the 6 to 12 weeks which is the usual duration of this manifestation. Sedation is necessary to control the involuntary movements. The simplest drug to use is phenobarbital, 15 to 45 mg, 4 times a day. In approximately one half of Bland and Jones's patients, chorea appeared at some stage of the illness.
5. Circulatory failure in children with acute rheumatic fever is primarily right-sided failure with hepatomegaly, puffiness of face, and unexpected weight gain. Pulmonary rales are not heard until late in the course. A diastolic gallop rhythm is commonly present. The treatment is salt restriction, diuretics, and digitalis. In the presence of acute carditis, myocardial irritability is increased and doses of digitalis ordinarily used may precipitate various arrhythmias.
6. Acute glomerulonephritis occurs in about 4 percent of cases of acute rheumatic fever.

REFERENCES

Feinstein, A. R., et al. The prognosis of acute rheumatic fever. Amer. Heart J. 68:817, 1964.

Johnson, E. E., et al. Rheumatic recurrences in patients not receiving continuous prophylaxis. J. A. M. A., 190:407, 1964.

Kuttner, A. G., and Mayer, F. E. Carditis during second attacks of rheumatic fever. J.A.M.A., 268:1259, 1963.

____ et al. A comparison of short-term intensive prednisone and acetylsalicylic acid therapy in the treatment of acute rheumatic fever. New Eng. J. Med., 272:63, 1965.

Massell, B. F., et al. Evolving picture of rheumatic fever. J.A.M.A., 188:287, 1964.

RHEUMATIC HEART DISEASE

The critical factor in the development of rheumatic heart disease is the presence of carditis during an attack of rheumatic fever. Polyarthritis alone or chorea alone, without coexistent carditis, is not followed by rheumatic heart disease. In a group of 441 patients studied by Feinstein, Stern, and Spagnuolo, 59 percent had carditis in the initial attack; 57 percent of these were left with definite residual heart disease; 8 percent of these died in a mean of 7.8 years. In the initial attack of rheumatic fever, severe carditis consisting of cardiac enlargement, congestive failure, or both, carries the worst prognosis.

For practical purposes the main emphasis in rheumatic heart disease is focused on the valvular lesions and their hemodynamic effects. Thirty-five years ago Cabot found the mitral valve involved in 85 percent, the aortic in 44 percent, the tricuspid in 10 to 16 percent, and the pulmonary in 1 to 2 percent of his cases. Wood has calculated the relative frequency of various valvular involvement in terms of the load against the different valves. If the mitral valve were involved in 80 percent of cases the calculated frequency of aortic, tricuspid, and pulmonary involvement would be 48, 12, and 5 percent respectively, figures that closely approximate Cabot's findings.

MITRAL INSUFFICIENCY

Mitral insufficiency is the major valvular lesion in 34 percent of patients with mitral disease. One half of these have combined but minor mitral stenosis. The more severe and recurrent types of rheumatic fever are more likely to produce major mitral insufficiency which develops early in the course of active carditis. Insufficiency has a longer symptom-free interval than stenosis, but once symptoms appear the course is more rapidly downhill.

The most prominent symptom of mitral insufficiency is dyspnea followed by signs of left ventricular failure.

SIGNS. The apex beat is forceful and displaced to the left. The first sound is normal or soft in intensity. A holosystolic murmur is present at the apex and transmitted laterally to the axilla. A loud third heart sound due to rapid ventricular filling may be present. A short diastolic apical murmur due to the same mechanism may be heard. A long diastolic murmur is not compatible with a high degree of insufficiency for it indicates prolonged ventricular filling due to valvular obstruction. The rhythm is generally related to the age of the patient. One third of all patients with mitral insufficiency and the majority of those over the age of 50 fibrillate.

Radiologically the left ventricle is enlarged. Massive enlargement of the left atrium and appendage is more common than in mitral stenosis. In the lateral view the posterior aspect of the heart may appear as a smooth unbroken curve resembling a shallow letter C continued down to the diaphragm. In the PA view the left border of the heart is straightened. Generally the heart of mitral insufficiency enlarges earlier in its transverse diameter because of increased left ventricular work than the heart of mitral stenosis.

MITRAL STENOSIS

Stenosis accounts for 64 percent of all mitral valve disease. It is more likely to occur following an isolated clinical episode of rheumatic fever or chorea (Wood).

Unlike mitral insufficiency, in which the primary effect is on the left ventricle, in mitral stenosis the effect is due to an obstructive lesion, the stenotic valve, interposed between the left atrium and ventricle. The orifice of the *normal* mitral valve is about 5 cm^2. The pressure in the left atrium normally is about 8 mm Hg (range 6 to 12) and the normal cardiac output is between 5 and 6 liters per minute (range 4 to 8). With increasing stenosis over a 20-year period the mitral orifice gradually narrows. When it reaches a size of *less than 1.0 cm*^{2} all patients are symptomatic. The pressure in the left atrium will have risen to 25 mm Hg, and the cardiac output will have fallen below 4.0 to 4.5 liters per minute. The rise in the left atrial pressure is transmitted to and accompanied by a similar rise in pressure in the pulmonary capillaries, pulmonary arteries, and the right ventricle. When the pulmonary capillary pressure rises above the osmotic pressure of the plasma, which is from 25 to 30 mm Hg, fluid transudes from the capillaries to the alveoli. With a valve area of less than 1.0 cm^2 pulmonary markings are prominent, but except for the left atrium the heart may be of normal size. Persistence of this degree of narrowing inevitably produces pulmonary vascular changes and a second obstruction to the circuit of blood from the right side of the heart to the left ventricle. Vasoconstriction and thickening of the walls of the arterioles and smaller arteries of the pulmonary tree are the cause of the sequential obstruction which follows critical narrowing of the mitral orifice. With a valve orifice of 0.9 cm^2 or less all patients are symptomatic in that they are dyspneic and may have hemoptysis and pulmonary edema. With obstruction in the pulmonary tree a further decline of cardiac output favors further narrowing of the mitral orifice. Only by a rise in pulmonary artery pressure at the expense of increased right ventricular work can blood be forced through to the left side of the heart. Eventually the right ventricle hypertrophies, dilates, and finally fails. At this stage the transverse diameter of the heart enlarges. The left ventricle and the aorta do not contribute to the enlargement and in fact are generally smaller than normal.

SYMPTOMS. Dyspnea due to increased pulmonary rigidity and chronic interstitial edema is the outstanding manifestation of mitral stenosis. Pulmonary edema occurs in about 10 percent of cases before the development of high pulmonary vascular resistance. With the onset of increased pulmonary resistance paroxysmal dyspnea occurs. It differs from pulmonary edema in that transudation into the pulmonary alveoli is prevented by a capillary alveolar barrier. Rales are not present and expectoration of frothy white or pink fluid is absent. Orthopnea, though it may be less alarming to the patient, is a late manifestation of severe pulmonary changes.

Five types of pulmonary bleeding may occur in mitral stenosis. The most striking is *pulmonary apoplexy,* which appears rather early in the course of the disease. It is due to rupture of intrapulmonary bronchial or pleurohilar veins before the walls thicken as a result of increased pressure over several years. With the continuance of increased pressure in the pulmonary circuit, hypertrophy of the walls occurs and pulmonary apoplexy ceases. The commonest precipitating causes of this type of hemorrhage are pregnancy and physical exertion. The hemorrhage may last from a few hours to two weeks. During pregnancy, it has been considered an indication for valvulotomy, but in practically all cases the bleeding will stop spontaneously with rest and sedation.

Pulmonary bleeding also occurs in the blood-stained sputum of *paroxysmal cardiac dyspnea,* as frank hemoptysis in, *pulmonary infarction,* as pink-stained frothy sputum in *pulmonary edema,* and as blood-streaked sputum in *"winter bronchitis."* This last cause of bleeding apparently is more common in Britain than in the United States.

SIGNS. The apex beat is diffuse over the left precordium in mitral stenosis. The beat is not forceful.

The first heart sound is accentuated unless the valve is calcified. Accentuation is due to the high atrial pressure that forces the cusps to remain open almost throughout diastole until the left ventricle contracts and snaps them together. In atrial fibrillation with varying length of diastole the first sound may vary in intensity.

The opening snap is probably the most persistent sign of mitral stenosis in the absence of heavy calcification of the valve. It is best heard at the lower left sternal border and at the apex. In character it is high-pitched and in time occurs after aortic valve closure. The sound is caused by the high atrial pressure snapping the aortic cusp of the mitral valve into the left ventricular cavity.

The next sign in the sequence of the cardiac cycle is an apical diastolic murmur. It begins just after the opening snap. It is low-pitched in character and not influenced by calcification of the valve or atrial fibrillation. The length of this murmur is of great significance. Its duration depends on the length of time it takes for left atrial and ventricle pressures to equalize. In mild stenosis this level is reached early, and the murmur is short. In severe stenosis the pressures may not equalize at all, and the murmur will extend up to the first sound.

A mitral presystolic murmur is practically a constant finding in mitral stenosis with normal rhythm. Like other auscultatory findings it is best brought out with the patient in the left lateral position after exercise.

Radiologically the cardiac silhouette depends on the degree of stenosis, its duration, the presence of concomitant valvular lesions, the pressure in the pulmonary circulation, and to a lesser degree the cardiac rhythm.

The aorta and left ventricle are small due to decreased ventricular filling and cardiac output. Left atrial enlargement appears early with significant degrees of stenosis. In the PA view the left atrial appendage forms a prominence between the pulmonary artery and the left ventricle. On the right the left atrium appears as a double shadow behind the right atrium. A giant left atrium, however, is more common in mitral insufficiency than in stenosis. Generally the atrium is larger in the presence of atrial fibrillation. The hilar areas are prominent because of interstitial edema and dilated hilar veins. With increasing pulmonary vascular resistance the pulmonary artery dilates and forms a prominent hump on the upper left cardiac border. In the lateral view the enlarged left atrium projects into the retrocardiac space displacing the esophagus backward. The displacement is high on the posterior cardiac border and usually does not extend down to the diaphragm. If the retrosternal space is obliterated by the right ventricle for 50 percent or more of the way up, this is considered radiologic evidence of right ventricular hypertrophy.

COMPLICATIONS

EMBOLI. Systemic embolization occurs in from 9 to 30 percent of cases of mitral stenosis. About 9 percent with normal sinus rhythm embolize. The higher percentage represents the incidence in those with atrial fibrillation. Wood believes that it is one and one-half times more common in stenosis than in insufficiency because of more stasis in the left atrium in the former than in the latter. In a postmortem study Wallach, Lukash, and Angrist found thrombi in the cardiac chambers in 26.9 percent of cases. They attribute thrombus formation in the atrium to a regurgitant jet of blood striking the same small area on the left atrial wall with each ventricular contraction. Over a period of time this trauma leads to collagenous thickening of the atrial endocardium ("bird nesting") high on the posterior wall, which is the usual location of thrombus formation and attachment. The most favorable combination of valvular lesions to produce such a mechanism is mitral insufficiency with stenosis. Stasis may explain thrombus formation in the atrial appendage, but it cannot account for the localization of the thrombus in the atrium proper. Wood states that embolization is cerebral in 60 percent, peripheral in 30 percent, and visceral in 10 percent of cases. In nonsurgical cases peripheral embolization is more common than is cerebral in our experience.

PULMONARY HYPERTENSION. There are two types of pulmonary hypertension in mitral stenosis.

1. Passive, due to transmitted pulmonary venous pressure from the left atrium. To maintain pulmonary artery flow the pressure must be at least 10 mm Hg higher in that vessel than a mean left atrial pressure of between 20 to 30 mm Hg at rest and 40 to 50 mm Hg during exercise in the presence of mitral stenosis.
2. Active, due to pulmonary vasoconstriction. This does not occur until

the valve orifice becomes critically narrowed to less than 1.0 cm^2 and the left atrial pressure is above 20 mm Hg with a cardiac output of 4 to 5 L/min and a normal heart rate. These factors will produce a mean pulmonary artery pressure of over 30 mm Hg at rest. Though they are important accompaniments of active pulmonary vasoconstriction, they are not the causes. Such vasoconstriction can raise the pulmonary vascular resistance to 480 to 800 dynes/sec/cm^{-5} (the normal resistance is less than 160 dynes/sec/cm^{-5}). The resistance is not due to sclerotic changes in the pulmonary arteries secondary to long-maintained passive pulmonary hypertension because it develops rapidly and falls gradually following a successful valvulotomy. The vasoconstrictive type of pulmonary hypertension is the most important form in mitral stenosis and is the direct cause of functional pulmonary and tricuspid insufficiency. High degrees of reactive hypertension are less common in mitral insufficiency.

PULMONARY INFARCTION. Pulmonary infarction in mitral stenosis is overwhelmingly due to embolism from phlebothrombosis of the leg or pelvic veins which is favored by the low cardiac output, increased venous pressure, and restricted activity. In only a small percentage of cases pulmonary infarction results from thrombosis in situ.

CONGESTIVE FAILURE. Congestive failure rarely occurs in mitral stenosis with regular rhythm in the absence of high pulmonary resistance (more than 560 dynes/sec/cm^{-5}). The common cause of failure is uncontrolled atrial fibrillation. Since this can be controlled by digitalis it is much less serious than failure due to high pulmonary resistance. The statement is made frequently that digitalis is of no use and may be actually harmful in mitral stenosis with regular rhythm. This belief is based on the reasoning that, with pulmonary resistance remaining constantly elevated, increasing the force of right ventricular contraction will not, or will only to a slight degree, increase the cardiac output and renal blood flow. The factors responsible for failure will still obtain.

ATRIAL FIBRILLATION. Atrial fibrillation in mitral disease is related directly to the increasing age of the patient and is not influenced by the degree of stenosis. Early in the course of fibrillation practically all patients can be converted to regular rhythm, but the greater the age of the patient the less likelihood of regular rhythm persisting.

INDICATIONS FOR COMMISSUROTOMY IN MITRAL STENOSIS

In general any patient with symptomatic (class 2B or more)

pure mitral stenosis should have a mitral commissurotomy. Unfortunately the issue is seldom so clear-cut because of the hemodynamic and technical problems posed by coexistent valvular lesions.

Minor degrees of mitral insufficiency are not a contraindication to surgery. However, in pure mitral stenosis some degree of insufficiency was created by closed or "blind" surgery in 30.5 percent of Bailey's cases. In patients with coexistent mitral insufficiency the leak was further increased in 27 percent.

Open mitral commissurotomy is the ideal surgical approach to mitral stenosis. Only by direct inspection can accurate incision of fused commissures be effected, subvalvular fusion of chordae be released, and atrial clots be safely evacuated. Only open commissurotomy with extracorporeal circulation permits total valve replacement by prosthesis, which is the indicated procedure for the correction of significant mitral insufficiency or extensive fibrosis or calcification of the mitral valeve.

All "reoperations" for mitral valve disease should be done "open." All patients with calcified valves and with atrial clots or history of recent embolization should be done "open."

Aortic stenosis is associated with mitral disease in about 20 percent of cases. Whether it is dynamically significant can be determined reliably only by left heart catheterization. The correction of mitral stenosis in the presence of significant aortic stenosis serves only to increase the left ventricular work against the aortic obstruction, with eventual earlier left ventricular failure. In such cases both stenotic lesions must be corrected at the same time.

Tricuspid insufficiency is most often functional, and if it responds to medical measures it will respond to correction of the mitral stenosis.

Tricuspid stenosis can be corrected at the same time as mitral stenosis when a right-sided approach to the mitral valve is employed.

Atrial fibrillation per se is not an indication for operation. About 25 percent of patients with normal sinus rhythm will have transient atrial fibrillation postoperatively. Five percent with previously normal sinus rhythm will develop persistent atrial fibrillation following surgery. On the other hand, only about 6 percent of chronic atrial fibrillation can be corrected to normal sinus rhythm following operation. In general the preoperative rhythm tends to remain the same. The operative mortality in patients with atrial fibrillation in Bailey's series of 1,000 cases was about three times that of those with normal sinus rhythm.

This is to be expected, since the arrhythmia represents a later stage of the disease. Other factors that influence mortality are age over 40 and cardiac enlargement of more than 2 plus on a scale of 4.

"Irreversible" *pulmonary hypertension* has been cited by some as a contraindication to mitral valve surgery. This probably exists only when mitral stenosis is complicated by primary pulmonary disease.

Following mitral valvulotomy *restenosis* is said to occur at a rate of about 2 percent per year. Whether this truly represents restenosis or failure to perform adequate commissurotomy is debatable.

AORTIC INSUFFICIENCY

Rheumatic valvulitis is three times more common as a cause of aortic insufficiency than syphilis. As an isolated lesion or combined with mitral valve disease the aortic valve is involved in about 40 percent of rheumatic carditis. Aortic insufficiency dates from the initial attack of carditis.

Symptoms depend on the appearance of left ventricular failure and consist of dyspnea, orthopnea, and paroxysmal cardiac dyspnea. With free regurgitation angina pectoris may occur.

Hemodynamically aortic insufficiency increases the diastolic stretch of the left ventricle by the quantity of blood that leaks back from the aorta during diastole. During systole the pressure is higher than normal, the ejection phase is shortened, and pressure falls away abruptly.

SIGNS. Left ventricular enlargement displaces the forceful and localized apex beat downward and to the left. The characteristic murmur is decrescendo and diastolic in time, beginning immediately after the first sound. It is heard best at the base and along the left sternal border with the patient erect and leaning forward. The Austin Flint diastolic murmur may be heard inside the apex. It differs from the aortic diastolic murmur by beginning appreciably after the second sound. Instead of being decrescendo it is rumbling in character and may be accentuated in presystole. The murmur is most likely due to the regurgitant jet of blood from the aorta striking the aortic cusp of the mitral valve.

The peripheral signs of aortic insufficiency are due partly to reflux from the aorta and partly to peripheral vasodilation.

These signs are modified markedly by the presence of concomitant mitral stenosis, which significantly decreases left ventricular filling and cardiac output.

AORTIC STENOSIS

Aortic stenosis is predominantly a disease of the elderly, though it does occur in childhood. As an isolated lesion it occurred in 34 percent of Hall's cases with the highest incidence between the years of 60 and 69. The diagnosis is not often made before the age of 40. Males are affected four times more often than females.

The causation of "pure" aortic stenosis is still being debated. When found as an isolated lesion in the aged it may be on the basis of a congenital bicuspid valve, be purely sclerotic, or be due to rheumatic fever. When found with other valvular lesions it is considered to be rheumatic in origin. Bean obtained a history of rheumatic fever in 50 percent of cases. Karsner and Koletsky believed that 98 percent of their autopsy cases were basically rheumatic. In Hall's series the mean age of the first attack of rheumatic fever was 18, and the first symptom of heart disease appeared at 55. Frank heart failure occurred at the age of 58, with an average age of 62 at death. Only 10 percent of Hall's cases survived more than one year after the advent of heart failure.

The outstanding symptoms of aortic stenosis, in addition to the usual breathlessness and eventual frank congestive failure with edema, are angina pectoris and syncope. Angina due to low mean blood pressure and decreased coronary filling occurs in 25 percent of cases. Syncope due to low fixed cardiac output appears in 20 percent of cases of aortic stenosis.

SIGNS. The apex beat is displaced downward and to the left. The apical impulse is forceful. A harsh basal systolic murmur, best heard over the aortic area, is the commonest sign. It is of greatest intensity in midsystole, rising to a gradual crescendo after the first sound, gradually diminishing and ending before the second sound. On the phonocardiogram the murmur has a characteristic diamond shape. A systolic ejection click often precedes the murmur. Transmission of the murmur depends on its loudness more than on the course of the great vessels. It may be heard over the carotid arteries and at the apex. The aortic sound is diminished or completely absent depending on the degree of immobilization of the calcified valve. The aortic sound, when present, is delayed due to prolonged left ventricular systole and is heard after the pulmonic second sound. Paradoxical splitting occurs, with the split widening during expiration rather than during inspiration.

Depending on the intensity of the murmur a systolic thrill, best elicited with the patient leaning forward, may be palpated.

Radiologically the left ventricle is enlarged, though not as much as in aortic insufficiency. There may be poststenotic dilation of the aorta. In most cases beyond middle age calcification of the aortic valve can be demonstrated.

TRICUSPID INSUFFICIENCY

Tricuspid insufficiency is most often functional in origin, due to right ventricular dilation following pulmonary hypertension secondary to mitral stenosis. It has been recognized in 17 percent of patients during mitral valve surgery by Bailey. If the symptoms and signs of tricuspid insufficiency occurring with mitral stenosis are reversed by medical means, the lesion is functional rather than organic.

Symptoms include swelling of the abdomen with the appearance of edema and ascites. The patient may be aware of pulsations in the neck and abdomen.

SIGNS. The right ventricular systolic pulsation is palpable parasternally in the third and fourth left interspaces. The rhythm is almost invariably atrial fibrillation. A holosystolic murmur is present between the left sternal border and the apex. As in the case of mitral insufficiency a short functional diastolic murmur may be present. Systolic pulsation of the liver is best demonstrated by lateral expansion of the upper abdomen.

The murmur of tricuspid insufficiency is markedly diminished in expiration. The murmur of mitral insufficiency changes little.

Radiologically the right border of the heart is prominent due to enlargement of the right atrium, which extends downward to meet the diaphragm at an obtuse angle.

TRICUSPID STENOSIS

Trisucpid stenosis is practically always associated with mitral stenosis and in many instances also with aortic valvular disease. It occurs in 15 percent of mitral disease. This lesion, interfering with right ventricular filling, relieves pulmonary congestion due to the associated mitral stenosis, and as a result hemoptysis and pulmonary edema are absent when the combined lesions are present. As in mitral stenosis, tricuspid stenosis is more common in the female.

Fatigue due to reduced cardiac output, hepatomegaly, edema, and ascites are the outstanding symptoms.

SIGNS. The apex beat is faint. A presystolic or diastolic murmur increased in intensity during inspiration is present at the fourth left intercostal space at the sternal border. The usual increase in the pulmonic second sound noted in mitral stenosis is absent when the two valvular lesions are associated.

Radiologically the right atrium is enlarged, but more impressive are the relatively hypovascular lung fields.

REFERENCES

Arnott, W. M. The lungs in mitral stenosis. Brit. Med. J., October 5, 1963.

Bentivoglio, L., Uricchio, J., and Goldberg, H. Clinical and hemodynamic features of advanced rheumatic mitral regurgitation. Amer. J. Med., 30:372, 1961.

Bleifer, S., Dack, S., Grishman, A., and Donoso, E. The auscultatory and phonocardiographic findings in mitral regurgitation. Amer. J. Cardiol., 5:836, 1960.

Dack, S., Bleifer, S., Grishman, A., and Donoso, E. Mitral stenosis. Amer. J. Cardiol., 5:815, 1960.

Hugenholtz, P. G., Ryan, T. J., Stein, S. W., and Abelmann, W. H. The spectrum of pure mitral stenosis. Amer. J. Cardiol., 10:773, 1962.

Selzer, A., et al. The syndrome of mitral insufficiency due to isolated rupture of the chordae tendineae. Amer. J. Med., 43:822, 1967.

Szekely, P. Systemic embolism and anticoagulant prophylaxis in rheumatic heart disease. Brit. Med. J., May 9, 1964.

RHEUMATOID ARTHRITIS

Rheumatoid arthritis is a general disease with heart, lung, muscle, nerve (peripheral neuropathy), and other system involvement, due to the local presence of rheumatoid nodules and/or arteritis. The usual age of onset is 25 to 50. Women are affected three times as often as men.

CRITERIA FOR DIAGNOSIS

(American Rheumatism Association)

1. Morning stiffness.
2. Pain on motion or tenderness in at least one joint.

3. Swelling (soft tissue thickening or fluid, not bony overgrowth alone) in at least one joint continuing for 6 weeks.
4. Swelling of at least one other joint (intervals free of joint symptoms between the two joint involvements of not more than 3 months).
5. Symmetrical joint swelling with simultaneous involvement of the same joint on both sides of the body (bilateral involvement of the midphalangeal, metacarpophalangeal, or metatarsophalangeal joints is acceptable, without absolute symmetry).
6. Subcutaneous nodules over bony prominences, on extensor surfaces, or in juxta-articular regions.
7. Roentgenographically visible changes typical of rheumatoid arthritis (which must include at least bony decalcification localized to or greatest around the involved joints and not just degenerative changes). Degenerative changes, however, do not exclude the diagnosis.
8. Positive result demonstrating the "rheumatoid factor" by any method which, in two laboratories, has been positive in not over 5 percent of normal controls, or positive result of the streptococci agglutination test. Generally accepted positive titers are sheep cell agglutination (Rose-Waaler) of 1:32, bentonite flocculation of 1:32, and latex fixation of 1:20 (see below).
9. Poor mucin precipitate from synovial fluid (with shreds and cloudy solution).
10. Characteristic histologic changes in synovial membrane with three or more of the following: marked villous hypertrophy; proliferation of superficial synovial cells, often with palisading; marked infiltration of chronic inflammatory cells (lymphocytes or plasma cells predominating) with tendency to form "lymphoid nodules"; deposition of compact fibrin, either on surface or interstitially; or foci of cell necrosis.
11. Characteristic histologic changes in nodules showing granulomatous foci with central zones of cell necrosis surrounded by proliferated fixed cells, and peripheral fibrosis and chronic inflammatory cell infiltration, predominantly perivascular.

The diagnosis of definite rheumatoid arthritis must fulfill five of the above eleven criteria. In criteria 1 through 5 the joint symptoms must be continuous for at least 6 weeks. The diagnosis of probable rheumatoid arthritis requires three of the above. In at least one of criteria 1 through 5, the joint symptoms must be continuous for at least 6 weeks.

DIFFERENTIAL DIAGNOSIS

The following conditions are frequently associated with joint manifestations.

Systemic lupus erythematosus
Polyarteritis nodosa
Hypertrophic pulmonary osterarthropathy

Dermatomyositis
Scleroderma
Rheumatic fever
Gout
Acute infectious arthritis
Tuberculous arthropathy
Reiter's syndrome
Hand-shoulder syndrome
Temporal arteritis
Psoriatic arthritis
Neuroarthropathy
Alkaptonuria
Sarcoidosis
Multiple myeloma
Erythema nodosum
Leukemia or lymphoma
Agammaglobulinemia
Rubella polyarthritis
Allergic reactions

THE RHEUMATOID FACTOR

The rheumatoid factor appears in 70 to 90 percent of cases of rheumatoid arthritis if the disease has been present for 6 months or more. This factor is associated with a macroglobulin with a sedimentation of about 18.7 Svedberg units (S20). The factor is not affected by steroids or other drugs. Its presence is associated with a more active disease and the prognosis is favorable in its absence. The sensitized sheep cell test while not as positive as the latex fixation test is more specific for rheumatoid arthritis.

The rheumatoid factor may be positive in many conditions other than rheumatoid arthritis. The latex fixation test, for example, was found to be positive in the following:

Normals	0-5%
Systemic lupus erythematosus	50%
Hepatic diseases	25%
Viral infections	20%
Syphilis	10%
Subacute bacterial endocarditis	50%

FELTY'S SYNDROME

This variant of rheumatoid arthritis occurs most frequently in young females of 25 to 30 years of age. In addition to the arthritis, hepatosplenomegaly and leukopenia occur. Anemia and fever may also be present. Treatment consists of steroids initially; if the patient is poorly responsive splenectomy may be of value.

TREATMENT

Anti-inflammatory agents, especially high doses of aspirin with bed rest and rehabilitative medical procedures. If the disease is progressive gold salts therapy has been recommended.

REFERENCES

Bartfeld, H. Incidence and significance of seropositive tests for rheumatoid factor in non-rheumatoid diseases. Ann. Intern. Med., 53:5, 1960.

Brannan, H. M., et al. Pulmonary disease associated with rheumatoid arthritis. J.A.M.A., 189:914, 1964.

Decker, John (ed.). Primer on the rheumatic diseases. J.A.M.A., 190:509, 1964.

Talbott, J. A., and Calkins, E. Pulmonary involvement in rheumatoid arthritis. J.A.M.A., 189:911, 1964.

SARCOIDOSIS

Sarcoidosis is a systemic granulomatous disease of unknown origin involving the pulmonary hilar and peripheral lymph nodes, skin, lungs, liver, eyes, salivary glands, cardiac and voluntary muscles, and the phalanges and other bones. Sarcoidosis involves the hilar nodes in 90 percent of patients and the lungs in 65 percent.

DIAGNOSIS

Diagnosis rests upon the combination of a suggestive clinical picture and a positive biopsy or a positive Kveim test. The scalene node biopsy is positive in about 60 to 80 percent of patients, and the Kviem test in 75 to 85 percent of cases. Liver biopsy is positive in about 60 to 70 percent of patients. Biopsy of the gastrocnemius muscle is also positive in a fair percentage of cases (30 to 50 percent).

Other laboratory tests of value include the following:

1. Proteinemia (over 7.9)	30%
2. A/G ratio (less than 2:1)	88%
3. Serum calcium over 11 mg %	35%
4. Alkaline phosphatase over 5 Bodansky units	30%
5. Leukopenia (less than 5,000)	30%
6. Eosinophilia (over 7%)	15%

In an analysis of 123 patients, the following pulmonary findings were present (see table page 390).

	PATIENTS	REGRESSED	PROGRESSED
Early			
Bilateral hilar nodes	62	25	13
Miliary	33	7	13
Patchy infiltrates	14	4	6
Transitional	7	0	7
Late fibrotic	7	0	7

The death rate was found to be 5 to 10 percent within 5 years. The usual causes are cor pulmonale and active pulmonary tuberculosis.

EPIDEMIOLOGY

In the United States, most cases are reported from the Southeast and the Gulf States with a Negro to white ratio of 10 or 20 to 1. Of note are some data obtained from Sweden. There sarcoidosis occurs at a rate of 42/100,000 (about ten times the rate in the United States). Tuberculosis in Sweden occurs at a rate of about 90/100,000 population, and is constantly declining, while the sarcoidosis rate has remained steady.

In this country the usual case occurs in rural areas in the so-called pine-pollen belt.

TREATMENT

Steroid therapy is absolutely indicated in the following circumstances.

1. Involvement of the eye.
2. Alveolar-capillary block.
3. Severe CNS symptoms.
4. Myocardial involvement.
5. Hypersplenism.
6. Hypercalcemia with renal damage.

A relative indication for steroid therapy exists in the following four circumstances.

1. Increasing pulmonary lesions.
2. Disfiguring skin lesions.
3. Continuing facial palsy.
4. ENT lesions.

Because of the frequency with which tuberculosis occurs in

patients with sarcoid (20 to 30 percent) INH prophylaxis may be of value when

1. Steroid treatment is used, or
2. Tuberculin conversion occurs.

Chloroquine has been found of value in sarcoidosis of the skin. Colchicine is reported to be useful in sarcoid arthritis.

REFERENCES

Israel, H. L., and Sones, M. Selection of biopsy procedure for sarcoidosis diagnosis. Arch. Intern. Med., 113:255, 1964.

Sharma, O. P., Colp, C., and Williams, M. H., Jr. Course of pulmonary sarcoidosis with and without corticosteroid therapy as determined by pulmonary function studies. Amer. J. Med., 41:541, 1966.

Stone, D. J., and Schwartz, A. A long-term study of sarcoid and its modification by steroid therapy. Amer. J. Med., 41:528, 1966.

GRAM-NEGATIVE BACTEREMIC SHOCK

(Endotoxic Shock, Septic Shock)

Gram-negative bacteremia is the second most common cause of shock on the medical service; it is only surpassed in frequency by myocardial infarction. With better understanding and management the mortality of this type of shock has been reduced from 80 percent to 50 percent. Approximately 25 percent of patients with gram-negative bactermia will develop endotoxic shock. The mortality of bacteremia alone is 25 percent.

The organisms commonly cultured during bactermia are: *E. coli* 40 percent, Klebsiella-Aerobacter 30 percent, Proteus species 20 percent, Pseudomonas species and other gram-negative (Paracolobactrum, Salmonella, etc.) 10 percent. *E. coli* shows the lowest incidence of shock and the lowest mortality; Proteus and Pseudomonas produce the highest mortality.

Excluding septic abortion, endotoxic shock is rarely found in patients under 40 years of age and is twice as frequent in males. The average age is usually 60 years. The high-risk population are patients with genitourinary tract infections, cirrhosis, septic abortion, pneumonia, uremia, burns, and neoplasms. Patients being treated with steroids, cytotoxic and immunosuppressive drugs for malignancies of the hematopoietic system are especially susceptible. The most common source of bacteria is the genitourinary tract which is involved in 60 to 80 percent of cases and is precipitated by manipulative procedures, (i.e., catheterization, cystoscopy). Other inciting causes are gastrointestinal surgery, cholecystectomy, cholangitis, and intravenous cannulation.

Shock for practical purposes is defined as a blood pressure of less than 80 mm/Hg systolic with the clinical signs and symptoms of the shock state. The hemodynamic alterations are due to the release of complex lipopolysaccharide endotoxins from the bacterial cell wall. One of the currently held hypotheses states that endotoxin utilizing complement in an "antigen antibody like" reaction causes the release of vasoactive substances such as histamine, norepinephrine, bradykinin and serotonin. These stimulate the precapillary arterioles and muscular venules resulting in an immediate increase in peripheral vascular resistance which in turn causes peripheral pooling in the microcirculation and leads to a decrease in the effective circulating volume, a decrease in venous return, and a reduction of central venous pressure. The cardiac output usually falls and hypotension ensues, but a normal or high cardiac output can be seen. This is the reversible stage of shock. If the vasoconstriction is not relieved, blood will be shunted away from the capillary beds causing a decrease in tissue perfusion leading to hypoxia and disruption of oxidative metabolism with lactic acidosis. In the face of the resultant acidosis precapillary sphincter tone is lost while postcapillary or venular tone is maintained. Blood entering the arteriolar side can not escape; hydrostatic pressure rises and transudation of fluid into the extravascular space takes place. This is the irreversible stage of shock.

This outline has been offered as a working model in order to aid in the management of shock. It is important to realize that many observations made in the experimental animal may not be applicable clinically.

The initial clinical manifestations of bacteremic shock "warm shock" are chills, fever, dry skin, mental confusion, full pulses, hyperventilation, and adequate urine output. If untreated "cold shock" ensues with cold, clammy, mottled skin, and weak pulses and oliguria.

Laboratory studies show early leukopenia followed by leukocytosis with a shift to the left. The BUN is elevated early in the course, with subsequent rise in SGOT, and amylase in the later stages. Serum bicarbonate is decreased. The ECG shows nonspecific ST-T changes.

Since 50 percent of patients die within 48 hours, early diagnosis and treatment are imperative.

TREATMENT

1. The therapeutic approach should be tailored according to the monitored values obtained, i.e., C.V.P. central aortic pressure, peripheral vascular resistance, urine output, and arterial blood gases.
2. A recommended antibiotic regimen without isolation of an organism is as follows:
   a. Kanamycin: 0.5–1.0 g I.M. q 12 h. plus Colistin: 2.5 m 5 mg/kg I.M. per day in divided doses.
   b. Colistin plus ampicillin 6-12 g a day in divided doses or aqueous penicillin, 20 million units per day.
   a. and b. are adequate coverage for all the aforementioned pathogens. Regimen b. will not be effective against Proteus strains other than *P. mirabilis*. (See section on antibiotics.)
3. Dynamic alteration of the C.V.P. with increments of fluid replacement should serve as a guide to effective circulating volume and cardiac competence. a. If the C.V.P. is normal or less than 5 cm H_2O administer a fluid "challenge" of 250 ml D/W in 10 minutes; if the C.V.P. does not rise more than 2 cm H_2O in 10 minutes the patient is considered to have adequate cardiac function and one may proceed with expansion of intravascular volume with incremental challenges until a C.V.P. of 15 cm H_2O is attained. Volume may be replaced with plasma, low molecular weight dextran or saline. b. If C.V.P. is greater than 10 cm H_2O or a fluid challenge elevates the C.V.P. more than 5 cm H_2O diminished cardiac reserve is suggested and institution of digitalization or isoproterenol is indicated in the dose of 2 to 5 mg in 500 ml D/W at the rate of 1 to 2 μg per minute. If isoproterenol in the presence of adequate circulating volume fails to maintain a mean aortic pressure of 80 mm Hg levarteranol may be indicated in doses of 2 to 4 mg in 500 cc D/W for maintenance of a mean aortic pressure of 80 mm Hg.
4. Steroids in the form of hydrocortisone 3 to 6 g daily or its equivalent should be given early in the course of treatment.
5. Chlorpromazine may be used to overcome persistent vasoconstriction, after adequate volume expansion and a mean aortic pressure of 80 mm Hg is obtained. Five milligrams I.V. q. 10 minutes to total dose of 25 mg may be used.
6. For assisted ventilation and management of oliguria see the section on cardiac shock and renal disease.

REFERENCES

Laib, H. S., et al. Haemodynamic studies in shock associated with infection. Brit. Heart J., 29:883, 1962.

Rahal, J. J., Jr., MacMahon, H. E., and Weinstein, L. Thrombocytopenia and symmetrical peripheral gangrene associated with staphylococcal and streptococcal bacteremia. Ann. Intern. Med., 69:35, 1968.

Spink, W. Endotoxic shock. Ann. Intern. Med., 57:538, 1962.

Weinstein, L., and Klainer, A. S. Management of emergencies. IV. Septic shock – pathogenesis and treatment. New Eng. J. Med., 274:950, 1966.

SJÖGREN'S SYNDROME

Sjögren's syndrome is probably a variant of generalized vascular disease (rheumatoid arthritis, etc.) associated with dryness of the mouth and of the mucous membranes. There is aptyalia, deficient lacrimation, and hoarseness.

REFERENCES

Bloch, K. J., et al. Sjögren's syndrome: A clinical pathological and serological study of 62 cases. Medicine, 44:187, 1965.

Denko, C. W., and Bergenstal, D. M. The Sicca syndrome (Sjögren's syndrome). Arch. Intern. Med., 105:849, 1960.

Tu, W., Shearn, M., Lee, J., and Hopper, J. Interstitial nephritis in Sjögren's syndrome. Ann. Intern. Med., 69:1163, 1968.

SPLENOMEGALY

Splenomegaly may occasionally occur as an isolated finding. Usually, however, other findings coexist. The following tabulation lists some of the more frequent combinations.

1. Isolated splenomegaly in the absence of other findings.

Gaucher's disease	Primary splenic neoplasm
Sarcoid	

2. Splenomegaly and fever.

Infectious mononucleosis	Leukemia
Subacute bacterial endocarditis	Hodgkin's disease
Brucellosis	Systemic lupus erythematosus
	Periodic disease

3. Splenomegaly with pallor and icterus.
   Hemolytic anemias
   Cirrhosis

4. Splenomegaly and generalized lymphadenopathy.
   Infectious mononucleosis
   Chronic lymphatic leukemia
   Lymphosarcoma
   Hodgkin's disease
   Sarcoid

5. Splenomegaly with petechiae and ecchymoses.
   Acute leukemia
   Terminal chronic leukemia
   Lymphosarcoma with metastases to bone marrow

6. Splenomegaly and plethora is found in polychthemia vera.

7. Splenomegaly and bone changes.
   Severe thalassemia
   Gaucher's disease
   Myelofibrosis with myeloid metaplasia
   Multiple myeloma
   Amyloid disease
   Metastatic carcinoma

8. Splenomegaly and cytopenia (especially leukopenia or thrombocytopenia).
   Typhoid
   Malaria
   TBC
   Histoplasmosis
   Granulomas
   Syphilis
   Portal hypertension
   Splenic neoplasms (incl. hemangiomas, cysts)
   Systemic lupus erythematosus
   Rheumatoid arthritis (Felty's syndrome)
   Paratyphoid

9. Splenomegaly with leukocytosis.
   Pyogenic infections (SBE, abscess)
   Infectious mononucleosis
   Measles
   Leukemia
   Polycythemia vera
   Myeloid metaplasia
   Thrombocytopenia
   Hemolytic anemia

REFERENCE

Dameshek, W. Splenomegaly – a problem in differential diagnosis. Med. Clin. N. Amer., 41:1357, 1957.

STEROID DOSAGES

The normal adrenal cortex secretes approximately 15 to 30 mg of cortisol (hydrocortisone) daily.

The following doses are approximately equivalent in antirheumatic activity to 25 mg of oral cortisone.

Hydrocortisone (P.O.)	20 mg
Prednisone and prednisilone (P.O.)	5.0 mg
Methylprednisiolone (P.O.)	4.0 mg
Triamcinolone	4.0 mg
Fluprednisilone	2.5 mg
Dexamethasone	0.75 mg
Fludrocortisone†	0.1 mg

†Fludrocortisone (9-alpha-fluorohydrocortisone), because of powerful salt and fluid retaining effects, is limited in use to adrenocortical insufficiency states.

REFERENCES

Boland, E. Chemically modified adrenocortical steroids. J.A.M.A., 174:835, 1960.

Danowski, T. S., et al. Probabilities of pituitary-adrenal responsiveness after steroid therapy. Ann. Intern. Med., 61:11, 1964.

Reed, P. I., et al. Adrenocortical and pituitary responsiveness following long-term, high dosage corticotropin administration. Ann. Intern. Med., 61:1, 1964.

STROKES

Each year in the United States over 500,000 persons are stricken by a cerebrovascular accident (CVA) of some form. With increasingly available and accurate diagnostic techniques, and with advances in therapy, a significant percentage of this group can be helped, if not indeed cured.

The approach to a CVA should be as dynamic and complete as the approach to, say, a fever of unknown origin. Standing alone the clinical diagnosis of cerebrovascular accident tells no more of the underlying pathology than does the temperature chart of the fever of unknown origin.

Clinically, one hemiplegic looks more or less like another, yet "strokes" are really a heterogenous group of disorders, each responsive to its own therapy.

The *causes of "strokes"* are as follows:

1. Spasm, thrombosis, embolism, or rupture of a cerebral artery	60% of cases
2. Basilar and/or vertebral artery "insufficiency" 3. Carotid artery "insufficiency"	25% of cases
4. Ruptured cerebral artery aneurysm 5. AV anomaly 6. Subdural hematoma 7. Primary or metastatic tumors	10% of cases

Rarer causes include cerebral arteritis produced by infections or by drugs and the collagen group of diseases. Combined lesions of the cerebral and carotid-vertebral-basilar systems occur frequently.

DIAGNOSIS

In addition to routine initial evaluation (history, physical, and lumbar puncture) skull and chest x-rays should be obtained in an attempt to eliminate fractures with subdural hematoma and bronchogenic carcinoma with cerebral metastases as the cause (10 to 15 percent of bronchogenic carcinomas metastasize to the brain). Initially, careful carotid palpation should be performed; later ophthalmodynamometry is done.

Serial cerebral angiography offers the only sure diagnostic approach in the majority of cases, and should be performed far more frequently than it is at present. In addition to providing precise anatomic diagnosis, it frequently suggests the proper medical or surgical approach.

THERAPY

1. Anticoagulation remains a subject of dispute. However, our experience correlates with studies suggesting its usefulness in the nonhypertensive patient demonstrating insufficiency of the carotid or vertebral-basilar artery system, cerebral artery embolism, and in those with the multiple "little stroke" syndrome of cerebral artery origin. The ultimate place of anticoagulant therapy in cerebral spasm and throm-

bosis remains to be determined. Anticoagulation is contraindicated in demonstrated hemorrhagic strokes.

2. Surgical techniques are available for demonstrated carotid artery disease. These include grafts to replace narrowed or occluded segments as well as endarterectomy. Evacuation of the subdural hematoma, removal of the primary or metastatic tumor, and clipping the aneurysm are accepted procedures.

After evaluation as indicated, in particular cerebral angiography, a significant number of stroke victims can be cured or salvaged without progression of the disease.

REFERENCES

Gurdjian, E., et al. Analysis of occlusive disease of the carotid artery and the stroke syndrome. J.A.M.A., 176:194, 1961.

Siekert, R., et al. Anticoagulant therapy in intermittent cerebrovascular insufficiency. J.A.M.A., 176:19, 1961.

Wolf, G. Current status of therapy in cerebral vascular accidents. J.A.M.A., 172:562, 1960.

SYNCOPE

Syncope is temporary loss of consciousness. It may occur in three ways.

1. Change in blood composition.
   a. Critical decrease in O_2, sugar, or CO_2 (hyperventilation).
   b. Increase in CO_2.
2. Reflex cerebral dysfunction.
   a. Epilepsy.
   b. Brain tumor.
3. Cerebral ischemia.
   a. Loss of peripheral resistance.
      Vasovagal syncope.
      Carotid sinus syncope.
      Orthostatic hypotension.
   b. Decreased cardiac output.
      Adams-Stokes attacks.
      Aortic stenosis.
      Angina pectoris.
      Myocardial infarction.
   c. Cerebrovascular disease or spasm.
      Arteriosclerosis.
      Thrombosis.

In an analysis of over 500 patients with syncope, the most common causes were as follows.

Vasovagal syncope	60% of cases
Orthostatis hypotension	6%
Epilepsy	5%
Cerebral vascular disease	5%
Unknown	4%
Postmicturition	3%
Adams-Stokes attacks	3%
Hyperventilation	3%
Carotid sinus	3%
Tussive	2.5%
Aortic stenosis	2%
Paroxysmal tachycardia	2%

Accounting each for 1 percent of cases or less were angina pectoris, hysteria, myocardial infarction, pulmonary hypertension, migraine, and hypertensive encephalopathy.

REFERENCE

Wayne, H. Syncope. Amer. J. Med., 30:418, 1961.

SYPHILIS

(The Biologic False Positive Reaction)

Biologic false positive (BFP) reactions are defined as positive serologic tests for syphilis but negative *Treponema pallidum* tests.

Positive results will occur in both groups of tests with syphilis, and with yaws, pinta, and bejel (the last three are also spirochetal diseases). In addition, one case of a false positive *Treponema pallidum* test has been reported in herpes zoster.

Biologic false positive reactions occur in the following circumstances.

1. Technical errors.
2. Acute BFP reactions (due to infections listed).

	Percent BFP
. Pneumococcal pneumonia	2-5
. Streptococcal pharyngitis	5

SBE	5
Chancroid	5
Leptospirosis (Weil's disease)	10
Rat bite fever	20
Relapsing fever	30
Malaria (acute)	100
Varicella	5
Infectious hepatitis	10
Infectious mononucleosis	20
Lymphogranuloma venereum	20
Measles	5
Atypical pneumonia	20
Upper respiratory infections	20
Vaccinia	20
Typhus	20

Reactions may also occur in mumps and postimmunization states.

	Percent BFP
3. Chronic BFP reactions	
Due to infections	
Tuberculosis	3-5
Leprosy	60
Due to other diseases	
Systemic lupus erythematosus	10-20
Rheumatoid arthritis	5-10
Liver disease	5-10
Rheumatic heart disease	5-10
Diabetes mellitus	5
Myocardial infarction	5
Sarcoidosis	5

In addition a large number of other conditions may cause BFP reactions. These conditions include congenital hemolytic anemias and a wide range of other blood dyscrasias. Many patients exhibiting BFP reactions, but entirely asymptomatic and not falling into any of the above categories, may in long-term follow-up go on to develop SLE.

REFERENCES

Fiumara, N. J. The treatment of syphilis. New Eng. J. Med., 270:1185, 1964.

Rockwell, D. H., et al. The Tuskegee study of untreated syphilis. Arch. Intern. Med., 114:792, 1964.

TETANUS

Tetanus is an acute intoxication caused by *Clostridium tetani.* The disease is characterized by stiffness of the skeletal muscles of all parts of the body, tonic spasms and convulsions, and episodes of laryngospasm. A frequent initial complaint is that of inability to open the jaw. The symptoms are produced by an exotoxin which affects the neuromuscular end plate and the motor nuclei of the central nervous system.

Although the illness is generally associated with a contaminated traumatic wound, cases are seen in large metropolitan areas due to the use of contaminated syringes by drug addicts. Hence the illness may be acquired by intravenous injection of the organism, and in these circumstances there is no local wound. In situations such as this, the mortality rate is high and approaches 75 percent. The illness lasts 6 to 8 weeks. During the first 3 or 4 weeks the symptoms become increasingly worse, then begin to abate.

TREATMENT

1. Provide an open airway.
2. Sedation.
3. Meticulous nursing care.
4. Antibiotic and antitoxic therapy.
5. Hyperbaric oxygen therapy.

1. *Tracheotomy.* If the patient has had one episode of cyanosis due to a generalized spasm, or has one episode of laryngospasm, a tracheotomy must be performed promptly.
2. *Barbiturates* should be administered in a sufficient dose to keep the patient in a semistuporous state. This may require as much as 400 mg of phenobarbital every 4 hours. Phenothiazine tranquilizers are useful in addition to the barbiturate in preventing muscle spasms. Very large doses are required (Sparine in doses to 200 to 400 mg every 6 to 8 hours may be necessary). Meprobamate and other muscle relaxant drugs are not as useful as the above-mentioned drugs.
3. *Meticulous nursing care* is the sine qua non for recovery. Careful recording of the vital signs, observation of the state of sedation, and careful attention to the tracheotomy are necessary. Without the proper nursing care survival is unlikely.
4. *Penicillin,* in doses of 4,000,000 units per day, and *tetanus antitoxin,* 200,000 units are given intravenously. If there is a local wound,

200,000 additional units of antitoxin are given in the region of the wound.

REFERENCES

Kloetzel, K. Clinical patterns in severe tetanus. J.A.M.A., 185:559, 1963.

Pascale, L. R., et al. Treatment of tetanus by hyperbaric oxygenation. J.A.M.A., 189:408, 1964.

THYROID DISEASES

The thyroid gland is a specialized organ which "traps" circulating iodides and incorporates the iodide and tyrosine by a series of reactions into organic iodine compounds (chiefly thyroxin). Hamolsky and Freedberg have reviewed the steps involved in this process in detail.

DIAGNOSIS

LABORATORY TESTS

1. *Basal metabolic rate* (BMR). In essence the BMR may be considered to measure the effect of thyroid hormone on all the tissues of the body. Because of the multiplicity of factors thereby involved, the diagnostic accuracy of the test is low (50 to 70 percent). At present it is perhaps best employed to follow response to thyroid hormone therapy. A normal test is good evidence against the presence of hyperthyroidism.
2. The protein-bound iodine (PBI) measurement offers better diagnostic accuracy (80 to 90 percent).
3. Thyroxine-iodine by column chromatography – unlike the PBI, the T_4-B_4 by a column is not influenced by excessive amounts of inorganic iodine, iodoproteins, or iodotyrosines. The values are comparable to the butanol-extractible iodine (BEI). Normal range, 2.9-6.4 mg per 100 ml.
4. Radioactive iodine (I^{131}) uptake (RAI uptake) studies offer a diagnostic accuracy of 85 to 95 percent. The red cell uptake of I^{131}-labeled triiodothyronine avoids the administration of I^{131} to the patient, and is generally unaffected by prior administration of iodine-containing compounds.
5. In vitro I^{131}-labeled triiodothyronine (T_3) uptake of red blood cells on resin. The test avoids the administration of I^{131} to the patient and is generally unaffected by prior administration of iodine-containing compounds.
6. Achilles reflex test (photomotogram) – reflex delayed in hypothyroid-

ism and quickened in hyperthyroidism. *The serum cholesterol* level determination is of value in hypothyroid states and in following the response to thyroid medication.

The following table outlines some of the factors capable of influencing the BMR, PBI, and RAI levels.

	NORMAL	INCREASED	DECREASED
Basal metabolic rate	+20 to −20	Hyperthyroidism; anxiety; fever; heart failure; hypertension; anemia; carcinoma; perforated eardrum	Hypothyroidism; technical errors
Protein-bound iodine	4-8 μg%	Hyperthyroidism; thyroiditis; I^{131} administration in therapeutic doses; pregnancy; hepatitis; some cases of cretinism; administration of thyroid, organic or inorganic iodine-containing compounds and estrogens	Hypothyroidism; nephrosis and other hypoalbumenemic states; mercurial diuretics; administration of ACTH, cortisone, triiodothyronine, and cobalt chloride
RAI^{131} uptake	15-40% in 24 hr	Hyperthyroidism; some renal diseases including nephrosis; some cases of heart failure and liver disease; low dietary iodine; pregnancy	Hypothyroidism; some renal diseases; acute thyroiditis; administration of thyroid, triiodothyronine, Butazolidin, iodides and cobalt chloride; congestive heart failure
T_3 red blood cell uptake	11-19%	Hyperthyroidism	Hypothyroidism
Resin uptake (trisorb)	25-35%	Hypoproteinemic states; severe metastatic malignancy; anticoagulant therapy; Dilantin, Butazolidin, salycylates (large dose); thyroxine and desiccated thyroid therapy	Pregnancy; estrogen therapy (oral contraceptives)

REFERENCES

Grayson, R. R. Factors which influence the radioactive iodine thyroidal uptake test. Amer. J. Med., 28:397, 1960.
Hamolsky, M., and Freedberg, A. The thyroid gland. New Eng. J. Med., 262:23, 70, 129, 1960.
McAdams, C. B., and Reinfrank, R. F. Resin sponge modification of the I^{131}-T_3 test. J. Nucl. Med., 5:112, 1964.
Solomon, D. H., Bennett, L. R., Peter, J. B., Pollack, W. F., and Richards, J. B. Hyperthyroidism. Ann. Intern. Med., 69:1015, 1968.

TREATMENT OF HYPERTHYROIDISM

General measures in the treatment of hyperthyroidism include rest, a good dietary intake, especially of protein, and sedation when necessary. Symptoms such as nervousness, palpitation, and anxiety can be controlled satisfactorily by reserpine, which does not affect the underlying disorder. The effective dose is from 0.5 to 1.0 mg daily. To control the symptoms of thyroid storm the dose is increased to 4.0 to 8.0 mg, parenterally, daily for 3 to 4 days.

There are three specific means available for the treatment of hyperthyroidism.

1. Antithyroidal drugs, which include a) propylthiouracil, b) methylthiouracil, c) methimazole, d) carbimazole, and e) perchlorate.
2. Surgical resection of the gland.
3. Radioactive iodine therapy.

Antithyroid drugs may be used either as preparation for surgery or as the sole form of treatment of hyperthyroidism. Generally the age group under 40, including children, would be considered for prolonged antithyroid drug therapy.

The two most widely used antithyroid drugs are propylthiouracil (available in 50 mg tablets) and methimazole (Tapazole, available in 5-mg and 10-mg tablets). The initial dose is 100 to 200 mg of propylthiouracil which is comparable to 10 to 20 mg Tapazole, orally t.i.d. Improvement may be noted in about 3 weeks, though a euthyroid state may not be reached for 2 to 3 months. Therapy should be continued for one to one and a half years. A permanent remission is achieved in about 50 to 60 percent of patients.

Early in the course of propylthiouracil treatment increasing enlargement of the gland is often noted. A favorable sign of a sustained remission is the reduction of the gland to normal size. The addition of thyroid hormone to regimen with antithyroid medication will usually bring about a reduction in the size of the gland.

Minor reactions to the drug are dermatitis and urticaria. Alopecia has been reported. Major reactions include leukopenia, agranulocytosis, and lupus-like reactions. White cell counts of 5,000 to 6,000 mm^3 are not uncommon in hyperthyroidism. In 10 percent of untreated cases the white cell count is below 4,000 mm^3. A decrease in the total white cells below this level, or in the granulocytes below 50 percent, calls for close observation. A continuing fall necessitates stopping the drug.

A lupus-like reaction may follow long-term treatment with propylthiouracil. It consists of fever, serositis, joint pains and swelling, leukopenia, and enlargement of the liver and spleen.

The antithyroid drugs may be used during pregnancy. However, since they readily cross the placenta, thyroid hormone is added to the regimen to prevent the development of a goiter in the fetus. Triiodothyronine (Cytomel) may cross the placenta more readily than the T_4 compounds and should be given in a dose of 100 g orally daily. Mothers using antithyroid drugs should not breast feed, since the antithyroid drugs are found in high concentration in the breast secretions.

Radioactive iodine (I^{131}) may be used in the adult population and is generally now used in the treatment of most hyperthyroid patients over the age of 40, provided that the gland is not so large as to cause pressure symptoms. It is especially indicated in debilitated individuals, cardiac patients, and diabetics.

The initial dose generally ranges between 3 and 6 millicuries and about two-thirds of patients are cured by the initial dose. The initial response to radioactive iodine may not be seen for 3 to 6 weeks or even longer. Since it has been recognized that the incidence of hypothyroidism is significant, and may be delayed, a second therapeutic dose may be withheld for a period of 6 months. If the patient is symptomatic from the hyperthyroidism, antithyroid drugs or iodides may be used until a better therapeutic effect from the I^{131} is achieved or until the administration of an additional dose of I^{131}. Radioactive iodine should not be used during pregnancy, since the fetal thyroid can concentrate iodine by the twelfth to sixteenth week of pregnancy and iodine readily crosses the placenta. The use of radioactive iodine in children should generally be avoided, since there may be increased susceptibility to development of carcinoma of the thyroid following radioactive exposure in this age group.

Surgery is indicated in large pressure-producing goiters and in large adenomatous goiters, which because of their size are unlikely to shrink under propylthiouracil or which would require excessive radioactive iodine for control. If surgery is elected the euthyroid state is first achieved with propylthiouracil, then stable iodine (Lugol's solution, 0.3 ml) is administered three times daily for 2 to 3 weeks preceding operation in order to decrease the vascularity of the gland.

The adverse effects of surgery are hypoparathyroidism, which is transient in the majority of instances, vocal cord paralysis, myxedema, and recurrent hyperthyroidism. Following proper preoperative management the mortality should be under 0.5 percent.

Though iodine has a beneficial effect on thyrotoxicosis, its use should be limited only to the preparation for surgery.

REFERENCES

Brown, Josiah, et al. Adrenal steroid therapy of severe infiltrative ophthalmopathy of Graves' disease. Amer. J. Med., 34:786, 1963.

Dunn, J. T., and Chapman, E. M. Rising incidence of hypothyroidism after radioactive iodine therapy in thyrotoxicosis. New Eng. J. Med., 271:1037, 1964.

Hirshman, J. M. The treatment of hyperthyroidism. Ann. Intern. Med., 64:306, 1966.

Lipman, L. M., Green, D. E., Snyder, N. J., Nelson, J. C., and Solomon, D. H. Relationship of long-acting thyroid stimulator to the clinical features and course of Graves' disease. Amer. J. Med., 43:486, 1967.

Solomon, D. H., moderator. UCLA inter departmental conference. Hyperthyroidism. Ann. Intern. Med., 60:1015, 1968.

THYROID STORM

Thyroid storm is usually of abrupt onset characterized by fever, marked weakness, and tachycardia, a well-maintained blood pressure initially and even transient diastolic hypertension. Tremors, agitation, confusion, and psychosis are the central nervous system manifestations. Diarrhea, abdominal pain, nausea, and vomiting may be other features. Finally, apathy, stupor, coma, and shock may develop.

Thyroid storm is now most commonly seen when the thyrotoxic state is complicated by infection, trauma, or surgical emergencies. With adequate preparation with antithyroid medication for subtotal thyroidectomy, surgical storm is less commonly seen.

TREATMENT

1. 1 to 2 g of sodium iodide by slow intravenous drip.

2. Reserpine, 2.5 mg I.M. q. 6 h. in the agitated phase of storm, or in less urgent cases 40 to 140 mg by mouth daily.
3. Intravenous fluids, saline, and B-complex vitamins.
4. Oxygen.
5. Cooling with wet packs or induced hypothermia.
6. Glucocorticoids (300 mg hydrocortisone the first day and tapering thereafter).
7. Treatment for heart failure if this supervenes (digitalis, diuretics).
8. Large doses of antithyroid drugs. Propylthiouracil, 800 to 1,000 mg by mouth or Tapazole, 80 to 100 mg daily by mouth or gastric tube.

REFERENCE

Ingbar, S. H. Management of emergencies. IX. Thyroid storm. New Eng. J. Med., 274:1252, 1966.

TREATMENT OF HYPOTHYROIDISM

The exact mechanisms responsible for hypothyroidism may be obscure and complex, but the treatment of the hypothyroid state is simplicity itself, consisting of the administration of sufficient thyroid hormone to raise the oxygen consumption of the tissues to a normal level.

Primary hypothyroidism is due to the effect on the gland of one or more of the following.

1. Hashimoto's thyroiditis (chronic thyroiditis), most common.
2. I^{131} therapy for hyperthyroidism – increasing incidence.
3. Following subtotal surgical resection for hyperthyroidism – incidence after 10 years may be from 5 to 40 percent.
4. Destruction from radiation.
5. Antithyroid drug.
6. Congenital defects in hormone synthesis.
7. Iodine deficiency.
8. Excessive iodine intake.

Secondary hypothyroidism is due to lack of the thyroid-stimulating hormone which may result from:

1. Sheehan's disease (postpartum pituitary necrosis).
2. Surgical hypophysectomy.
3. Primary or metastatic tumors in the gland.

Regardless of the cause of hypothyroidism the treatment is the same: administration of thyroid hormone. The normal maintenance dose is between 90 and 180 mg of desiccated thyroid daily, which is equivalent to 150 to 300 mg of thyroxin or 50 to 100 μg of triiodothyronine. Thyroid hormone may be given in any of the above forms.

The PBI is generally not too valuable in following the patient on therapy. Thyroid extract preparation may have variable effect on PBI, thyroxine may elevate the PBI, and triodothyronine may lower the PBI. Clinical judgment remains the best way of determining dose, though the serum cholesterol and Achilles reflex test are helpful objective parameters.

In hypothyroidism it is important to initiate therapy with small dosages such as 50 to 10 μg triiodothyronin, or sodium l-thyroxine 0.05 mg, or 15 mg of thyroid extract. With the more rapidly acting T_3 compound (triiodothyronine), the dosage may be increased by 5 μg every 5 days, while with the T_4 compounds (thyroxine) the dose may be increased by 0.05 mg every two weeks. Although in most instances thyroid extract is adequate therapy, its potency may be variable and sometimes the preparation may be biologically inactive. For this reason it is preferable to use the crystalline compounds, such as triiodothyronine or sodium l-thyroxine.

Thyroid hormones are also used in the treatment of simple nontoxic goiter. In one series desiccated thyroid caused 87 percent to decrease in size, and in another series treated with triiodothyronine 25 percent of the goiters disappeared. The use of these hormones is also an effective method of demonstrating the possible presence of nodules obscured by general enlargement of the gland.

MYXEDEMA COMA

Patients with untreated hypothyroidism may progress into increasing stupor or coma. This may be precipitated by exposure to cold, trauma, surgery, or infections. Emergency treatment is necessary as the prognosis worsens the longer the patient is left untreated. One can draw blood for PBI, T_3 uptake, cholesterol electrolytes, and then initiate therapy as follows:

1. T_3-triiodothyronine, 10 mg by mouth or gastric tube q. 6 to 8 h.
2. Hydrocortisone, 50-100 mg I.M. q.6 h. and rapidly tapering dose.
3. Restriction of fluid, 1,500 ml with part saline (may have inappropriate ADH syndrome).
4. Do not rapidly rewarm patient.

Patients with hypothyroidism may have electrocardiographic change and enzyme changes of SGOT, but particularly CPK, which may be differentiated from acute ischemia only with difficulty.

REFERENCES

Catz, B., and Russell, S. Myxedema, shock, and coma. Arch. Intern. Med., 108:407, 1961.

Green, W. L. Guidelines for treatment of myxedema. Med. Clin. N. Amer., 52:431, 1968.

Lerman, J. The treatment of hypothyroidism. Med. Clin. N. Amer., 42:1305, 1958.

THYROID NODULES

("Nodular Nonsense"*)

The nontoxic thyroid nodule presents as a most difficult diagnostic and therapeutic problem. Opinions range the entire gamut from surgical removal in all cases to medical treatment in all cases. A few outstanding facts are available.

1. In the United States, thyroid carcinoma occurs at the rate of about 4,000 cases per year, with a death rate about 1,000 per year.
2. In the same population best estimates suggest a total of at least 5,000,000 nontoxic nodular goiters.
3. Thyroid carcinoma occurs in less than 1 case per 1,000 individuals with nodular goiter, and death in 1 case per 5,000.
4. Therefore, to find (not necessarily cure) 1 thyroid carcinoma over 1,000 patients must come to surgery. One must assume an operative mortality of less than 0.1 percent to come out even on these statistics, presuming cure of the 1 carcinoma.
5. Finally, the best evidence suggests that thyroid carcinoma arises de novo and does not develop from a benign adenoma.

Concluding then that surgery provides few answers, some further points are available.

1. A solitary thyroid nodule is more likely to contain carcinoma than a multinodular gland (approximately 2 to 1). However, the accuracy of clinical determination of the number of nodules by palpation is notoriously poor. Very often the uninodular gland is found to be multinodular.
2. Nodularity may be determined by I^{131} scan, and further, the hot and cold (the latter presumably potentially malignant) nodules may be differentiated.
3. The toxic nodule (hot nodule) suppressing activity of the remainder of the gland may be treated surgically if the patient is thyrotoxic. The incidence of malignancy is low; however, they are not generally suppressed by thyroid hormone.
4. Cold nodule activity over the nodule is relatively less than over the

rest of the gland. If present in a young adult (20 years), particularly in a male, the incidence of malignancy is significant, 20 to 40 percent, and hence surgery is advisable. In a female above this age a 3 to 4 month course of suppression therapy may be tried, but if suppression is not achieved surgery may be performed. The patients should be maintained on thyroid medication indefinitely following surgery. Local lymph node involvement, nodule fixation, hoarseness with vocal cord fixation and tracheal compression call for more immediate surgical intervention.

REFERENCES

Eller, M., et al. The treatment of toxic nodular goiter with radioactive iodine: 10 years experience with 436 cases. Ann. Intern. Med., 52:976, 1960.

Meadows, P. M. Scintillation scanning in the management of the clinically single thyroid nodule. J.A.M.A., 177:229, 1961.

Mustacchi, P., and Cutter, S. Some observations on the incidence of thyroid cancer in the U.S. New Eng. J. Med., 255:889, 1956.

Sokal, J. The problem of malignancy in nodular goiter – recapitulation and a challenge. J.A.M.A., 170:405, 1959.

Woolner, L. B., et al. Classification and prognosis of thyroid carcinoma. Amer. J. Surg., 102:534, 1965.

SUBACUTE THYROIDITIS

Thyroiditis may occur in an acute, subacute, or a chronic form.

Subacute thyroiditis presents with fever and a swollen, tender thyroid gland. The pain often radiates to both ears. Typically the PBI and BMR are elevated and the RAI uptake is decreased.

The disease responds well to salicylate therapy, though prednisone may be necessary for the more severe case.

CHRONIC THYROIDITIS

Chronic thyroiditis (Hashimoto's disease) usually presents clinically as a slow growing goiter, though occasionally more rapid enlargement of the thyroid and even pain and tenderness may occur. Laboratory results may be variable. The RAI uptake may be low, normal, or elevated, but does not increase with TSH stimulation. The PBI may also be variable but the difference between the PBI and BEI is abnormally large. Thyroid antibodies in high titers can usually be demonstrated. Thyroid hormone is the treatment of choice.

REFERENCES

Hall, R. Immunologic aspects of thyroid function. New Eng. J. Med., 266:1204, 1962.

Rose, E., and Royster, H. Invasive fibrous thyroiditis (Reidel's struma). J.A.M.A., 176:224, 1961.

Vickery, A. L., and Hamlin, E. Struma lymphomatosa (Hashimoto's thyroiditis). New Eng. J. Med., 264:226, 1961.

TRANSFUSION OF BLOOD

REACTIONS

Reactions occur in from 1 to 10 percent of all transfusions.

FEBRILE REACTIONS. These are the most common reactions. Chills and fever begin usually in the first few minutes. Aspirin or sublingual nitroglycerine usually suffices to control the reaction.

HEMOLYTIC REACTIONS. Hemolysis is the most serious of transfusion reactions and may present a problem in differentiation from the uncomplicated febrile reaction. Symptomatically, pain in the lumbosacral area, legs, and chest is most suggestive. Diagnosis is confirmed by the presence of hemoglobin in the plasma and urine. Treatment is directed toward preventing shock. Urinary output should be followed carefully.

ALLERGIC REACTIONS. This group presents with hives, angioneurotic edema, and, rarely, asthma. Epinephrine and Benadryl are of value.

CIRCULATORY REACTIONS. Circulatory overload in the elderly patient with compensated arteriosclerotic heart disease may result in pulmonary edema and may present as an allergic reaction with asthma. In these patients the danger of overload may be minimized by the use of packed red cells infused at a rate of not more than 1 ml/lb/hr.

TRANSMITTED INFECTIONS. Viral hepatitis, syphillis, malaria, and brucellosis may be transmitted from contaminated blood.

MISCELLANEOUS. These include citrate toxicity with hypocalcemia, air embolism, thrombophlebitis, and, with long-term transfusion therapy, hemosiderosis.

TO BE NOTED

1. It is rarely useful to give less than 1,000 ml of whole blood to an adult. Don't give a "single" pint. If a transfusion is necessary, at least two pints are necessary.
2. Attempts to raise the hematocrit above 30 by transfusion are generally not necessary and may be dangerous.

REFERENCES

Duke, M., et al. Hemodynamic effects of blood transfusion in chronic anemia. New Eng. J. Med., 271:975, 1964.

Grove-Rasmussen, M., et al. Transfusion therapy. New Eng. J. Med., 264:1092, 1961.

TUBERCULOSIS

Tuberculosis is an infectious disease caused by one of several closely related mycobacteria. It usually involves the lungs, but also involves other organs and tissues. The clinical and pathologic findings may range from acute to chronic.

PATHOLOGY

Primary tuberculosis as seen in children is usually situated in the lower parts of the upper lobes or upper part of the lower lobes, just beneath the pleura. The primary lesion is usually a single focus of tuberculous pneumonia, which undergoes caseation. The regional bronchopulmonary lumph nodes are commonly involved. The *primary complex* consists of the pneumonic parenchymal focus and the regional lymph node focus.

Primary tuberculosis in the adult resembles the reinfection type with respect to location of the pulmonary lesion. The enlargement of the regional lymph nodes is much less striking than in children, and may be absent in x-ray examination.

REINFECTION TUBERCULOSIS

The progress and healing of the primary infection may be followed by chronic tuberculosis after a latent period of months or years. This may be the result of exogenous or endogenous reinfection.

Lesions may be nodular with discrete foci or may be pneumonic, fibrotic, cavitary, and calcified.

Dissemination occurs by the hematogeneous, bronchogenic, lymphatic, direct extension, or pleural dissemination.

BACTERIOLOGY

MYCOBACTERIUM. Nonmotile, nonsporulating, aerobic, acidfast rods.

Saprophytes (including potential parasites):

1. *M. phlei* – timothy hay bacillus, found in soil, dust and plants.
2. *M. smegmatis* – includes bacteriola, butyrecum, ranae – found in soil, dust and water.
3. *M. fortuitum* – found in soil, cattle, cold-blooded animals, may cause human disease.
4. *M. marinum* – causes TBC in salt-water fish.

Parasites in Warm-blooded Animals:

1. *M. ulcerans* – causes skin ulcers in men.
2. *M. tuberculosis* – (*M. tuberculosis* var. *hominis*) } known as mammalian tubercle bacilli
3. *M. bovis* – (*M. tuberculosis bovis*) } known as mammalian tubercle bacilli
4. *M. microti* – the vole bacillus, causes generalized TBC in voles, and localized disease in guinea pigs, rabbits, and calves.
5. *M. avium* – causes TBC in birds and pigs.
6. *M. paratuberculosis* – causes a chronic diarrhea in cattle.
7. *M. leprae* – (Hansen's bacillus) causes human leprosy.

UNCLASSIFIED SPECIES.

Also known as atypical or anonymous mycobacteria.

1. Photochromogens – (*M. kansasii, M. luci flavum,* the yellow bacillus, Runyon Group I).
2. Scotochromogens (Runyon Group II) – yellow-orange pigment is seen regardless of the presence or absence of light.
3. Nonchromogenic strains – (the "Battey" type, Runyon Group III) – pigmentation is variable, little or no pigment, not light conditioned.
4. Rapid growers (Runyon Group IV) – rapid growing, photochromogens, usually in three to four days.

DIFFERENTIAL CHARACTERISTICS

1. Rate of colony growth.
2. Virulence for various animals.
3. Niacin production: Only *M. tuberculosis* var. *hominis* produces enough niacin to give a positive reaction.
4. Catalase activity: Present in all mycobacteria except in INH-resistant strains.

5. Peroxidase activity: In mammalian bacilli except in INH-resistant organisms, absent in saprophytes and unclassified organisms.

VIRULENCE FOR VARIOUS ANIMALS.

M. TBC	AVIAN TBC	UNCLASSIFIED MYCOBACTERIA	SAPROPHYTES
Guinea pigs + (except INH-resistant strain)	–	–	–
Mice +	±	Photochromogens usually +, others negative	M. fortuitum +, others negative
Rabbits: Human ± Bovine +	+	None	None
Chickens, none	+	None	None

DRUG SUSCEPTIBILITY.

	MAMMALIAN TBC	AVIAN TBC	UNCLASS. MYCOBACT.	SAPROPHYTES
INH	Susceptible	Resistant	Resistant	Resistant
Streptomycin	Susceptible	Sl. to mod. resistant	Same	Highly resistant
PAS	Susceptible	Highly resistant	Highly resistant	Highly resistant
Cycloserine	Susceptible	Susceptible	Susceptible	Susceptible to slightly resistant

DRUG CONCENTRATIONS FOR SUSCEPTIBILITY TESTS: NOW IN USE

INH	1.0 and 10.9 u per ml
Streptomycin	10 and 100 u per ml
PAS	10 and 100 u per ml
Viomycin	10, 20 and 100 u per ml
Cycloserine	20, 40 and 80 u per ml
Pyrazinamide	10, 50 and 100 u per ml

DIAGNOSTIC METHODS

1. History:
   Personal
   Family exposure
   Social contacts
   Occupational contacts (hospitals and sanitation), silica and asbestos
   Past medical history – pleurisy
   Diabetes
   Peptic ulcer
   Postgastrectomy status
2. Physical Examinations:
   Pulmonary
   Extrapulmonary
3. Skin Tests:
   Tuberculin:
      Tine = 5 tuberculin units
      PPD intermediate = t tuberculin units
      OT – 1:2,000 = 5 tuberculin units
      PPD 2nd
      OT 1:100 = 250 tuberculin units
4. Induration over 5 cm – considered positive.
5. Induration above 10 mm – more serious and likely to develop acute disease.
6. Chest x-ray, routine, lordotic; tomography; Bucky.
7. Bronchoscopy.
8. Gastric washing.
9. Sputum.
10. Pleural biopsy: needle, open thoracotomy.

BASIC CLASSIFICATION OF TUBERCULOSIS

1. Extent of disease.
2. Status of clinical activity.
3. Bacteriologic status.
4. Therapeutic status.
5. Exercise status.

Example: Moderately advanced, active, postgastric culture, antimicrobial Rx, semiambulatory.

CHEMOTHERAPY

Basic drugs are streptomycin, para-aminosalicylic acid and isoniazid. Secondary drugs are cycloserine, viomycin, pyrazinamide, kanamycin, and ethioniamide.

May start with streptomycin 1 g q day for 2 months, INH 100 mg t.i.d., and PAS 12 g/d. Then after, may eliminate streptomycin and continue INH and PAS.

May start with INH and PAS without streptomycin for 2 years. May use streptomycin 1 g b.i.w. or t.i.w. in place of INH. In seriously ill patients and hematogenous TBC, use all three plus corticosteroids, e.g., 40 mg of prednisone daily, gradually reduced, and then discontinue by end of third month. Continue antimicrobial therapy for a minimum of two years.

Antimicrobial therapy plus steroid (prednisone) is effective in large pleural effusion, preventing fibrothorax and scoliosis in the young. Reduce and discontinue steroid by sixth or eighth week. Steroids are also used in TBC meningitis, pericarditis, miliary TBC, and in terminal TBC patients.

NOTES

1. TBC is found in 5 to 10 percent of silicotic patients.
2. TBC unresponsive to chemotherapy may suggest infection with anonymous mycobacteria (photochromogens and nonphotochromogens) or coexistent carcinoma of the lung. Fifteen cases of coexistent TBC and carcinoma have been reported.
3. TBC occurs with increased incidence postgastectomy. In England 5 percent of all new TBC cases were found in postgastrectomy males. INH prophylaxis may be of value in these patients.
4. INH prophylaxis is indicated in patients with sarcoidosis who are on corticosteroid therapy, or who show tuberculin conversion.
5. INH prophylaxis for 1 year is indicated in infants with tuberculin conversion, even in the absence of roentgenographic evidence of TB.
6. Bacille Calmette-Guérin (BCG) administration in this country remains an unsettled question. Except possibly in the high-risk groups, the value of BCG is questionable inasmuch as its use converts the tuberculin reaction to positive for approximately one year as a rule.

REFERENCES

Johnston, R. F., and Hopewell, P. C. Diagnosis and treatment: Chemotherapy of pulmonary tuberculosis. Ann. Intern. Med., 70:359, 1969.

Johnston, R. N., Smith, D. H., Ritchie, R. T., and Lockhart, W. Prolonged streptomycin and isoniazid for pulmonary tuberculosis. Brit. Med. J., June 27, 1964.

Pfuetze, K. H., and Pyle, M. M. Recent advances in treatment of organ tuberculosis. J.A.M.A., 187:805, 1964.

ULCERATIVE COLITIS

Chronic ulcerative colitis is world-wide in distribution, affects both sexes equally, and is more common in the northern, white, higher income, and Jewish population. The true incidence is low but is not known exactly, since mild cases may be missed in the absence of sigmoidoscopy. The cause of ulcerative colitis is unknown. Psychologic factors and autoimmune mechanism involving cell destruction and altered vascular proliferation are present theses. Necrosis begins as crypt abscesses, then diffusely involves the mucosa. Ulcer formation takes place and burrows into the submucosa to erode the friable, proliferating small arteries.

CLINICAL PICTURE

Clinically, ulcerative colitis is manifested by rectal discharges of blood, mucus, and pus ("red mud"). Most often, this is preceded by a long period of mild, nonspecific bowel complaints, slowly increasing in severity. Less frequently onset is abrupt, with rapid progression to bleeding, tenesmus, abdominal tenderness, fever, with weight loss and dehydration.

In less than 10 percent of patients the disease presents in fulminant form. Here there is evidence of severe vasculitis of the colon, with the necrotic process extending farther into the muscular layer, and finally penetrating through the serosa. The patient is in imminent danger of death from perforation, hemorrhage, fluid and electrolyte imbalance, and toxicity.

DIAGNOSIS

"No blood, no ulcerative colitis" is a reasonably reliable dictum. *Diagnosis is made primarily by sigmoidoscopy.* This is done gently, without a prep., and no attempt is made to advance the instrument up the diseased, friable bowel, once the pathology is visualized. The rectum is involved in at least 80 percent of the cases. The earliest change seen is petechiae on the mucosa with slight bleeding after rubbing with a cotton swab. Later, the mucosa appears hyperemic and granular with more bleeding on swabbing. Ulcers may or may not be present.

In the next stage is found marked hyperemia, edema, granulation, bleeding without swabbing, spasm, and adherent exudate. Ulcers are widespread, with no normal mucosa seen. In the fulminant stage, there is a thick purulent exudate, active bleeding, marked edema, granulation, and diffuse ulceration.

Stool culture and mucosal biopsy will rule out infectious or amebic etiology of bloody diarrhea.

X-ray flat plate and upright of the abdomen should be done in acute cases to observe dilatation or obstruction.

Barium enema is best postponed in the fulminant or acute severe cases. The diagnosis is made by the proctoscope picture. In less sick patients, it is done without prior laxative or cathartic, but a gentle saline enema may be administered. In the early stages the films may appear normal. Later, loss of haustral markings and many small serrations of the mucosa are seen. Areas of hyperemia or regenerating tissue surrounded by diffuse ulceration will present as pseudopolyps. If inflammation progresses to fibrosis, there will be narrowing of the lumen, smoothing of the mucosa, and shortening of the colon. Stricture, fistulas, or carcinoma may be seen.

COURSE OF THE DISEASE

The disease usually flares up for weeks or months, then subsides, frequently to exacerbate at a later date. Persistence of symptoms, continuous for over six months, occurs in one third of patients. Prognosis is worse in children, the elderly, and those with severe abrupt onset. Treatment, especially with steroids, will bring about symptomatic remission in 80 percent of cases, but an exacerbation occurs in the majority within two years, whether treated or not. Overall mortality rate is about 10 per cent in the first two years, and is due to the complications of hemorrhage, perforation, stricture, fluid and electrolyte imbalance, and attempts at surgery. Many other complications exist, including arthritis, skin rash, multiple vascular thrombosis, and pyoderma gangrenosa.

MANAGEMENT

The essence of the management is a close doctor-patient relationship. Frequent visits to the physician are necessary. During these visits the doctor must have the patient discuss his personal life and environment. A relationship between social conflicts and exacerbation of illness will become apparent. These must be discussed in order to avoid repetition of them. The attending physician must be willing to be available via telephone or office visit. Frequent short visits are better than longer visits infrequently placed.

STEROIDS. All patients with active ulcerative colitis should be taking steroids. At the beginning high doses (60-80 mg/d) are started. The dose is then rapidly reduced to 25-30 mg. This dose is continued for 2 to 3 months. It is then further reduced so that it can gradually be discontinued at 5 to 6 months.

DIET. A high caloric intake is mandatory. In this context any reasonable household can prepare a palatable, nourishing, and satisfying diet. With very severe symptoms more caloric intake is necessary. Caloric intake should not be sacrificed to give unattractive "soft," "low-residue" foods.

SEDATION. Most of these patients need and take phenobarbital. If more than this is needed, Librium is very useful in doses of 40-80 mg/d.

OTHER MEDICATIONS. Belladonna, antispasmodics, Lomotil, codeine, paregoric are all useful from time to time. The safest is probably small doses of paregoric. Chronic blood loss is best treated with parenteral iron (Imferon 2 ml daily for 5 days). Antibiotics are generally used if the patient is febrile. These should only be given for short courses, as they possibly are not necessary, and when combined with steroids result in resistant infections.

SURGERY. Some patients with ulcerative colitis will need surgery for 1) massive hemorrhage, 2) stenosis, 3) perforation, 4) systemic complications, and 5) intractable symptoms. This last is very hard to define. However, both the patient and physician must be very patient, and certainly a year should go by before any irreversible surgery is attempted for "intractable disease."

CARCINOMA OF THE COLON IN ULCERATIVE COLITIS

Cancer occurs more often in these patients than in the random population. It is hard to detect. The mortality is high. The incidence of colon cancer in ulcerative colitis is in the area of 3 to 5 percent, which is within the range of operative mortality for elective colectomy.

"TOXIC MEGACOLON"

Fulminant ulcerative colitis is an urgent situation, which will end fatally unless effective treatment is instituted immediately. In the first day, often several liters of I.V. fluid with potassium are needed; also, several units of blood. Penicillin, 1.2 million units, and streptomycin, 1 g are given I.M. Parenteral steroid (100 mg of prednisone) is used. Abdominal flat plates are obtained to check on the ever present danger of silent perforation. A surgical opinion is called from the start; and in the face of perforation, abscess, persistent ileus, or severe deterioration over many days, the patient is operated upon. Total colectomy with ileostomy is performed as treatment for unresponsive fulminant disease. The rectal segment may be preserved for possible reanastomosis at a later date.

REFERENCES

Aylett, S. Ulcerative colitis treated by total colectomy and ileorectal anastomosis: A ten-year review (abridged). Proc. Roy. Soc. Med., 56:183, 1963.

Janowitz, H. D., Lindner, A., and Marshak, R. H. Granulomatous colitis. J.A.M.A., 191:825, 1965.

Kirsner, J. B. The immunologic response of the colon. J.A.M.A., 191:809, 1965.

Lepore, M. J. Emotional disturbances in ulcerative colitis. J.A.M.A., 191:819, 1965.

Stauffer, M. H., Sauer, W. G., Dearing, W. H., and Baggenstoss, A. H. Spectrum of cholestatic hepatic disease. J.A.M.A., 191:829, 1965.

Tumen, H. J. Toxic megacolon in fulminating disease. J.A.M.A., 191:838, 1965.

Welch, C. E., and Hedberg, S. E. Ulcerative colitis and colonic cancer. J.A.M.A., 191:815, 1965.

ULCER: PEPTIC

DUODENAL ULCER

Peptic ulceration of the duodenum is probably the most common nonmalignant serious disorder of the civilized population. It is estimated that 5 to 10 percent of adult males will have a peptic ulcer at some time during their lives. The usual manifestations of the chronic peptic ulcer syndrome are quite clearcut and predictable. The patient experiences burning epigastric pain relieved by food. The pain occurs 1½ to 3 hours after eating. The chronic pain, indigestion, and vomiting experienced by most people is at least a cause of great loss of time and efficiency, and may prove incapacitating. It is only rarely, however, that serious complications occur which threaten life. Although it is estimated that 10 percent of patients with peptic ulcer will require surgery, this is based on the hospitalized population and does not represent the usual person with benign duodenal ulcer. A great majority of patients with this illness never suffer any serious consequences.

The complications which occur are bleeding, perforation, and obstruction. The onset and exacerbation of symptoms are clearly linked to the environmental circumstances of the patient's life.

MANAGEMENT OF THE PATIENT WITH DUODENAL ULCER

The doctor must spend a considerable amount of time with the patient discussing the circumstances under which the ulcer has occurred, and in trying to help the patient understand himself in order to prevent recurrences. Unless the patient and the physician consider this aspect of the illness with great seriousness, very little is being done for the patient. During time of acute symptoms, patients are generally treated with diet and medication.

DIET. The essence of the diet is that the patient takes 6 feedings per day to keep his stomach from becoming empty. Some physicians prefer a bland diet. Others believe that the patient may take food which is part of a regular sensible household diet without reference to quality, other than that it be not unusually spicy.

MEDICATION.

1. A sedative such as phenobarbital 15-30 mg, 3 to 4 times daily is advised for most patients.
2. Antacids: Aluminum hydroxide gel, 20 to 30 ml, given 4 to 6 times daily, is effective and economical. When combined with magnesium compounds (such as Gelusil) it is more palatable and less constipating.
3. Anticholinergic drugs are reserved for those patients who do not do well on the above regime. Many anticholinergic compounds are available, all generally effective. Probanthine, 15 mg, t.i.d., is useful, effective, and safe. Tincture of belladonna or belladonna-phenobarbital is likewise useful, but generally not as powerful in the doses usually prescribed. Whatever the compound used, it must be given in doses that produce slight dryness of the mouth.

COMPLICATIONS

PERFORATION. The occurrence of perforation of an ulcer is a major catastrophe and requires immediate surgery. Although cases have been recorded in which nonsurgical therapy has been effective there has been very little experience with this in the United States. The results of early surgical intervention are so good that there seems little reason to avoid this procedure.

PYLORIC OBSTRUCTION. The important clinical aspect of this complication is persistent vomiting. Approximately two thirds of patients exhibiting this complication will require surgery. Persistent vomiting with x-ray verification of "outlet" obstruction is necessary for the diagnosis of pyloric obstruction. The diagnosis should be verified from time to time by gastric aspiration. There should be less than 100 ml present 3 hours after a meal.

Frequently this complication is due to an acute duodenal ulcer. Hence a trial of antacids and liquid feedings should be carried out. Nasogastric suction is also started. This suction is applied intermittently, depending upon the volume aspirated with the general purpose being to keep the stomach empty.

Under this therapy about half of the obstructions will "open up." If it does, conservative management is continued. Prophylactic surgery is not done. If obstruction persists (vomiting and x-ray evidence of a high degree of obstruction), surgery is necessary and generally quite successful. The long-term results of surgery from this complication are very satisfactory, and obstruction is a clear indication for surgery.

INTRACTABLE PAIN. By intractable pain is meant that despite all efforts by the patient and the physician the patient continues to complain of pain. Under these circumstances the physician must be certain that he is not dealing with a complication, i.e., a penetrating ulcer which has involved the pancreas and caused pancreatitis. There are patients who do not have a "complication" yet complain bitterly of pain, do not participate well in therapy, and are unable to change an unworkable set of values and standards. It is very likely that these patients are chronic complainers. No therapy will be effective for them. They do not do well, in general, with surgery. For those with penetrating peptic ulcer not responding to therapy, surgery should be performed after the doctor is convinced that adequate medical therapy has been attempted. The word adequate is difficult to define, but at least 6 months of intensive medical therapy should be employed prior to surgical intervention.

RECURRENT HEMORRHAGE. Surgery should not be performed simply because the patient has had one or more episodes of bleeding. It is unlikely that gastrectomy will prevent the recurrence of hemorrhage. This applies to those who have bled once, twice, or possibly three times. In patients who have bled more often than this there are very little data available upon which to base a decision for or against surgery.

MASSIVE HEMORRHAGE. Patients below the age of 45 years rarely, if ever, lose their lives from bleeding ulcer. Conservative therapy is indicated (treat as if an acute ulcer were present). Adequate blood replacement must be accomplished. An hour-by-hour record of the vital signs must be kept.

MORTALITY

High mortality is associated with the following:

1. Patients over the age of 45 with bleeding peptic ulcer have a mortality which increases with each decade of life. If the vital signs can be sustained by blood replacement at a rate which is below 3,000 ml of blood per 48 hours, conservative therapy should be continued. When the requirement for blood exceeds this rate of replacement, or where it is apparent from hematemesis and melena and failing vital signs that he is *going to require* more than 3,000 ml in 48 hours, the mortality rate approaches two thirds.
2. The physician must quickly determine the presence of serious complicating illness. These (heart failure, old or new myocardial infarction, serious valvular heart disease, cirrhosis of the liver, severe head trauma, or burns) almost double the mortality rate. When the rate of

blood replacement approaches 2,000 ml per 48 hours the mortality rate in such patients is very high.

3. If a patient with upper gastrointestinal hemorrhage stops bleeding while in the hospital, and then suddenly rebleeds (as indicated by a sharp change in the vital signs or the occurrence of melena) a high mortality rate is to be expected.
4. Constant falling of the hematocrit during hospitalization over a period of weeks in the absence of sharp changes in the vital signs also indicates continued bleeding. When the blood replacement in this circumstance approaches a total of 5,000 ml, a definitive step to stop bleeding must be taken.

Emergency gastrectomy under the above circumstances requires a very experienced surgeon. In the absence of considerable surgical experience the patient is probably best treated conservatively.

LOCAL GASTRIC HYPOTHERMIA FOR BLEEDING ULCER

Recently the use of gastric hypothermia for the control of hemorrhage from peptic ulcer has been applied, using a device which simplifies the technical aspects of maintaining a constant flow of ice water into and out of the stomach. Experience with this device is very encouraging. We urge a thorough trial of gastric hypothermia before emergency gastrectomy is attempted.

GASTRIC ULCER

THE ULCER-CANCER PROBLEM

Some patients with cancer of the stomach present with upper gastrointestinal complaints and radiographic findings indicative of benign peptic ulcer. Hence all patients who show radiographic evidence of gastric ulcer should be evaluated to rule out malignancy. In this situation the old adage "no acid, no ulcer" is remarkably reliable. In the absence of free acid in the stomach one should not temporize. Surgery is necessary. If the patient has free acid present he may have a peptic ulcer or he may have a gastric cancer. Optimal therapy for peptic ulcer should be instituted. After three weeks of treatment the ulcer should be 50 percent smaller by x-ray; otherwise surgery is indicated. Gastroscopy and gastric cytology should be done.

REFERENCES

Grace, W. J., and Mitty, W. Does subtotal gastrectomy in benign peptic ulcer prevent recurrence of bleeding? Amer. J. Dig. Dis., 7:69, 1962.

Harvey, H. D. A follow-up study of surgically treated peptic ulcer over forty-six years. Maryland Med. J., August, 1963.

____Twenty-four years of experience with elective gastric resection for duodenal ulcer. Surg. Gynec. Obstet., 112:203, 1961

____Twenty-five years of experience with elective gastric resection for gastric ulcer. Surg. Gynec. Obstet., 113:191, 1961.

Larson, N., et al. Prognosis of the medically treated small gastric ulcer. New Eng. J. Med., 264:119, 1961.

Mitty, W., et al. Factors influencing mortality in bleeding peptic ulcer. Amer. J. Dig. Dis., 6:389, 395, 400, 1961.

Wangensteen, S. L., Orahood, R. C., Voorhees, A. B., Smith, R. B., and Healy, W. V. Intragastric cooling in the management of hemorrhage from the upper gastrointestinal tract. Amer. J. Surg., 105:401, 1963.

VASCULITIS

(Arteritis)

The vasculitides may present clinically as a generalized syndrome in the presence of varied pathology and etiology. The etiology is not clear, though a hypersensitivity phenomenon is suspected. The prototype of the arteritides is polyarteritis or periarteritis nodosa, a systemic disease of fibrinoid degeneration of the medium and small-sized arteries.

Major variants of polyarteritis which are considered necrotizing arteritides include hypersensitivity angiitis, allergic granulomatous arteritis, arteritis of other connective tissues, cranial or temporal arteritis, and Wegener's granulomatosis. A wide spectrum of disease results, ranging from predominant arteritis to predominant granulomatosis.

The manifestations of vasculitis depend upon several factors: the location and distribution of the lesions, the location of the end organ vessel, the type and intensity of the reaction of the vascular wall, and the duration of the disease. In spite of these variables and modifications in the clinical picture of each polyarteritis variant, a predominant "vasculitis" syndrome may exist. Each variant will modify this syndrome to some degree.

VASCULITIS SYNDROME

(Modified from McCombs)

Systemic Signs (fever, weight loss)
Skin (purpura, erythematous rash, nodules, urticaria)
Musculoskeletal (arthritis, arthralgia, myalgia)
Pulmonary (asthma, pneumonitis – 25 percent of cases)
Renal (renal insufficiency, hypertension, proteinuria, hematuria, "telescoped" urine sediment, glomerulitis) 75 percent of cases
Cardiovascular (myocarditis, pericarditis, myocardial infarction, CHF, arrhythmias, peripheral vascular insufficiency)
Neurologic (neuropathy, encephalopathy) 8 to 25 percent of cases
Gastrointestinal (bleeding, mesenteric infarcation) 15 percent of cases
Hematologic (anemia, leukocytosis, eosinophilia)
Immunologic (elevated ESR, hypergammaglobulinemia)

Cardiac and renal involvement is most common; pulmonary, hepatic, splenic, gastrointestinal, adrenal, testicular, cerebral, and peripheral nerve involvement are also seen.

A definite diagnosis of vasculitis depends upon histologic evidence of arteritis. The common sites of biopsy include skeletal muscle, testis (the yield may be as high as 85 percent), liver, and sural nerve. If the clinical presentation suggests predominant renal involvement, renal biopsy will be diagnostic.

Management includes elimination of etiologic factors and administration of corticosteroids. Recently, immunosuppressive therapy has been employed in difficult cases. The prognosis is poor in the presence of polyarteritis and Wegener's granulomatosis.

REFERENCES

Alarcon-Segoyia, D., and Brosn, A. L., Jr. Classification and etiologic aspects of necrotizing angiitis: An analytical approach to a confused subject with a critical review of the evidence for hypersensitivity in polyarteritis nodosa. Mayo Clin. Proc., 39:205, 1964.

McCombs, R. P. Systemic "allergic" vasculitis. J.A.M.A., 194:1059, 1965.

Shulman, L. E., and Harvey, A. M. *In* Hollander, ed. Polyarteritis in Arthritis, and allied conditions, Philadelphia, Lea & Febiger, 1966.

Zeek, P. M. Periarteritis nodosa and other forms of necrotizing angiitis. New Eng. J. Med., 248:764, 1953.

VASOPRESSOR DRUGS

DRUG	MAJOR CAUSE OF PRESSOR ACTION	NET PERIPHERAL EFFECT	ROUTE OF ADMINISTRATION	DOSAGE
Ephedrine	Cardiac	Constrictor	All routes	15-50 mg
Epinephrine	Cardiac	Dilator	Parenteral	0.1-0.5 ml of 1:1,000 solution
Mephentermine (Wyamine)	Cardiac	Dilator	Parenteral	15-60 mg, I.M.; 15-30 mg, I.V.
Metaraminol (Aramine)	Peripheral	Constrictor	Parenteral	5-10 mg
Methoxamine (Vasoxyl)	Peripheral	Constrictor	Intramuscular or intravenous	10 mg, I.M.; 10-20 mg, I.V.
Norepinephrine (Levarterenol; Levophed)	Peripheral	Constrictor	Intravenous	4 mg or more in 500 ml of 5% g/w; dose adjusted to pressor response (can go as high as 60 mg/l)
Phenylephrine (Neo-Synephrine)	Peripheral	Constrictor	All routes	0.5-0.8 mg, I.V.; 5.0 mg subcutaneous; 50/200 mg, P.O.

In acute hypotensive states, Neo-Synephrine may be started first. If this fails, Levophed is employed.

The dose is a sufficient quantity to attain a systolic pressure of not less than 90 mm Hg in a patient known to be previously normotensive. In the presence of shock in a patient with antecedent hypertension, higher pressures may be required to prevent a "shock kidney."

Levophed is generally given only by indwelling venous catheter because of the danger of local extravasation and necrosis. The addition of 5 mg of phentolamine (Regitine) to the Levophed solution has been advocated to present sloughing.

REFERENCE

Bernstein, A. Treatment of shock in myocardial infarction. Amer. J. Cardiol., 9:74, 1962.

INDEX